HANYANE

A village struggles for eye health

QUESTIONS, DISCUSSION AND NOTES ON EYE CARE

by Erika Sutter, Allen Foster and Victoria Francis

The International Centre for Eye Health, London, are most grateful to the Royal Commonwealth Society for the Blind, Christoffel Blindenmission and Christian Blind Mission International for support given to the publication of this book.

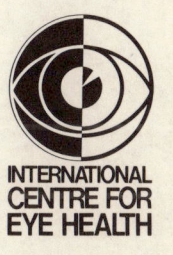

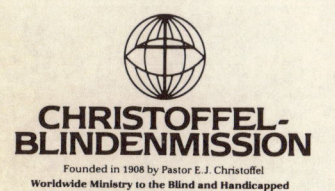

INTERNATIONAL CENTRE FOR EYE HEALTH

CHRISTOFFEL-BLINDENMISSION
Founded in 1908 by Pastor E.J. Christoffel
Worldwide Ministry to the Blind and Handicapped
International Headquarters:
Christoffel-Blindenmission e.V.
Nibelungenstrasse 124
D-6140 Bensheim 4, West Germany
Phone: 062 51 - 13 10. Telex: 468334 cbmb d

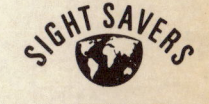

SIGHT SAVERS
ROYAL COMMONWEALTH SOCIETY FOR THE BLIND
Commonwealth House, Heath Road, Haywards Heath, West Sussex RH16 3AZ
Telephone: (0444) 412424 Telex: 87167 COMBLD

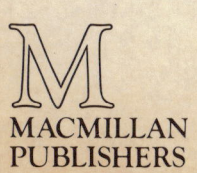

MACMILLAN PUBLISHERS

© International Centre for Eye Health – Text and Illustrations
Illustrations by Victoria Francis

Any parts of this book, including the illustrations, may be copied, reproduced, or adapted by individual persons as part of their own work or training without permission from the author or publisher, provided the parts reproduced are not distributed for profit.
For any reproduction by profit-making bodies or for commercial ends, permission must first be obtained from the publisher. Any person who does any unauthorised act in relation to this publication may be liable to criminal prosecution and civil claims for damages.

First published 1989

Published by *Macmillan Publishers Ltd*
London and Basingstoke
Associated companies and representatives in Accra, Auckland, Delhi, Dublin, Gaborone, Hamburg, Harare, Hong Kong, Kuala Lumpur, Lagos, Manzini, Melbourne, Mexico City, Nairobi, New York, Singapore, Tokyo

ISBN 0–333–51092–5

Printed in Hong Kong

A CIP catalogue record for this book is available from the British Library.

Contents

Foreword	iv
Acknowledgements	vi
Introduction	vii
PART 1: Community eye care	1
Section A: The roots of poor health	5
Section B: Action towards eye health	71
Section C: Village development leads to health	127
PART 2: Common eye diseases for village health workers	183
Section A: How to examine an eye patient	186
Section B: Making a diagnosis	190
Section C: How to work in your eye clinic	201
Section D: Health teaching to prevent blindness	204
PART 3: Lecture notes on common eye diseases for ophthalmic assistants	207
Section A: Examination of the eye	211
Section B: Basic sciences of the eye	213
Section C: Diagnosis of common eye diseases	222
Section D: Management of common eye diseases	258
Appendix:	
Recommended reading	262
Useful resource addresses	263

Foreword

The authors of this book address three important factors in eye health and its promotion.
- The belief (in line with Alma Ata) that all sections of health services should be responsible for developing and supporting health care within the community.
- That eye health is an essential part of primary health care.
- The need for health messages to be presented in a way that will be read, understood and absorbed. This is achieved in this book in the context of Joyce and Lerisa's story in the village of Hanyane – illustrated by lively drawings.

Eye health, in common with other health care, cannot be isolated from other activities in the community. As in all branches of medicine, knowledge of eye disease and treating acute conditions is not enough in providing eye care. It also requires an understanding of how people function and the ability to work with the local community and its existing power structure in a sensitive way. The authors bring their long experience of working in developing countries to show how health care workers need to get out of their 'box' and join with other sectors in working within and for the community (see the illustration opposite).

The competition for resources is such that disabled children are less likely to survive than other children. For instance, more than half of children blinded by measles die within the first year. Resources are important to eye health – adequate water, sufficient and appropriate food for children, and early identification and treatment of illness by those close to home – are all necessary to the promotion of eye health.

The authors in their story, which makes up Part 1 of this book, go through many of the problems in a community when new ideas and resources for looking after people with eye problems are brought into a village. Joyce, Lerisa and the better-off women in the story are allowed to make many of the common mistakes, and we can all learn from the way they overcome their difficulties. The authors emphasize simple and practical things that can be done to encourage all members of the community – from chief to the very poorest member – to work together to improve eye health and to increase resources for further improvement in health.

The great advantage and value of this book is that through experience and practice good methods are encouraged and understood, unlike many books on community health where theory is put before practice.

This is complemented in parts 2 and 3 of the book with systematic lecture notes on eye diseases, their diagnosis and management relevant to general health workers and more specialised ophthalmic assistants.

Professor David Morley
Institute of Child Health,
London

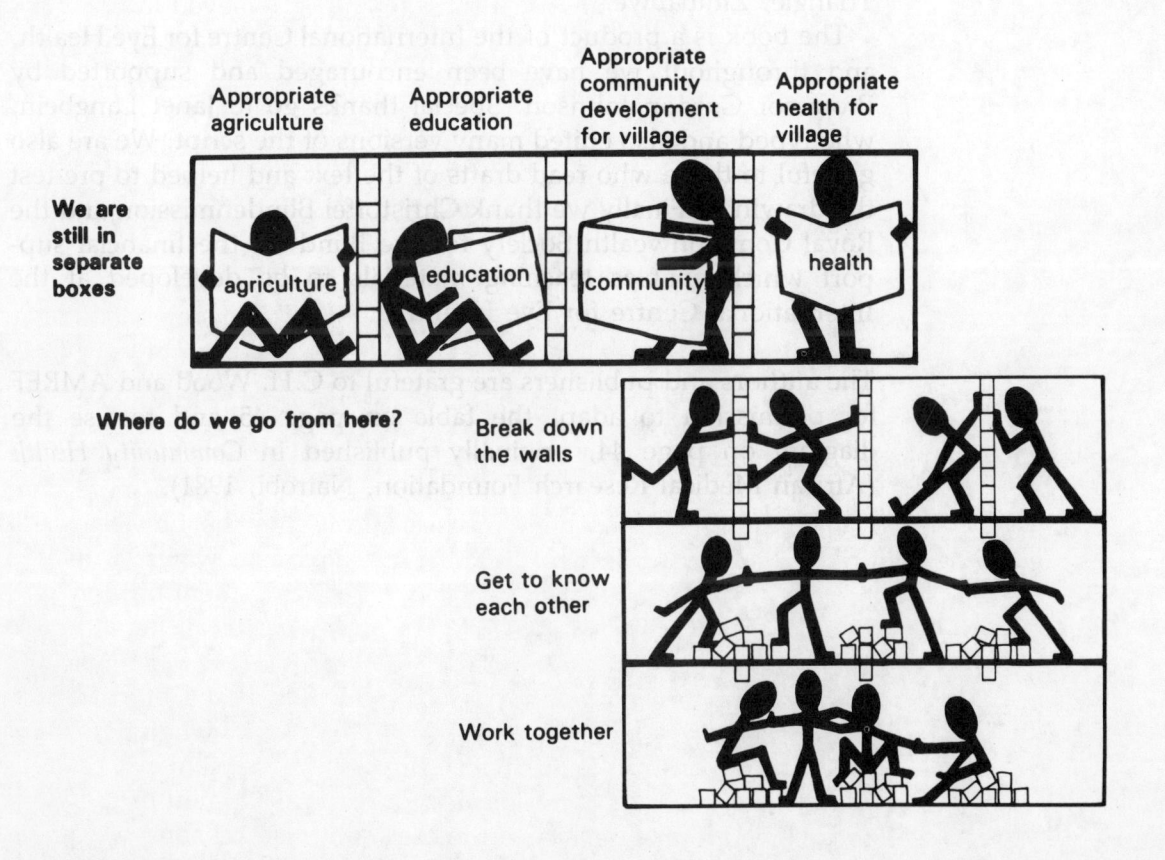

| | Appropriate agriculture | Appropriate education | Appropriate community development for village | Appropriate health for village |

We are still in separate boxes: agriculture | education | community | health

Where do we go from here?

- Break down the walls
- Get to know each other
- Work together

Acknowledgements

This book is a record of what African people have taught us about eye care and appropriate teaching methods. Our foremost thanks go therefore to those with whom we have worked and from whom we have learnt so much. They are too numerous to be mentioned individually, but include the staff and women of the Elim Care Group Project, the nurses and medical assistants from Mvumi hospital, Tanzania, and the health workers and communities of Triangle, Zimbabwe.

The book is a product of the International Centre for Eye Health, and throughout we have been encouraged and supported by Professor Gordon Johnson. Special thanks go to Janet Langbein, who typed and also edited many versions of the script. We are also grateful to those who read drafts of the text and helped to pre-test the drawings. Finally we thank Christoffel Blindenmission and the Royal Commonwealth Society for the Blind for the financial support which enables teaching materials to be developed at the International Centre for Eye Health.

The authors and publishers are grateful to C.H. Wood and AMREF for permission to adapt the table on page 45 and to use the diagram on page 44, originally published in *Community Health* (African Medical Research Foundation, Nairobi, 1981).

Introduction

This book is to help people involved in health care, particularly eye nurses, ophthalmic assistants and community health workers. It is divided into three parts.

Part 1 is based on the true story of how a group of villagers were encouraged to improve their own eye health. The problems they faced, the mistakes and the successes they made are discussed. There are 30 chapters, each one consisting of an illustrated narrative, and a set of questions and discussion notes. This section can be used in three different ways. First, individual health workers may read and study the principles involved. Second, teachers of health workers may use the narrative, drawings and questions in a classroom situation. And third, the story and illustrations may be used by health workers to stimulate discussion and activities within community groups.

Part 2 is written for health workers at the village level who, as well as preventing and treating general diseases, are required to know about common eye problems. This part explains how to examine an eye patient and to diagnose and manage the common eye disorders. There is also a section on the important health messages which can prevent eye disease and blindness.

Part 3 is a set of lecture notes for ophthalmic assistants and nurses. The lecture notes outline the basic sciences relevant to eye disorders, how to examine an eye patient and the diagnosis and management of the important eye diseases.

Together the three parts form a basis for teaching health workers at the primary and secondary levels about eye care. The book emphasises the two aspects of eye health and prevention of blindness. First, understanding how to work with communities in order to reduce eye disease and blindness. And second, knowing about eye disorders and their diagnosis and management.

This book is dedicated to those who started the Care Groups – Selina, Andrew and the women of Chabane, Mtsetweni and Nkuzana – and to all those who later joined them.

PART 1
Community eye care

Contents

Introduction to Part One   3

SECTION A: *The roots of poor health*   5
1. Will Musa see again? Roots of blindness   6
2. Vho-Mudau's wisdom; What is health?   14
3. Those people in white frighten me; Hospitals and health   21
4. We are not fit for visitors; Health and the poor   27
5. Visit to the chief; Health and village authorities   34
6. Who cares about reports? Health through statistics   40
7. Why draw a map? Knowing your village   48
8. Choosing a bag of beans; A random sample   55
9. Ten people with entropion; Interpreting the survey results   61
10. Disappointment with the survey; Where is the action?   66

SECTION B: *Action towards eye health*   71
11. Operation? No thank you; Inappropriate action   72
12. Where is the medicine? Health at a price   76
13. The best medicine; Keeping snakes away   82
14. The Tidy Ladies; Self-praisers or health carers?   89
15. Why has my child got trachoma? A community problem affects everybody   93
16. Becoming a health carer; Being alone is difficult   97
17. You must! Health Carers – Police or friends?   101
18. Refuse pits prevent trachoma; Working together   106
19. Treating trachoma; Medicine wins more community acceptance   111

20	Counting the beans; Self-evaluation	116
21	Don't wait until you are blind; Cataract and glaucoma	121

SECTION C: *Village development leads to health*   127

22	Musa is dying of diarrhoea; Ma-Anna becomes a Health Carer	128
23	The village fights for clean water; Health Carers activate the community	134
24	Joyce is sick; Coping by ourselves	141
25	Green vegetables prevent xerophthalmia; Gardening without water	147
26	Lerisa's new found knowledge; Acceptance or jealousy?	153
27	Starting a cooperative; Development and health	158
28	Who are we working for? The question of payment	164
29	Learning from the past; The Health Carers look back	170
30	Planning for the future; The struggle continues	176

Introduction to Part One

Hanyane derives its name from a Tsonga word, meaning 'let us live'. It expresses the spirit of a community struggling together to overcome the obstacles to health.

Although the characters are fictional, the story reflects the development – with its growing pains – of community groups and their leaders. The blindness prevention project in which we were involved is described. It is hoped that the events narrated and the questions asked will encourage the readers to draw their own conclusions and look critically at their own work with the people in their area.

The discussion, which follows the story, deals with one or more of the issues raised. Some questions are left unanswered to encourage independent thinking or to demonstrate that often there are no answers to community problems.

There are three sections to the story. In Section A the eye nurse, Joyce, meets Musa (who is blind from vitamin A malnutrition), his family and the whole village of Hanyane with its problems. We follow the people and Joyce as they find answers to questions such as:
1 Why is there so much disease and preventable blindness in poor areas?
2 How do we find out which health problems are most urgent and require action?

Section B shows how a group of interested women forms the basis of an innovative approach to community eye care. Both those in charge and the people themselves learn through experience how not to do things, and try new ways to reduce trachoma in their own community.

In Section C the Hanyane Health Carers grow in confidence and learn that together they can achieve much. They begin to work on other health problems. Realising that poverty remains the main obstacle to health, they start an agricultural cooperative. Other villages follow the example of Hanyane. A network of Health Carer groups is formed and the rural blindness prevention scheme becomes widespread throughout the area.

The experience of the Hanyane Health Carers provides an example for both health workers and communities of how to approach blindness prevention in a way which will also contribute to overall development.

PART 1 SECTION A
The roots of poor health

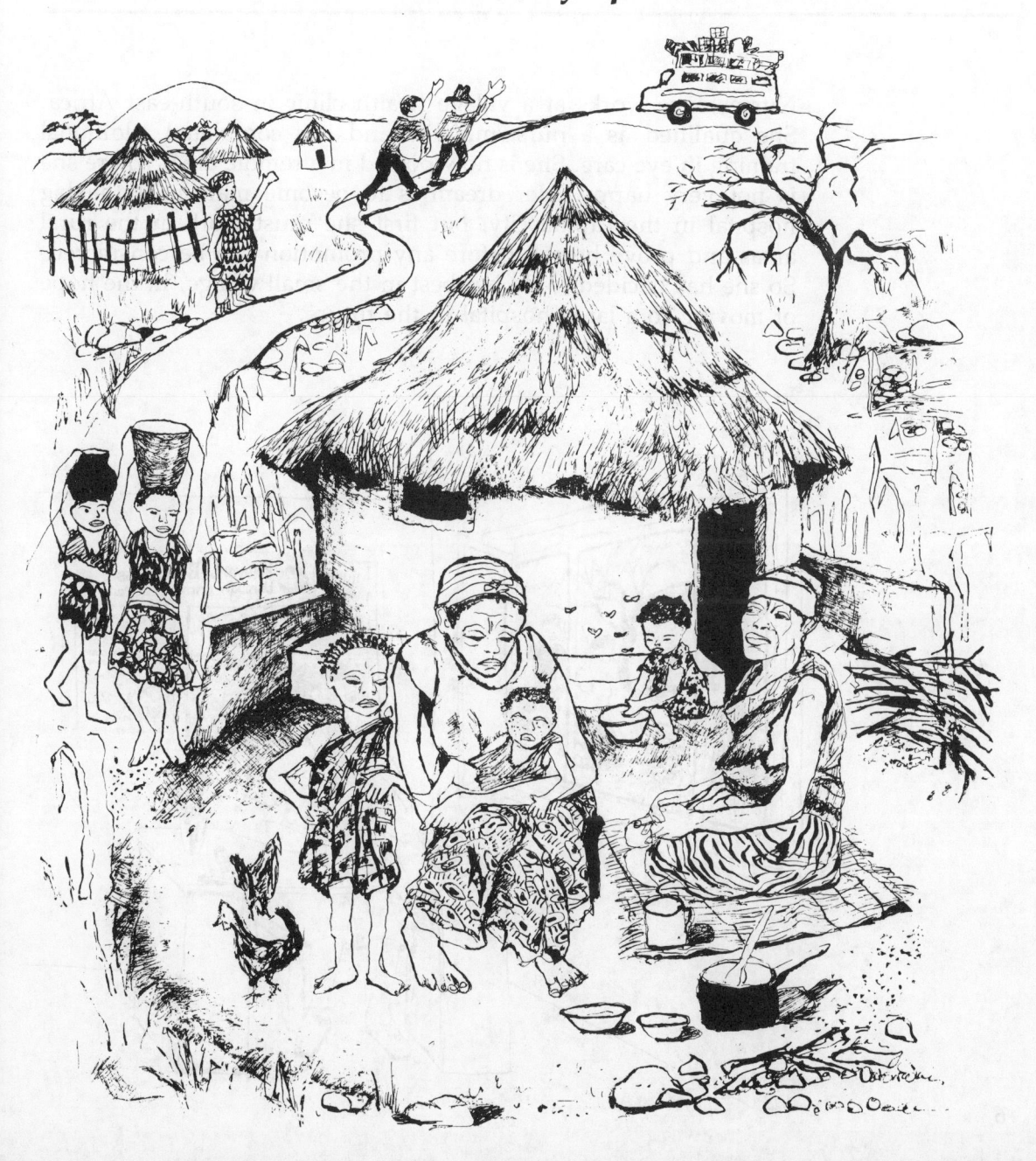

1

Will Musa see again?
– Roots of blindness

Nurse Joyce works at a village health clinic in south-east Africa. She qualified as a nurse/midwife and has completed additional training in eye care. She is now posted in a remote area, where she is not very happy. Her dream is to become matron at the big hospital in the capital city, but first she must work in the rural areas and prove herself before any promotion can be considered. So she has decided to do her best in the small village, in the hope of moving to a large hospital in the future.

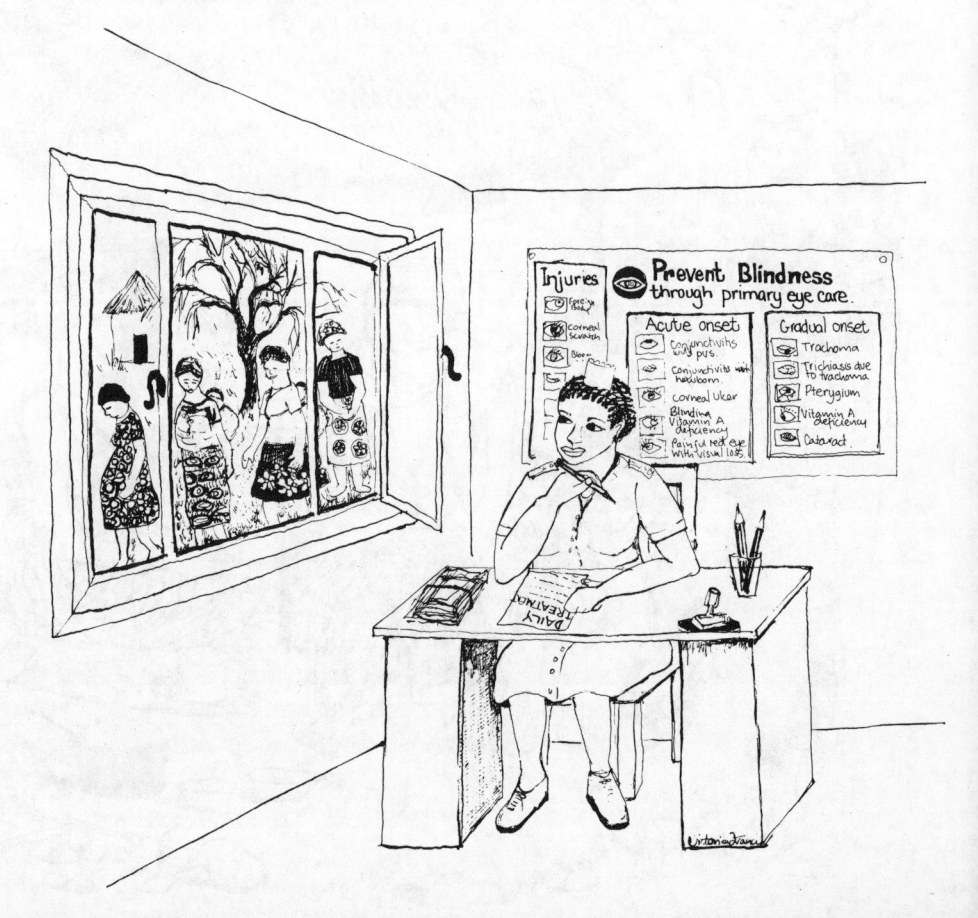

She is responsible for twelve settlements scattered over a wide area. One of them, Hanyane, is ten miles away and there is no public transport. The senior chief of the area lives in Kulani which lies midway between the clinic and Hanyane. In Kulani there are also a primary school, a secondary school and the office of the agricultural extension officer. It is the only place with piped water although, for most of the time, this is not working. Joyce can't understand why her clinic isn't in Kulani, where life is easier and less lonely, but she has little choice but to carry on.

From her clinic Joyce looks over the dry, flat countryside – the summer rains have not fallen for two years. Some grey thornbush is all that is left for the goats to eat. A few maize stalks stick out in a dusty brown field – planted in the vain hope of reaping some harvest.

In the village the round houses are clustered around small yards. The walls and floors have been smoothed and decorated with a mixture of cow dung and clay. There is little land to plough around the homesteads. The settlements resemble small towns with about 400–500 compounds, comprising a population of 1,000–2,000 people.

The area is poor – many people do not own land. There are very few job opportunities so the men are forced to leave their families and seek work in the city, on the big farms or in the mines. Most send some money home when they find a job. They return home to visit about once a year, and then go back to their work. Sadly, some forget their wives and children and start a new family in town.

It has not always been like this. The very old people still recall the tales of their fathers, remembering the times when the land was lush and fertile. People had lived well from the land which belonged to the whole community. Then foreigners from Europe arrived and took possession of the best pastures. The land left to the villagers is now too little to live from, and poverty and disease have taken over.

The hospital which supplies Joyce's clinic with medicines is far away. One of its two doctors, who is an eye doctor, visits her clinic about every two months. Joyce looks forward to his visits because he is willing to help her solve the problems she has with patients. Occasionally the matron turns up for an inspection, but she always finds something to criticise, and encouraging words are rare. It's as if clinic work is meant to be a punishment for a nurse like Joyce. One thing Joyce does enjoy is getting to know her regular patients.

One morning, when she opened her clinic and looked at the patients waiting under the big tree, she noticed a new face that struck her. Little did she know that this was the beginning of a great adventure which would change things, both for her and for the people of that poor area.

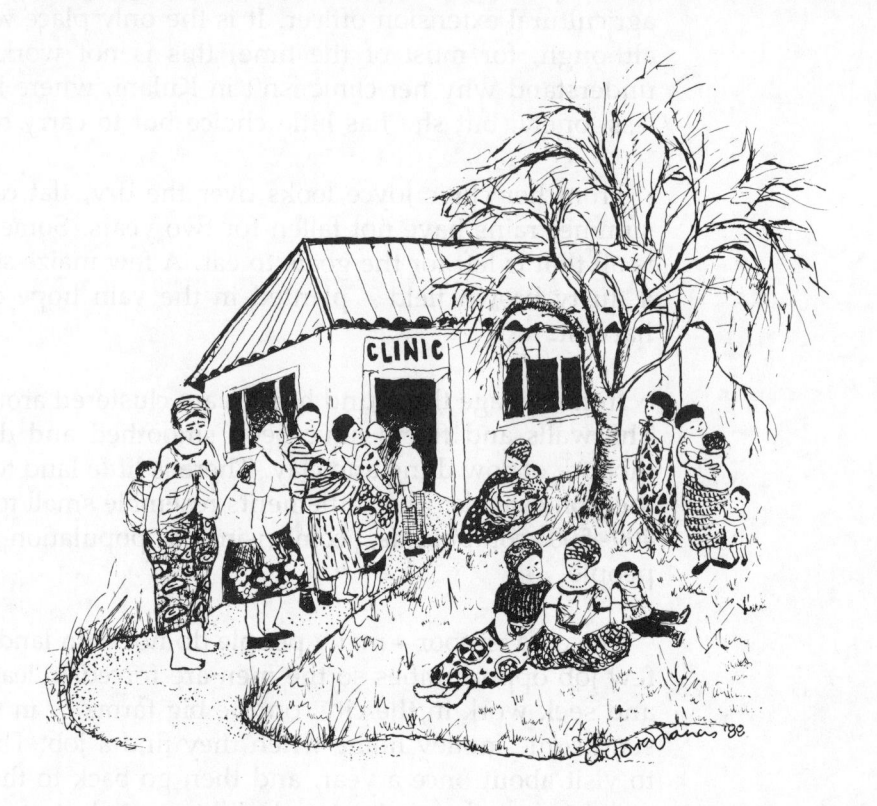

This new face belonged to a lean woman standing timidly at the end of the queue. She looked as if even the baby on her back was too much of a burden for her to carry. Her whole body expressed worry and hopelessness. Her name was Ma-Anna. She was from Hanyane village and she came because of her little boy Musa. It was quite difficult for Joyce to get information from Ma-Anna. After questioning her patiently she found out that the boy was about 18 months old. He had never been to the community health clinic and had no Road To Health Chart. Ma-Anna was worried about her son's eyes which 'went bad' the previous day.

On examination Joyce found that both eyes had extensive corneal ulcers.

'How long has it been like this?' asked Joyce.

'One day,' said Ma-Anna.

'Are you sure?'

'Yes. He was all right before. But when he opened his eyes yesterday they were grey.'

'Oh, has he been sick?'

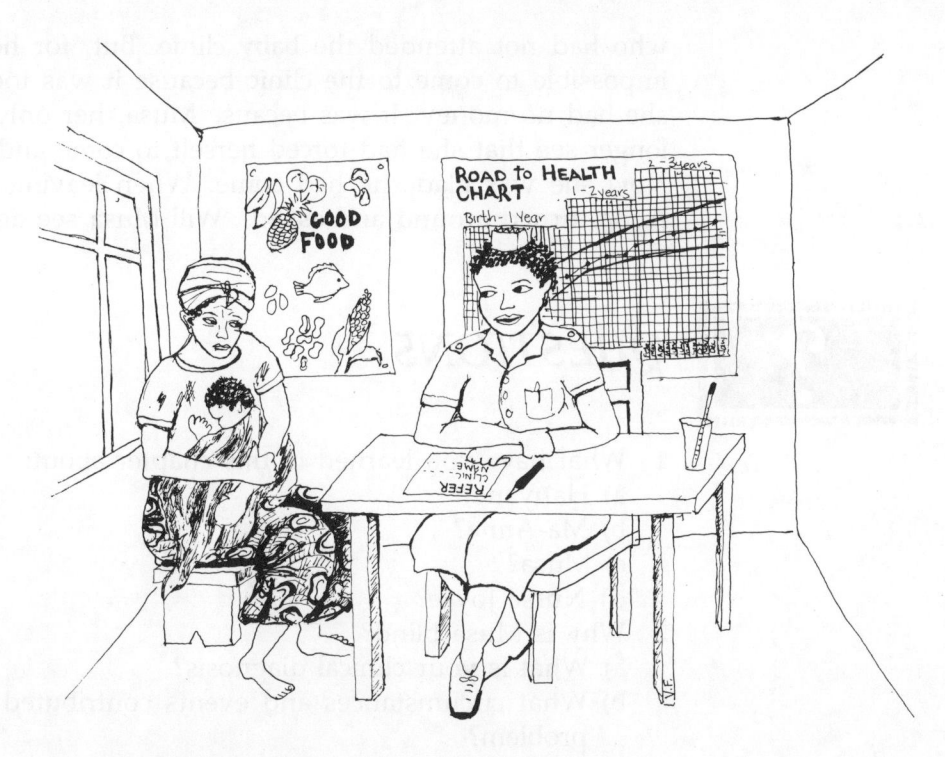

'We must send Musa to hospital. His eyes are very bad.'

'Yes, he had measles and hasn't opened his eyes since the day the children went back to school.'

Joyce estimated that to be about two weeks ago. Musa's weight was only 8 kg. He had been fed only maize and water.

Ma-Anna was no longer breast-feeding him – her milk had stopped long ago. There were no vegetables where she lived, and she had no money for powdered milk.

Feeling the nurse's readiness to listen, Ma-Anna gave more information. Bit by bit Joyce managed to join the pieces into a picture of Ma-Anna's situation: she had four children – the oldest, Anna, was about eight years old; Musa, the youngest, was the only boy. There had been another baby boy but he had had a bad cough and died. Her husband had gone to the city to find work. For a while he sent money home. However, for the last two years Ma-Anna had not heard from him. At the time her husband left to go to the city she was pregnant with Musa.

Joyce urged Ma-Anna to take Musa to hospital straight away. Fortunately, she knew of someone who would be driving that way the next day.

Ma-Anna thanked the nurse. She had been terrified of coming to the clinic, because she had heard that nurses chased away people who had not attended the baby clinic. But, for her, it had been impossible to come to the clinic because it was too far away and she had no money. It was because Musa, her only son, could no longer see that she had forced herself to come and see the nurse. Now she was glad she had come. When leaving the clinic, Ma-Anna turned around and asked, 'Will Musa see again?'

QUESTIONS

1. What have you learned in this chapter about:
   a) Hanyane?
   b) Ma-Anna?
   c) Musa?
   d) Nurse Joyce?
2. Why is Musa blind?
   a) What is your clinical diagnosis?
   b) What circumstances and events contributed to Musa's eye problem?
   c) Which factor do you think is the most important **root cause** of Musa's blindness?
3. Why is the Road To Health Chart important for the management of eye problems in children?
4. If Ma-Anna had come to you with Musa two months earlier, what would you have done to prevent his blindness?

DISCUSSION

Faced with Musa's problem you, as a health worker, will want to do more than just dispense some eye ointment to appease the child's mother. In order to respond sympathetically and appropriately you will first have to explore the situation. You need to know:
1. *What* happened to Musa? (Clinical diagnosis)
2. *Why* has it happened? (Root cause of health problem)
3. *What can be done* so that it will not happen again? (Prevention and health promotion)

1 Arriving at a clinical diagnosis

This is discussed in Part 3, Section C, page 222.

2 Finding the root cause of health problems

Here is a suggestion for a way to proceed:

Find out as much as possible about Musa, Ma-Anna and the conditions in which they live. You will find the required information scattered throughout the story. This is the way you usually get information. Patients never give you the facts in the logical order you would like to have them. You will have to fit the pieces together yourself.

Make a list of all the points you think are important. Having done that, you can ask yourself *why* things happened the way they did. For example: 'Why is Musa blind?'

Chain of events leading to Musa's blindness

a) *Why is Musa blind?*
Because he had measles and vitamin A deficiency, plus general malnutrition. This led to acute bilateral corneal ulceration, followed by perforation.

b) *Why did Musa not get a protective dose of Vitamin A at the time measles started?*
Because Ma-Anna was afraid to go to the clinic. She was afraid that the nurse would be angry with her for not having attended the clinic before. Ma-Anna was also reluctant to carry the child the long distance to the clinic.

c) *Why did Musa get such bad measles in the first place?*
Musa had not been vaccinated against measles, and his growth had not been monitored nor his nutritional state corrected. It was difficult for Ma-Anna to get these checked as the clinic is 15 km from Hanyane and there is no public transport to it.

d) *Why does Musa have vitamin A deficiency?*
Because there are no vegetables available.

e) *Why has Musa failed to gain weight?*
Musa is fed only maize porridge made with water, and Ma-Anna stopped breast feeding early because of ill health.

f) *Why does Ma-Anna have no money to buy milk for Musa?*
Because Musa's father has sent no money home – he has vanished.

g) *Why did Musa's father go to the city to look for work when Ma-Anna was already pregnant with Musa?*
Because Hanyane is a remote village with no job opportunities.

11

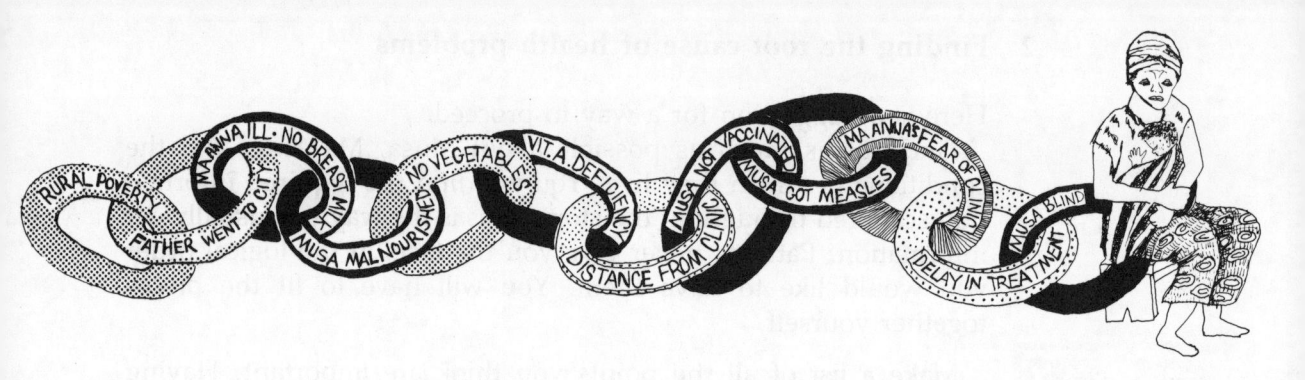

Now you see that a long chain of events led to Musa's problems.

This example illustrates how almost every aspect of village life influences the state of health of its people. The most fundamental factor is poverty which will be discussed in Chapter 4.

To understand Ma-Anna's situation better we would like to find answers to some more questions, such as:

h) Why did her husband not send any money?
  i) Has he taken another wife in town?
  ii) Did he spend all the money on himself?
  iii) Has he been the victim of doubtful 'friends'?
  iv) Has he been ill, or has he died?

i) Why are there no vegetables?
  i) Is there no land for planting?
  ii) Is the soil unsuitable?
  iii) Is there no water?
  iv) Are there no vegetables at the shop or in the market?
  v) Are vegetables too expensive for Ma-Anna?
  vi) Is it traditional practice not to give vegetables to young children?

j) Why has Musa not been vaccinated?
  i) Did Ma-Anna not know about vaccination?
  ii) Was the health service too expensive?
  iii) Was there no nurse at the clinic?
  iv) Did Ma-Anna mistrust western medicine?
  v) Have the nurses got a reputation for being rude to poor people?

3 What can be done?

In Musa's case treatment will not help him to recover his eyesight. The clinical diagnosis has come too late to be of any use to him. Action should have been taken long before Musa's disease had advanced so far.

Acting in order to overcome the root causes will prevent blindness in many young children who are at risk. This is why community eye care is so important.

Ideas on strategies to achieve better health in the community are illustrated in the story of Hanyane. Specific eye health promotion messages are summarised in Figure 27 on page 204, and Summary to Part 2 on page 205.

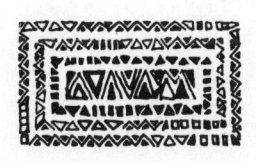

SUMMARY

1. Eye diseases are often the result of a combination of various factors such as poverty, insufficient food production, lack of education and inaccessible or inadequate health services.
2. Community eye care addresses these root causes of ill health in order to promote eye health and to prevent unnecessary blindness.

Vho-Mudau's Wisdom
– *What is health?*

Back home, Ma-Anna prepared herself for the journey to hospital. As Kokwana, her mother-in-law, was old, frail and almost blind, she didn't want to leave her too much work.

Ma-Anna collected wood to last for several days. Early next morning she cooked the mukapu (traditional soft maize porridge) for the day. Then she put on clean clothes, tied Musa on her back and left for the hospital.

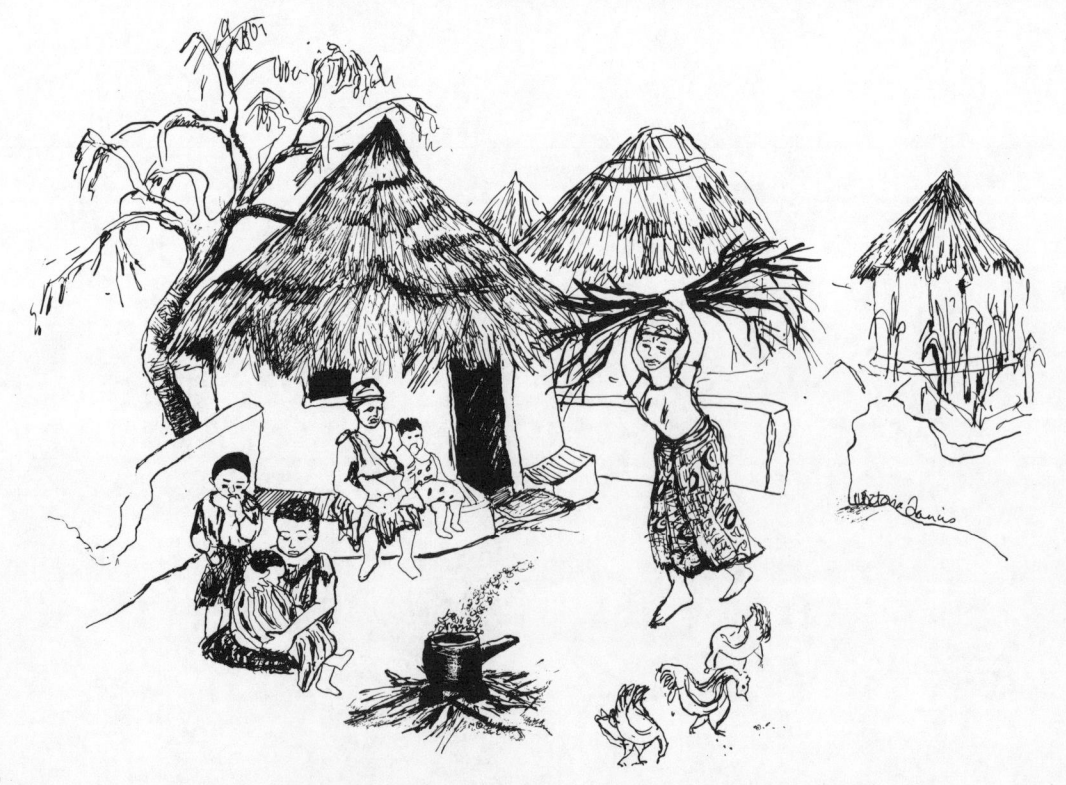

Kokwana watched Ma-Anna walk away until she disappeared. Then she filled a bowl with mukapu for the children. Soon afterwards, Kokwana's sister, Vho-Mudau, entered the yard – this being the usual time for her visit. They had hardly settled down for a talk when Ma-Anna's friend, Lerisa, arrived. Lerisa wanted to go with Ma-Anna to collect wood.

Kokwana told her about Musa's eyes and that Ma-Anna had taken him to the hospital. This angered Vho-Mudau. She asked, 'Why didn't you treat the child according to our old custom?'

'Of course we did everything', replied Kokwana. 'I know as well as you do about these things – our mother taught us. We smeared Musa with red clay and it worked well – the rash came out even stronger. But the chicken blood and goat's urine we put in his eyes didn't seem to help this time.'

The three ladies went on to discuss how things had changed for the worse in these modern times. They complained about people being sick more often now and that they had to bury too many young children. But each one had a different opinion about why this was so and what could be done.

Kokwana said, 'If there was a hospital here in Hanyane, people would be cured quickly. There are too few doctors to take sickness away from us.'

Vho-Mudau disagreed. 'I don't trust doctors. Why is there more disease since doctors and nurses are around? When I was young we listened to our ancestors and honoured the wisdom of our elders. Now people have lost all respect. Therefore the ancestors punish us and send disease.'

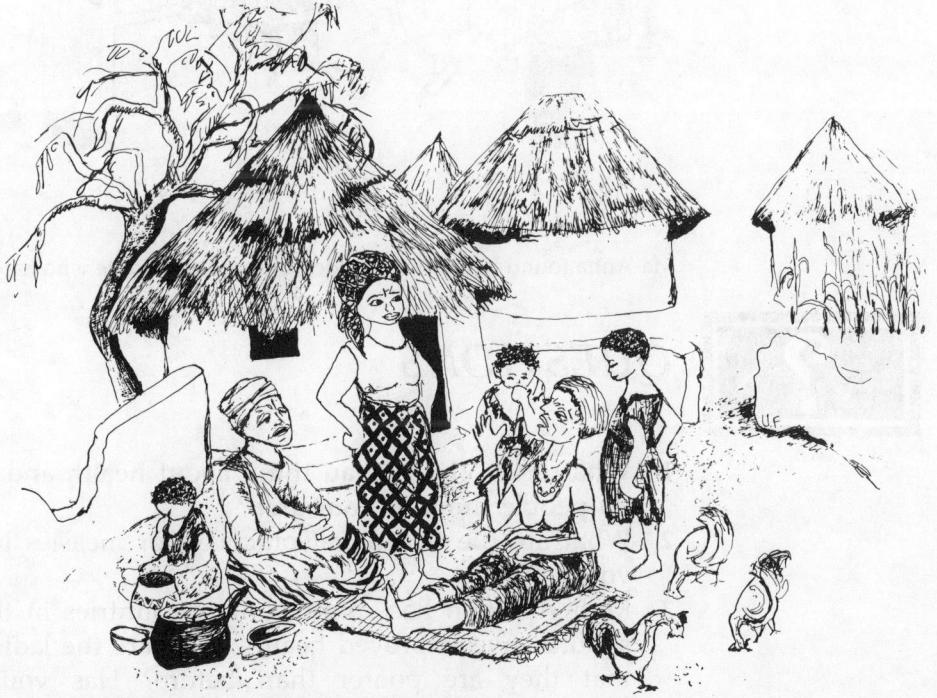

'I don't trust these doctors and nurses'

Lerisa reminded the two elderly ladies about other changes that had taken place. 'There used to be more land for everyone and people had enough to eat. Now many are hungry. Working hard in the fields doesn't help because the soil is too poor. Our men have left to find work elsewhere and some women are all alone – look at Ma-Anna, she can't cope any more.'

The three ladies went on arguing for a long time. In the meantime Ma-Anna had arrived at the district hospital and Musa had been admitted to the children's ward. He cried his heart out when he was put into the cot. Ma-Anna tried to comfort him although she herself felt threatened in the hospital which was so strange to her.

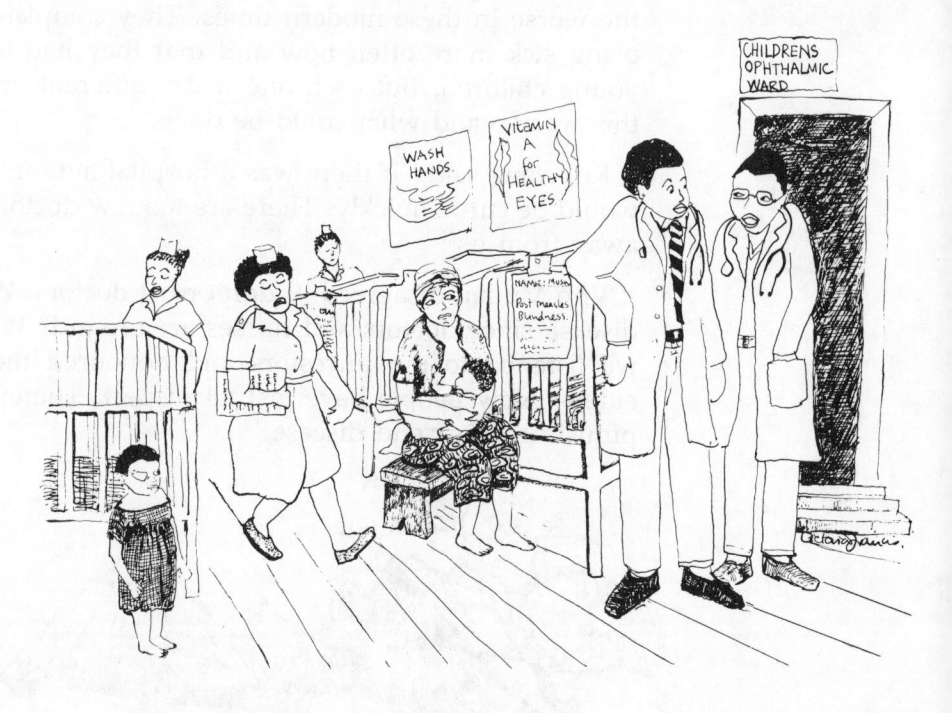

Ma-Anna found herself surrounded by people in white who hardly spoke to her

QUESTIONS

1. What does Vho-Mudau think about health and disease? What do people think in your area?
2. What are the traditional practices for measles infection where you work?
3. Modernisation has come to most countries in the world. This should have improved health. Why are the ladies complaining that they are poorer than before? Has your area similar problems? Why?

DISCUSSION

1 What is health?

The three ladies at Ma-Anna's home talk about disease, doctors and traditional remedies and practices. They know what 'disease' is, because disease causes pain and discomfort. Because health is much more difficult to define, most people describe it in negative terms, i.e. they say what health is *not*.

You will learn much about what people think of health when you listen to the three ladies.

For Kokwana health means not being sick

She wants doctors and a hospital to take disease away. Many people think like this. Even some doctors, politicians and welfare organisations share Kokwana's ideas. They believe that more and better equipped hospitals together with more doctors will improve health in the communities. But experience has shown that hospitals have not improved health because hospitals deal with disease, not with health.

For Lerisa health means having a good place to live

She believes that good health is impossible when living conditions are as bad as they are at Hanyane. In the past, people were healthier because, in those days, there was enough land to plough and there were enough cattle to provide milk and meat. All three ladies agree that disease and hunger go together.

It is easy to recognise shortages of food and water because hunger and thirst are acutely felt. Other health hazards, like poor hygiene or overcrowding, are seldom appreciated although they are quite as important as food.

For Vho-Mudau health is a matter of peace with the ancestors

She is sceptical of modern ways. You may have labelled her as ignorant and superstitious. But listen again, carefully and without prejudice, to what she has to say: disease is a punishment for offending the ancestors. Therefore, health depends on the harmonious relationship between man and the spiritual world. This idea is common to most religions. Disease is often considered a consequence of sin or misbehaviour, while healing miracles are linked with forgiveness and new life.

Translated into 'health language' the ideas of the three village ladies are that:

> HEALTH MEANS:
> NO DISEASE, PEACE OF MIND AND
> A FAVOURABLE ENVIRONMENT WITH ENOUGH GOOD FOOD

This is almost identical to the World Health Organization's definition of health:

> HEALTH IS A STATE OF COMPLETE
> PHYSICAL, MENTAL AND SOCIAL WELL-BEING

Lerisa made a last, very important, remark: 'Ma-Anna can't cope anymore'. The worries about her husband, her insecurity, Musa's illness, overwork and too little food have caused her to give up. Too much is asked of her, and she cannot see any sense in trying to do more, because things will never change.

Problems are part of everyone's life. A healthy person can face and overcome the hurdles. But when this capacity to *cope* breaks down, mental and physical illness follow.

Because 'coping' is such a vital element to health, it is important to include it in the definition. So,

> HEALTH IS:
> A STATE OF PHYSICAL, MENTAL AND SOCIAL WELL-BEING
> WHICH ENABLES ONE TO COPE WITH DAILY LIFE

Do you still attach the label of 'ignorance' to these three ladies who never went to school? Health workers often think people are ignorant. Those who take the trouble to sit and listen, especially to the old, find out how wise they are. Their knowledge is expressed in the language of their own culture and religious philosophy. This makes it difficult to interpret and is then taken as superstition and ignorance.

2 Traditional remedies and practices

Disease has always been with mankind and people have learned to deal with it. Healing plants were discovered, and various practices thought to be beneficial were developed. The acquired knowledge has been passed on from generation to generation. Old Kokwana treated Musa's measles with the methods she had learned from her mother.

When the Europeans settled in Africa and Asia they rejected traditional practices as being evil and harmful. They thought only white people were knowledgeable and that everyone else was ignorant. This attitude was upheld in schools, churches and hospitals. Many a health worker sneers at traditional practices to prove that s/he has left the 'dark ages' behind and is now educated. In this way, many beneficial practices are discarded together with the harmful ones. Not only is this a tragic loss, but it also affects the cultural confidence of the people.

As health workers we should take a new look at healing traditions. An exercise on practices in relation to measles in your area may help you. The example given here applies to Kokwana's tradition. Make a similar table for the traditional practices in your area.

Practice	Reasoning (if any)	Good	Bad	Harmless	Why?
Isolation of child	Prevent contact with 'bad' people	x			Reduces spread
Painting body with red mud	Provoke rash to come out			x	
Put goat's urine in eyes	Prevent blindness		x		Introduces infection to eyes
Add goat's milk to diet	Common practice for sick children	x			Prevents further malnutrition

Table 2.1

By encouraging beneficial practices you win the people's confidence and respect. Then you can go and demonstrate how harmful practices could be replaced by some medicine from your clinic, without hurting the people's feelings.

SUMMARY

1 You discover much wisdom when you listen carefully to people, especially the old folk.

2 People have always known that health depends on a favourable environment as well as social and spiritual harmony. This knowledge is expressed in various religious beliefs and practices.
3 Many traditional healing practices stem from observations made and passed on over generations. Some are good, some are dangerous. Good practices should be encouraged, bad ones replaced.

3

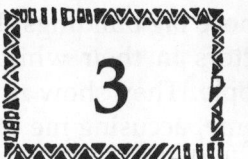

Those people in white frighten me – Hospitals and health

One week after arriving at the hospital Musa was discharged. Ma-Anna was given some eye ointment to take home and a letter for the clinic. Musa's eyes were still grey and he was still blind. Ma-Anna had been too scared to ask the doctor whether her child would see again. She would have to ask Joyce.

On her way home from the hospital, Ma-Anna called at the clinic. Joyce was glad to see her back. She asked all about the hospital. Ma-Anna told Joyce about her experience.

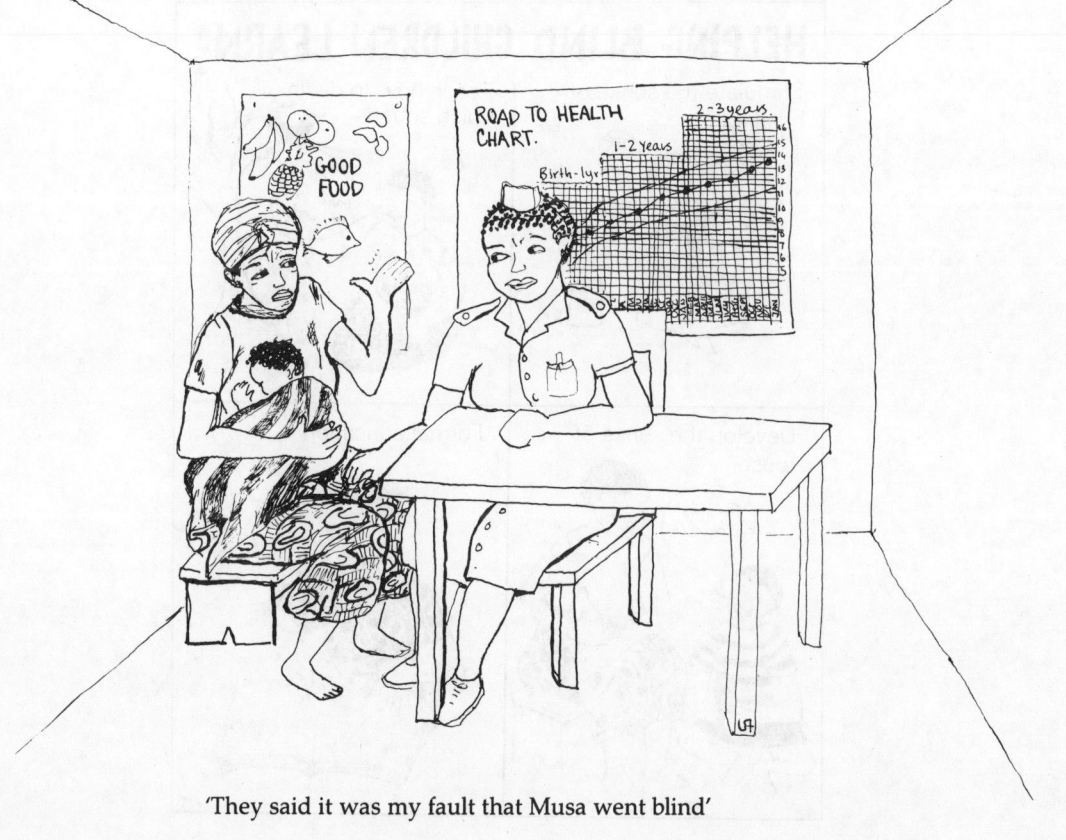

'They said it was my fault that Musa went blind'

'It was a very frightening place. I got lost in those big buildings. I couldn't understand all those nurses and doctors in their white coats. They behave differently from normal people. They show no respect towards older people. Some shouted at me, accusing me of being a bad mother. They said it was my fault that Musa went blind. Not all the nurses were like that. Some were good to me and they were especially good to Musa. They gave him medicines and very nice food, not just mukapu. But Musa is still blind.'

Joyce wanted to know what the doctor thought about Musa. But Ma-Anna couldn't tell her. He had only talked to the other doctor or to the nurse, not to her. She complained that he also talked in some strange language, using words she couldn't understand.

Joyce realised that Ma-Anna had not been told that Musa would always be blind. She had to break the bad news herself. She tried to comfort Ma-Anna by telling her about a school for blind children. She told her how they learned to read with their fingers. She also suggested that Ma-Anna could make some toys for Musa, such as putting stones in a tin to make a rattle.

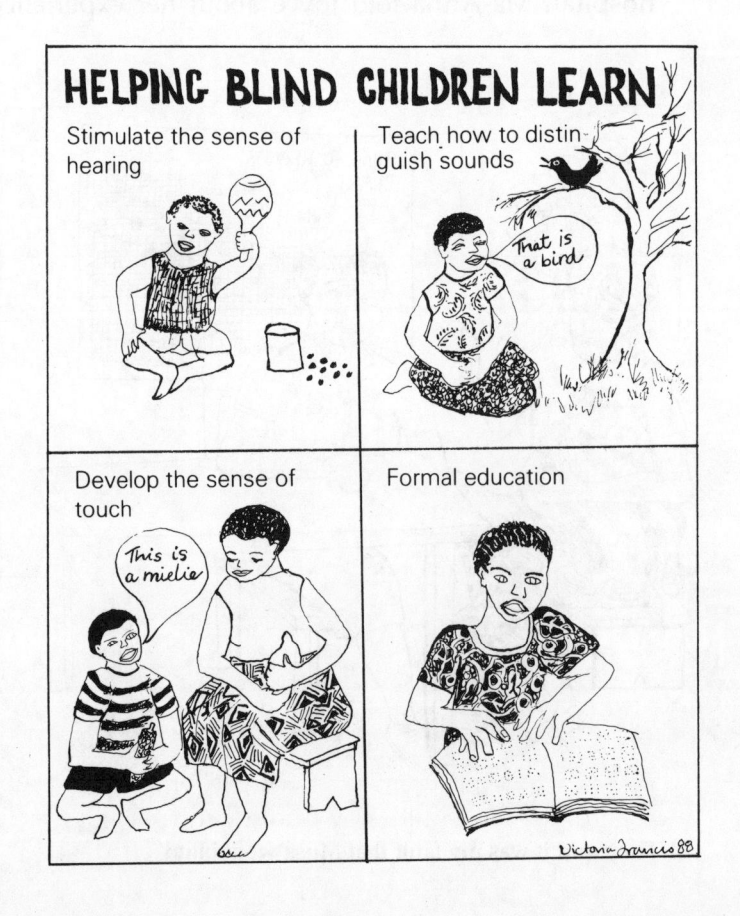

But Ma-Anna wasn't interested. She couldn't imagine how anybody could read with his fingers. In any case, Musa was far too young to go to school, even if there was a school for him. There were more important things to do in the immediate future. Joyce knew this. Musa must be fed properly from now on. Ma-Anna knew what food Musa should get. The nurses at the hospital had told her many times to give Musa eggs, milk, cheese and lots of dark green vegetables. She had listened to their lectures. But these things were not available in Hanyane. The few chickens she kept did not lay many eggs and the goats ate all the vegetables she planted because she had no money for fencing. Ma-Anna told Joyce that she did not want to argue with the nurses. They couldn't understand how difficult life was in Hanyane. She was afraid of offending them, as then they wouldn't care for Musa anymore. The best Joyce could do was to give Ma-Anna some powdered milk for Musa. She showed her how to mix it correctly.

After Ma-Anna had gone, Joyce returned to her desk to fill in the details on Musa's card. Her thoughts were not on her work. She watched the slow walk of this mother, with her child tied on her back, setting off on the long journey home, where she would be greeted by hungry children and little comfort. She asked herself why some people were so unlucky? Was it only a matter of luck?

Joyce took her diary and marked the day she would travel to Hanyane to see Musa in his home.

QUESTIONS

1. Look at the illustration on page 16. Does it look familiar?
   a) What is the attitude of the doctors and nurses?
   b) How do you think Ma-Anna feels?
   c) Describe what the same people would look like in your picture of an ideal children's eye ward.
2. What do you think of the health education given to Ma-Anna at the hospital?
3. What do hospitals do for the health of the people?
4. How might hospitals, doctors and nurses make people more sick?

DISCUSSION

Ma-Anna felt threatened by the big hospital buildings and the people in white uniforms. She found herself in an alien world where people could not understand each other. Her hopes that Musa would regain his health had been dashed. Why do people believe so much in hospitals? For her it has been a great disappointment.

In the eyes of your community you represent the hospital. People may come to you with requests for facilities and you have to answer them. It is thus worthwhile to take a critical look at hospitals and their effect on health and disease.

Hospitals are concerned with curative medicine

They are places where diseases are treated. Patients go to hospital when they notice that something has gone wrong – when there are *symptoms* of disease. By the time symptoms develop the disease may already have reached an advanced stage. For example, when a patient with glaucoma begins to notice visual loss, damage to the eye is already beyond repair. Doctors and nurses are most familiar with advanced *clinical disease* because this is what they see at the hospital or clinic. They are trained to help the patient to get back to normal – to *cure* him or her – if it is possible.

If hospitals are places for healing, why do they sometimes worsen a patient's illness? When many sick people are crowded together in one place, several things can go wrong. In the space below list five things you think can happen.

1 ....
2 ....
3 ....
4 ....
5 ....

Hospitals are sometimes described as 'Disease Palaces'. A *palace* is a large, expensive building of prestige. It stands alone, usually in the middle of a big park, remote from the dwellings of ordinary people. The owner may be rich and powerful, or he may just pretend to be rich and powerful. Does this apply to hospitals?

Expensive building

A hospital is not only expensive to build, but it is expensive to keep functioning. Equipment and medicines are costly, doctors' and nurses' salaries are high.

Prestige

Governments like to enhance their credibility by building a big hospital in the capital city, even if the country is too poor to pay

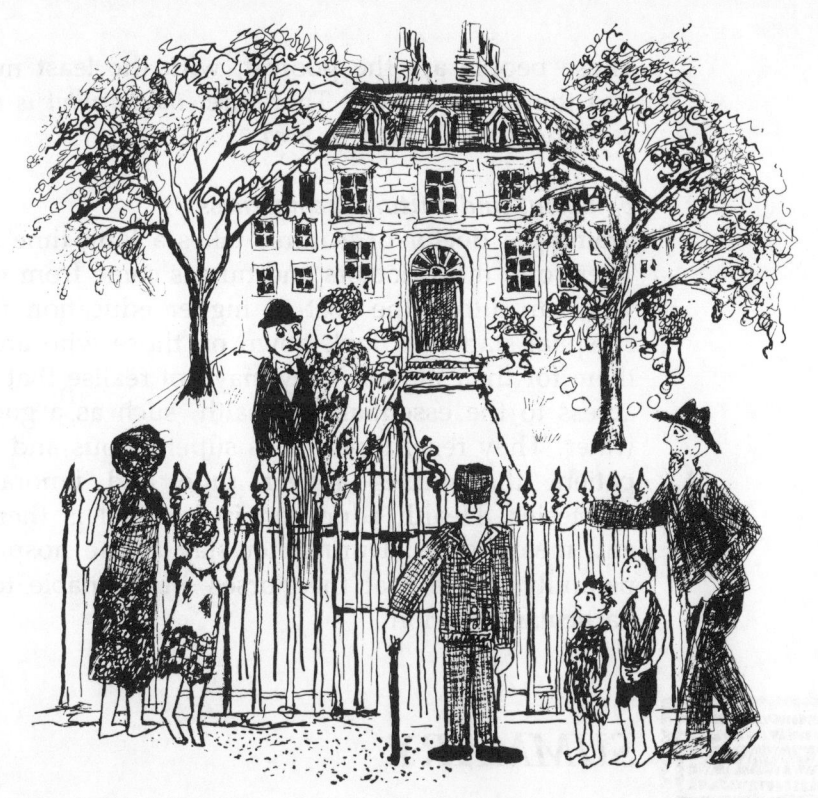

What has this palace in common with a hospital?

for it. A *single hospital may consume most of the health budget of a country*, leaving no funds for the promotion of health or for preventing disease. So, *governments usually spend a lot more money on disease than on health.*

Isolation
There is a danger for hospitals to isolate themselves from the communities they serve, because they are too much concerned about the smooth running of their institution. The hospital's aim is to provide good curative care, and most energy is directed towards the improvement of diagnostic techniques and treatment. This benefits those who go to hospital. Doctors and nurses are so involved in hospital routine that they are not aware that the events outside the hospital determine whether people will be sick or healthy. (See Chapter 1.)

Remoteness

Hospitals are remote from the people they serve – geographically, socially and culturally.

a) Geographical remoteness
Hospitals are usually situated in, or near, large cities. However, in developing countries 80% of the population live in rural areas.

These people are the poorest, with the least means of transport and the most disease. Therefore, *the hospital is out of reach for the majority of people most in need.*

b) Social and cultural remoteness
Training a doctor or a nurse takes a long time and is expensive. Therefore, most doctors and nurses come from well-to-do families who can afford the cost of higher education for their children. Hospital staff may look down on those who are poor and blame them for their illness. They may not realise that the poor have no access to the essentials of health, such as a good diet and clean water. They regard people as superstitious and backward. To the patient the nurses appear rude and ignorant of traditional courtesies. Health education in hospital is therefore often futile and meaningless. During her stay at the hospital Ma-Anna was painfully aware that the nurses were unable to understand her particular situation.

SUMMARY

1 Hospitals are good – and necessary – in order to *cure* diseases requiring special care, but do little to *improve health.*
2 Hospitals are expensive. If financial and staff resources are scarce, hospitals function at the expense of public health.
3 Hospitals are remote and inaccessible to those who need most care.
4 In order to improve the health of the people, the hospital staff must come out of their 'palaces' and go where the people in need live.

4

We are not fit for visitors – Health and the poor

Ma-Anna was walking home from the clinic. She kept repeating to herself what the nurse said about Musa's blindness. 'They did all they could at the hospital but, unless a miracle happens, Musa will stay blind.'

If the hospital couldn't help any more, thought Ma-Anna, maybe the mungoma (traditional medicine man) could. He had worked miracles before, why not for Musa?

And so Ma-Anna decided to borrow some money to open the mungoma's mouth. The mungoma chose some roots she should burn. The smoke would cure Musa's eyes. But the expected miracle didn't happen.

More than a week later, Vho-Mudau and Lerisa dropped in at Ma-Anna's home. As usual, they talked about Musa. Vho-Mudau was still confident that traditional treatment would eventually help. But Kokwana had given up hope. She was going blind herself, and no medicines helped her.

'It will be even worse with Musa,' Kokwana said. 'He will not learn anything. He will never work to support his mother. He will eat her food instead.'

Just then a car approached on the main road. The ladies got up to see. They watched the vehicle stop next to the footpath leading to their house.

The nurse stepped out. Vho-Mudau shouted, 'She comes our way! What does she want? I don't want to see her. I'm going.'

Kokwana was upset too. 'We are not fit for visitors,' she said and ordered Ma-Anna to sweep the yard. Lerisa hastily put sand over the diarrhoea stools the youngest girl, Rose, had just produced.

Joyce waited at a distance from the house, making her presence known according to local customs.

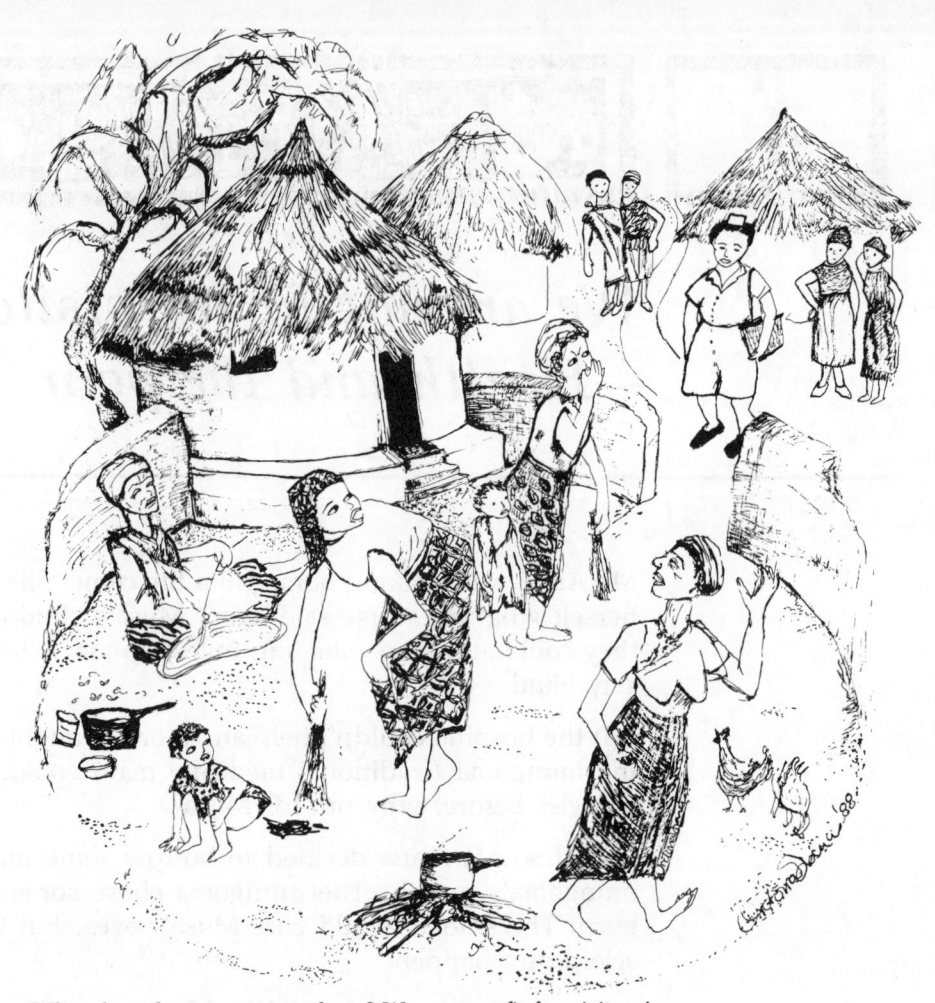

'What does that nurse want here? We are not fit for visitors'

Ma-Anna fetched a chair for the visitor. But Joyce insisted that she felt more comfortable on a mat. 'I have come to see how Musa is getting on and brought a toy for him. I also have a packet of powdered milk in case the first is finished.'

Joyce didn't seem to mind when Ma-Anna showed her the old packet which had hardly been used. She just asked for a mug and some water so that she could, once again, show how the milk was prepared.

Ma-Anna took the nearest mug, dipped it into the water container, rinsed it and gave it to the nurse. Then she took a jug of water from the same container. Joyce asked whether the water was clean. The three ladies were surprised.

'Of course! These days the river water is not as muddy as usual. Can't you see how clear it is?'

'But do you boil it?' asked Joyce.

'What? How can we boil it when there is so little wood?'

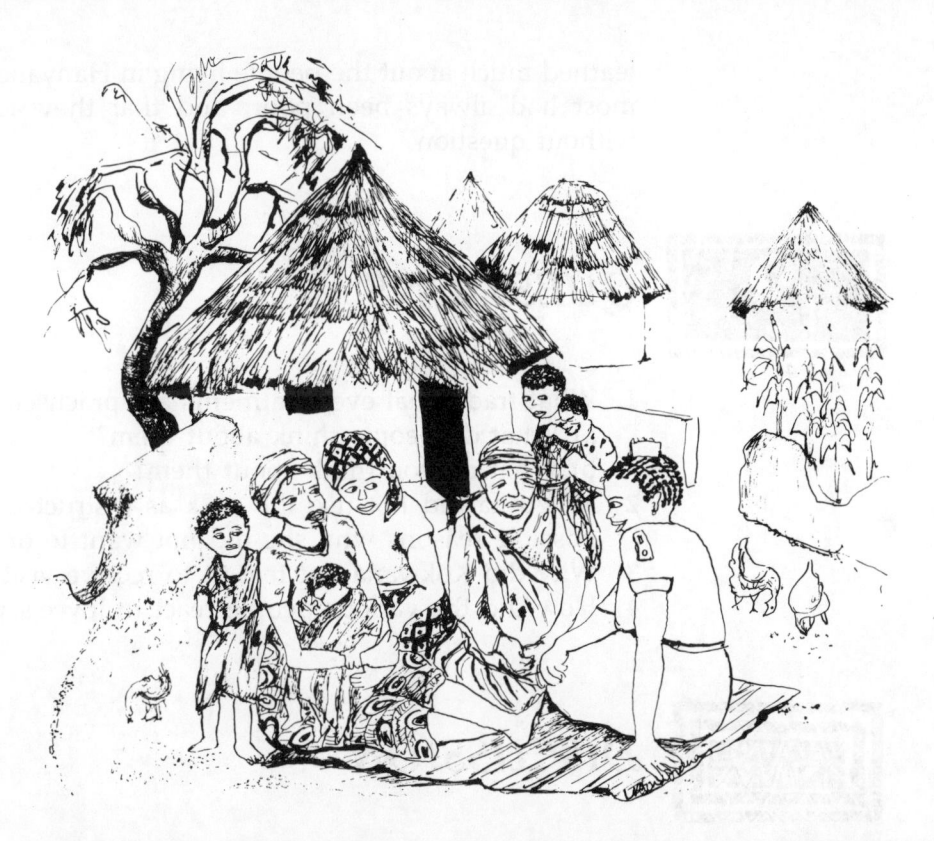

Joyce tried to explain that river water is polluted and could make people sick in the stomach. Lerisa was the only one who listened intently. She wanted to know whether this water could have caused Rose's diarrhoea. Joyce thought that this was quite possible, although there were many other causes as well. 'Food left standing for a long time before eating can also cause it,' she said, looking at the pots standing around with leftovers in them. Kokwana argued that food and wood could not be wasted. It was more economical to cook once a day.

Joyce was disheartened. Just about everything was wrong in this family. Kokwana was almost blind from trachoma; all the children seemed to be malnourished. Their discharging eyes were riddled with flies. She wouldn't be surprised either if Ma-Anna had TB.

'It seems you have a lot of problems in Hanyane. Why do you not have a village health worker?' Joyce asked.

Lerisa remembered that there had been some talk about it but nothing had come of it. It appeared that the chief was unhappy because some men from the city had proposed it.

Lerisa suggested that if Joyce spoke to the chief, she could explain it better to him. As Lerisa lived near the chief's place she could show Joyce the way. Joyce welcomed the opportunity to leave Ma-Anna's home and go and introduce herself to the chief. By the time they reached the chief's place, Joyce had already learned much about the people living in Hanyane. It appeared that most had always been poor, and that they accepted their fate without question.

QUESTIONS

1 What traditional eye treatments are practised in your area?
   a) What do people think about them?
   b) What do you think about them?
2 Ma-Anna did not use the milk as instructed. Try to find five possible reasons why she did not want to or could not do so.
3 Why did Kokwana not feel fit to receive visitors?
4 How did the various people react to Joyce's visit?

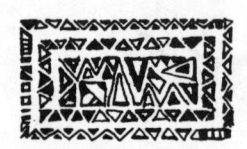

DISCUSSION

In the preceding chapters, Ma-Anna has told the nurse about her home situation. Now Joyce faces the shocking reality of poverty at Ma-Anna's home.

Many who have no personal experience of poverty tend to blame the poor for their fate. They say poor people are lazy, careless and stupid. This is not true. We find just as much, if not more, laziness and stupidity amongst the rich. What is often not realised is that poor people have everything against them, and that it requires toughness, hard work and imagination to survive.

Poor people are sick more often than others. Therefore we want to find out which aspects of poverty are responsible for poor health. According to Chambers poverty includes:
1 Material deprivation (food, land, money)
2 Isolation
3 Vulnerability
4 Powerlessness
5 Poor health.

1 Material deprivation

There are no job opportunities in Hanyane. Ma-Anna's husband, like most other men, had to seek work elsewhere. He found a job in the city. We do not know why he disappeared but, whatever happened, Ma-Anna has been left without any income. She has no land either to produce the food for her family. She cannot afford proper clothing or school education for her children.

In addition, Hanyane lacks essential infrastructures such as safe water or official transport facilities. Polluted water is one of the reasons why diarrhoea is so common. Also, the long distance to the clinic makes access to adequate health care difficult. Because Hanyane lacks clean water and is so remote, the whole village is poor. Ma-Anna's family is one of the hardest hit.

2 Isolation

Ma-Anna's home is on the outskirts of the village, far away from the shop, the school or the big tree, where most activities take place. General announcements, such as vaccination campaigns, often do not reach her or she does not understand that she is included. Being illiterate she cannot read any news, important notices or safety instructions. This may cause accidents or poisoning with insecticides or other dangerous substances.

The better off, with the exception of Lerisa, are not interested in Ma-Anna. When she receives visitors she feels embarrassed that she has no special food to offer them and that people see how poor she is. That is why Kokwana said 'We are not fit for visitors'.

3 Vulnerability

Odd expenses over and above the budgeted daily essentials pull Ma-Anna deeper into poverty. It becomes increasingly difficult to get out of it. Ma-Anna spent all her savings on the hospital fees and the mungoma. Now she is forced to borrow money, increasing her debts. She will spend even less on food, and she and her family will become weaker and more susceptible to disease.

4 Powerlessness

The better off in a community ignore poor people like Ma-Anna because of their low social status. The poor people's opinion carries no weight. Thus the poor feel they have nothing to say, or are not allowed to raise their voices. To participate in community and political activities is therefore useless. They also have less time to be involved because they have fewer time-saving conveniences like running water or electricity.

The land, by law due to Ma-Anna, has not been allocated to her. The chief knows that she is unaware of her rights and has taken advantage of this. Even if she were aware of them she would not know how to fight for her rights.

In the hospital she felt at the mercy of the nurses and therefore said 'yes' to everything, knowing well that she would never be able to follow their instructions regarding food for Musa.

The people of Hanyane have not taken any steps to request public transport to the clinic. It does not occur to them that it could be done. Thus, those who are most in need of health care are the least able to get it.

5 Poor health

All aspects of poverty discussed so far affect health. Material deprivation causes Musa to be malnourished and Ma-Anna to be weak; she is probably suffering from TB. Malnutrition weakens the body's defence mechanisms (the immune system) making it vulnerable to infections.

Through isolation and powerlessness Ma-Anna has little access to health services and hesitates to use them, for fear of verbal abuse from the nurse. She has not attended the child health clinic because she did not appreciate its importance and the clinic was too far away. Musa is therefore not vaccinated and his older brother has died of untreated broncho-pneumonia.

Ma-Anna has no husband. She therefore has to take the role of head of the family as well as the full-time job of mother. Increased physical and mental stress, together with an undernourished, weakened body, are too much for her. As Lerisa aptly remarks (Chapter 2), Ma-Anna cannot cope any more. She has to concentrate her efforts on the essentials: food for the family. She cannot afford to waste the little strength she has on 'luxuries' like household hygiene. This has to wait for better times. Ignorant outsiders believe this to be laziness. In some agricultural societies a tidy home is scorned upon. In these places, a woman who has time for her home is regarded as lazy because she is supposed to be working in the fields.

People seldom realise how heavy a price they have to pay for ignoring hygiene. For example, Kokwana is blind from trachoma and the children suffer from frequent bouts of diarrhoea. It is not Ma-Anna's fault because she does not know any better. She has not had the opportunity for education.

SUMMARY

1 Poverty causes poor health.
2 Most poor people are trapped into poverty against their will. It is not true that poor people are lazy and stupid. Poverty often

results from those in control drawing the best from the community and putting little back into it. It is therefore unjust to blame the poor for their poverty and illness.

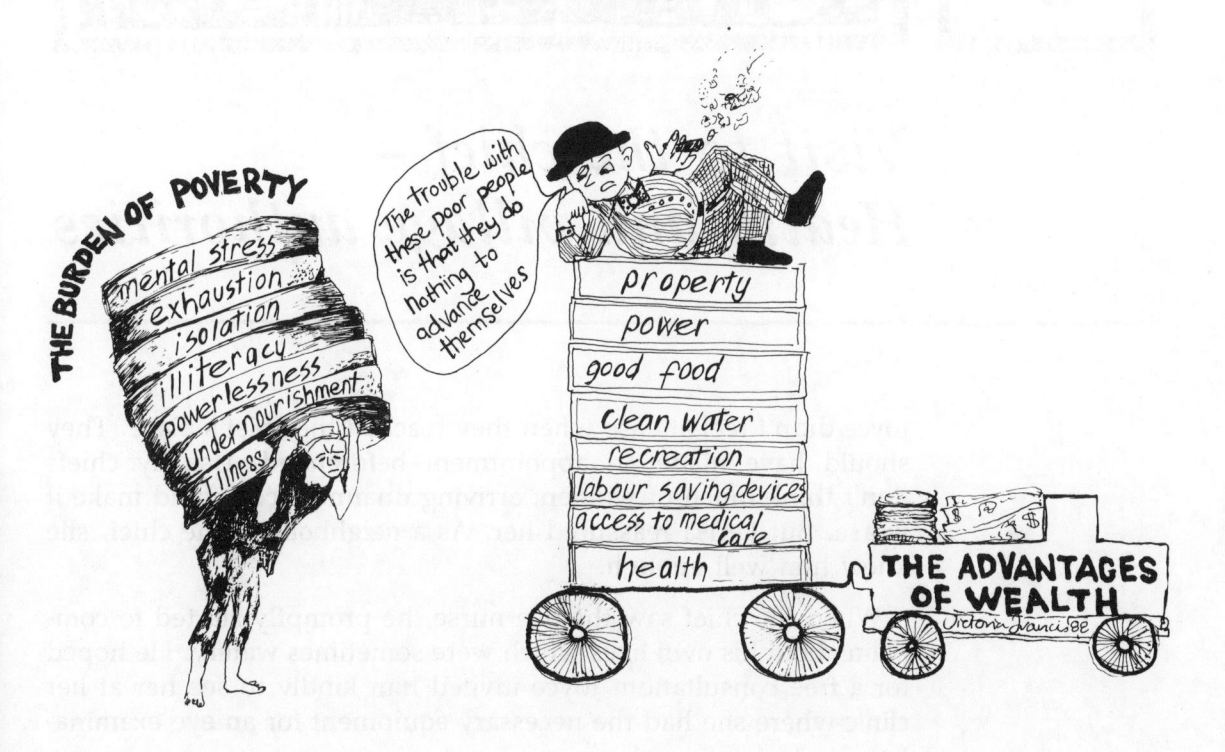

Reference
Chambers, R., *Rural Development* (Longman, 1983)

5

Visit to the chief – Health and village authorities

Joyce didn't feel at ease when they reached the chief's place. They should have made an appointment beforehand. Usually chiefs don't think much of women; arriving unannounced could make it worse. But Lerisa reassured her. As a neighbour of the chief, she knew him well enough.

When the chief saw the eye nurse, he promptly started to complain about his own eyes which were sometimes watery. He hoped for a free consultation. Joyce invited him kindly to see her at her clinic where she had the necessary equipment for an eye examination.

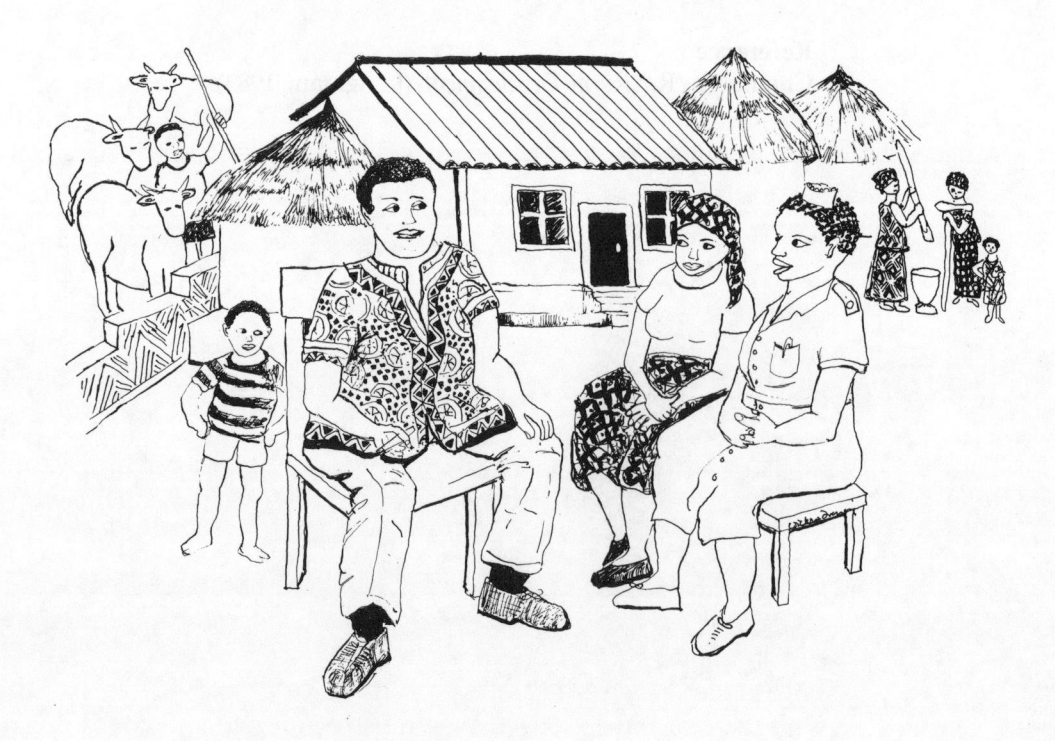

Joyce and Lerisa visit the chief

'How are things here in Hanyane? Do you have any health problems?' asked Joyce.

'Oh yes,' he replied. 'People refuse to build toilets. It is a government order, you know. We fine all those who have no toilets. But it doesn't help. People are lazy and stubborn.'

He got up to fetch the government notice and showed it to Joyce. It read:

> To all administrative offices of district . . . .
> Order:
> It has come to the notice of this office that typhoid cases are on the increase in your area. It is therefore deemed essential that all households are equipped with an adequate toilet within six months of date of issue of this notice. Village authorities will be held responsible for the implementation of this order.
>
> Signed: District Chief Medical Officer

Joyce noticed that there was no toilet at the chief's compound either. She remarked that toilets are difficult to install because skills and money are required to build them.

The chief changed the subject. He complained about the long distance to the clinic. He wanted a clinic and a nurse in Hanyane. This was the occasion to take up the issue of the village health worker. Both Lerisa and Joyce tried to convince the chief of the idea, but he didn't want to commit himself. He had to discuss the matter first with his councillors.

'And,' he added, 'the people won't agree. They are very stubborn and many want a proper nurse here.'

Joyce bade farewell to the chief and thanked Lerisa for arranging the meeting. Then she hurried back to the clinic – she had been away much longer than planned. The encounter with the chief had not been very encouraging. She got the impression that it was he who was reluctant to change things, although he wasn't a bad man either. Maybe developing a good relationship slowly would help.

A week later Joyce received an invitation from the chief to attend a village gathering in Hanyane. He wanted her to talk about toilets. Joyce happily went to the meeting. She spoke about the importance of toilets, but people did not seem to be interested.

After the meeting Lerisa told Joyce what had happened with the toilets in Hanyane. The government notice had been pinned up in the shop and in the school. Many of the educated who could read the notice already had a toilet and didn't need to worry. Those who did not have a toilet were mostly illiterate and could not read the order. So, finally, no one cared.

Then a new order went out. People were given one month to start building their toilets. Each month the chief's officials visited every home. They fined all those who hadn't made any progress. One old lady eventually got tired of paying her fine every month. She built a neat little house with a toilet seat in the middle. It looked just like a nice toilet, but there was no pit underneath. Of course, this toilet was never used. When the officials came back for their monthly fine, they were surprised to find the little house. When they opened the door, they saw the seat and left satisfied. The old lady was no longer fined.

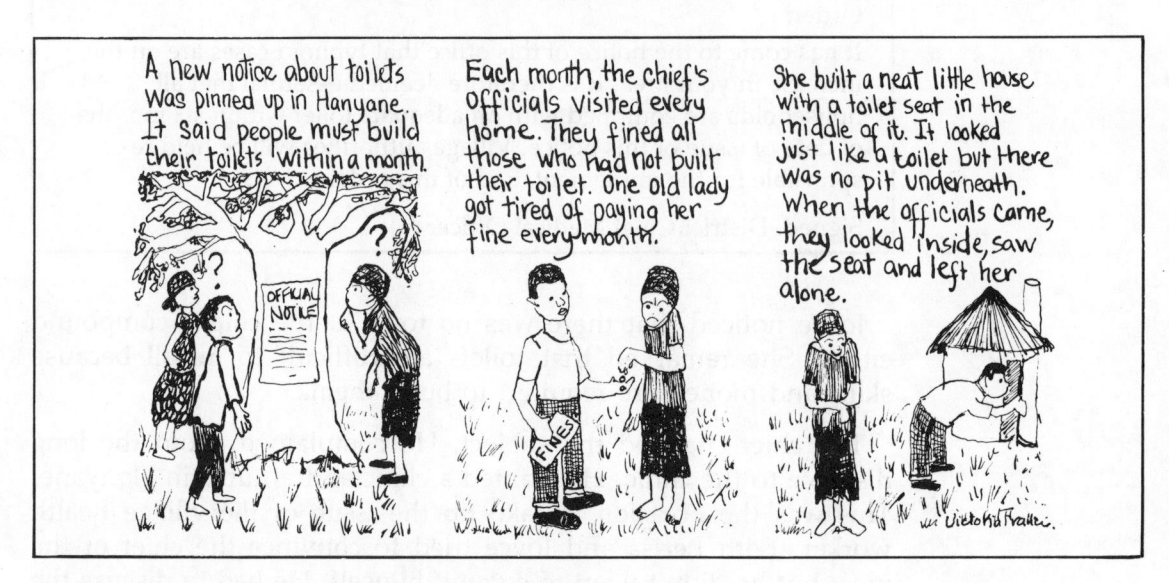

The story of toilets in Hanyane

QUESTIONS

1. What does the chief want from Joyce?
   What does Joyce want from the chief?
2. What should be the role of the village authority in promoting health?
3. Toilets are a problem in Hanyane. How would you motivate the people to build them?

DISCUSSION

The chief of Hanyane has not understood the government's order. He cannot see the link between typhoid and toilets. But he had to carry out the instructions. When the deadline drew nearer and many people still had no toilet, he felt pressurised by his authorities and resorted to fines. It is also possible that he introduced fines to fill his own pocket. Whatever his reasons, the fines were not helpful.

1 Approaches to community health management

The story of the toilets illustrates a common practice in public health administration. Village authorities have to implement instructions coming from above. Health workers are expected to motivate people 'for their own good' to carry out the instructions. People may resist orders of which they do not see the point. The reason for this is not so much people's 'stubbornness', but the style of health management.

According to A. Hope, traditional health management often functions like this:
a) Health management organises a programme to achieve a particular aim (e.g. toilets for all households to reduce typhoid).
b) People need to be directed, motivated and controlled (e.g. the chief gives orders to build toilets and then checks for compliance).
c) People need to change their behaviour to meet the aims of health management (e.g. use the toilets instead of the bush).
d) People, therefore, must be persuaded (health indoctrination), rewarded or punished (e.g. fines), and supervised closely.

This method is based on the following beliefs about human nature:
a) The average person is, by nature, lazy.
b) The average person lacks ambition, dislikes reponsibilities and prefers to be spoonfed.
c) The average person is self-centred.
d) The average person is resistant to change.
e) The average person is not very bright and can be easily led.

Therefore, officials generally have a low opinion of people. The chief of Hanyane is no exception.

It is very discouraging for people to be judged in such negative terms. A wise man once said: 'By thinking the best of a person you enable that person to be better'. The same applies to communities. We may encourage communities to take care of their own health if we assume that:
a) People are not, by nature, passive. (They have become so because of their previous experience of 'traditional health management'.)
b) Decisions in health policy can be shared by the community (e.g. Hanyane people could have decided, together with the chief, how to introduce toilets).

c) People are able, and like, to take responsibility (e.g. Hanyane could have formed a 'toilet committee').
d) People have many skills which can be tapped (e.g. some people in Hanyane may be good builders and know how to use the available local resources).
e) If people are aware of the importance of a communal issue (e.g. the need for toilets) – they are willing to work together towards a common goal.

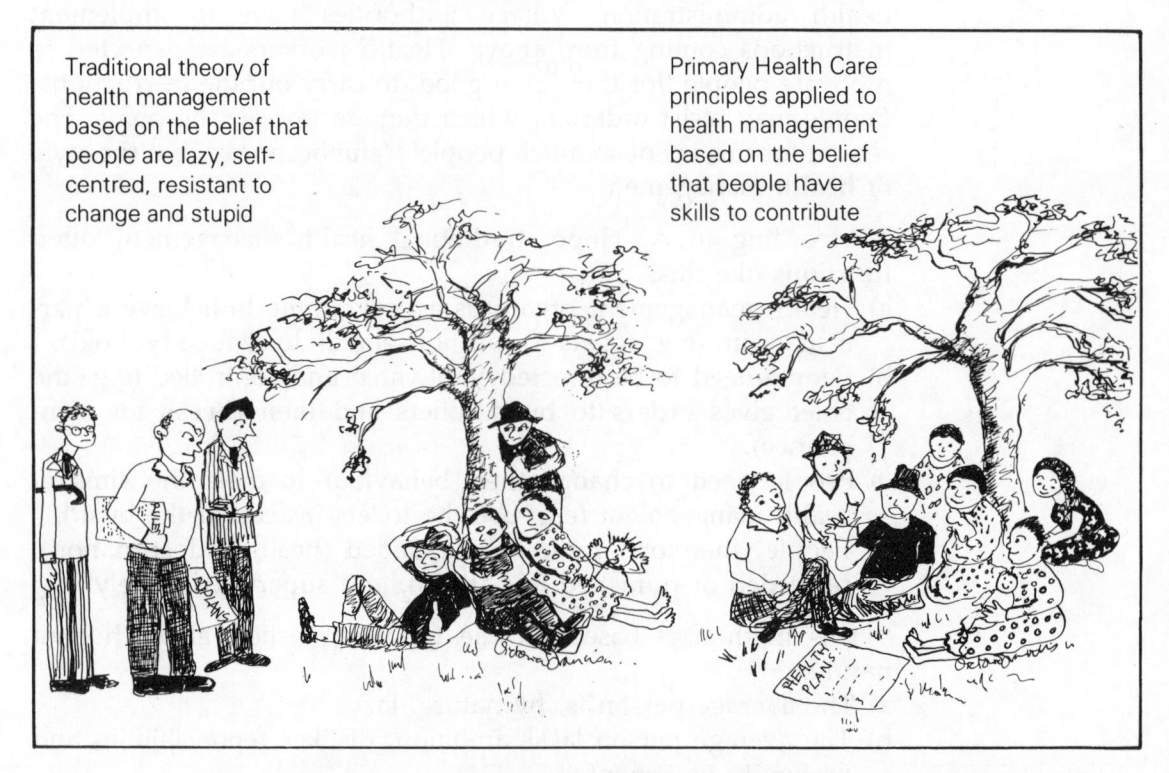

Traditional theory of health management based on the belief that people are lazy, self-centred, resistant to change and stupid

Primary Health Care principles applied to health management based on the belief that people have skills to contribute

The story of Hanyane village illustrates that these principles can become reality in a community programme.

2 Is community participation a threat to authority?

The story of Joyce's encounter with the chief demonstrates some aspects of power. There are many kinds of power: a village chief or a state president holds *political power*; a wealthy person has an advantage over the poor, so he has *financial power*; the well-educated, clever person has an advantage over the less gifted, so he has *intellectual power*.

All these forms of power can be used for good or bad purposes. A village government uses its power well if it caters for the people's needs and respects the rights of each inhabitant. The manager of a factory who pays his labourers a proper living wage and takes care that working conditions are safe has made good use of his money power.

Unfortunately, few people can resist the temptations of power:
a) People may use their position of power for their own and their friend's benefit, making the poor poorer.
b) Powerful people often enforce rules for others, but not for themselves, e.g. the chief of Hanyane did not build a toilet for his own home. Therefore the people did not take him seriously and treated the orders as a joke.

The powerful live in constant fear of losing their power. They feel threatened when people from the community take initiatives for change. Therefore the chief of Hanyane is reluctant to introduce a village health worker. After training, this person might bring new ideas and challenge his authority.

People in authority believe that it is a sign of weakness to listen to the people and work *with* them. In reality, being open to other people's ideas is a sign of strength.

How could Joyce motivate the chief to assist health promotion in Hanyane instead of blocking it?

One good way for Joyce to win the chief's cooperation is to make him party to her health projects. Instead of telling him what to do she could ask him for advice – even if she thinks she does not need any. The chief will feel flattered and offer his assistance.

Joyce should also explain the reasons behind health instructions which come from the district office. Once the chief understands their purpose he can discuss, with his councillors, sensible ways of implementing them. The more insight people are allowed, the more support they will offer.

SUMMARY

1 Traditional health management teaches that people are passive and need to be persuaded, directed and controlled. This attitude makes people worse than they are.
   If health management believes in people's skills and initiatives, it helps them to discover and use their best qualities.
2 Power, if used wisely and unselfishly, can be to the benefit of the people. Few can resist the temptation to misuse power for selfish ends. Then power corrupts.

Reference
Hope, A. and Timmel, S., *Training for Transformation* (Mambo Press, 1984)

6

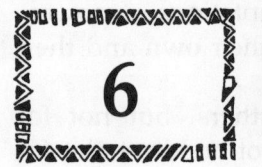

Who cares about reports? – Health through statistics

At the end of the month it was time to write the clinic report for matron. Joyce hated statistics. Arithmetic wasn't her strong point. There were always mistakes somewhere when she added the numbers of patients seen, ailments treated or medicines used. The matron was often cross with Joyce when the medicines in stock didn't tally with her figures. In Joyce's opinion, these statistics were a waste of time. She was convinced they just ended up in a drawer in matron's office and were never looked at again.

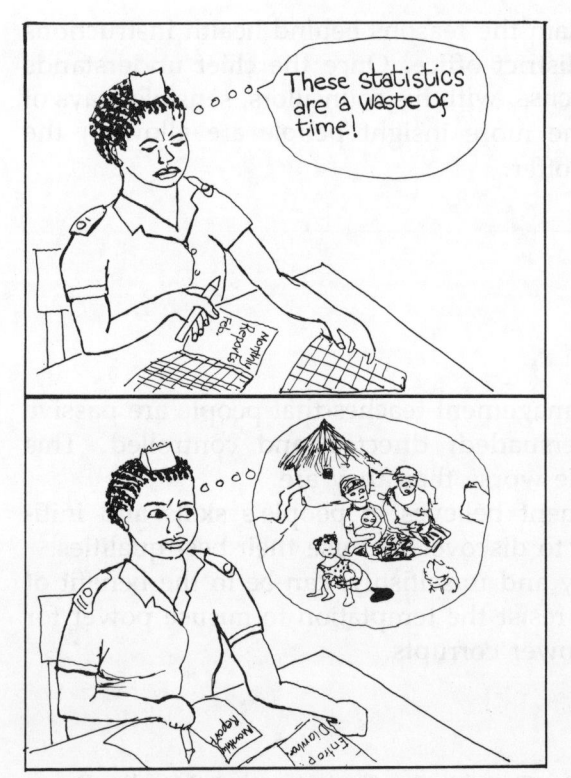

On a hot afternoon, her sweaty hand stuck to the paper as she wrote. She seemed to be writing the words 'diarrhoea', 'purulent conjunctivitis', 'scabies', 'measles' and 'trachoma' hundreds of times. As she mechanically wrote down the figures, her thoughts wandered back to the day she visited Ma-Anna's home. In her mind she saw Musa sitting helplessly in a corner and Rose soiling everywhere with her uncontrollable diarrhoea. The children rubbed their sticky eyes and Kokwana was half blind with her in-turning eye lashes. It appeared everyone had trachoma.

Suddenly it dawned on Joyce: the list of figures in her report was a summary of what happened in her area. It stood for many Musas, Roses and Kokwanas and for hundreds of families struggling to cope with life. Joyce realised for the first time that these families lived right on her doorstep. She quickly added up the last figures.

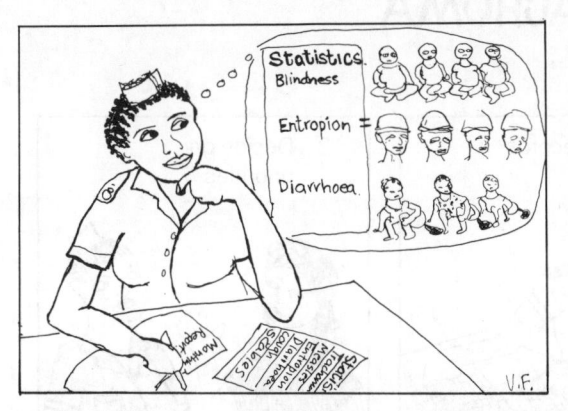

Joyce realises for the first time what statistics mean

Next day the doctor visited. Joyce was glad it was the eye doctor who came. The other doctor was always in a hurry and often angry when she had many patients to see. The eye doctor usually had time for her and listened to her problems.

'Everybody is sick at present with conjunctivitis or diarrhoea. It is always like this in summer. It is the season of the flies,' Joyce told him.

The doctor looked at the monthly report and praised her for her good observation. He wanted to know how she dealt with this problem.

Joyce complained that she tried hard with health education, but it was useless. People were not very interested in it. At Hanyane they didn't listen at all when she talked about toilets. They asked for jobs, water and wood – things she was unable to provide. Only when she asked specifically about their health problems did some mention eyes or diarrhoea. But only a few talked.

'There are too many problems here, doctor. I can't cope with them all on my own. I need some help,' Joyce burst out. She told him about Ma-Anna, Musa and the whole family.

The doctor listened intently and then said, 'Joyce, I understand your problem. Unfortunately there is no other nurse to help you. And there are no village health workers in the area yet. We must find another way to decrease your workload. At present you are overworked with treating unnecessary diseases. Most of them could have been prevented.'

Joyce replied, 'I know that. But how can we prevent these diseases when the people don't change?'

'Exactly,' said the doctor. 'This is why we should help the people to become more aware of what is wrong and what they can do to put it right. You, too, should find out exactly what is wrong. Perhaps we should do a health survey of your community. You could then plan your actions on the basis of your findings. It might

FINDING OUT ABOUT TRACHOMA
What is the problem?

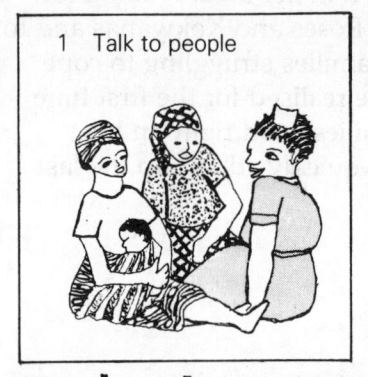

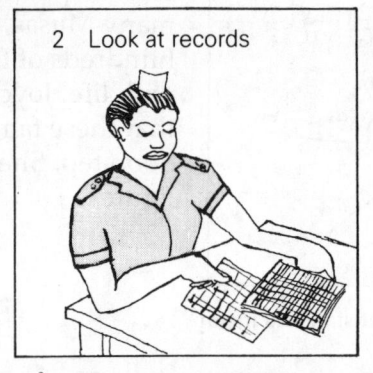

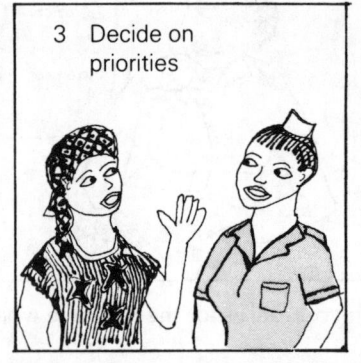

1. Talk to people
2. Look at records
3. Decide on priorities

Find out more – plan a survey

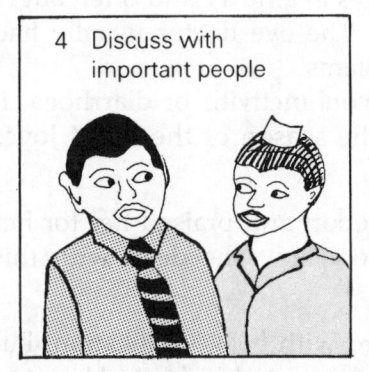

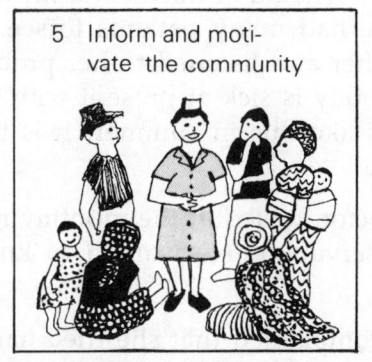

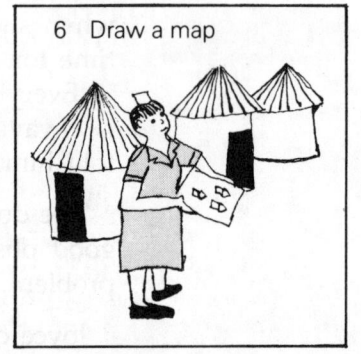

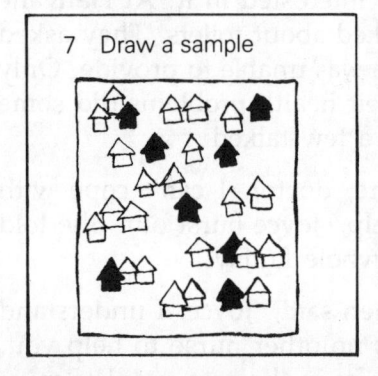

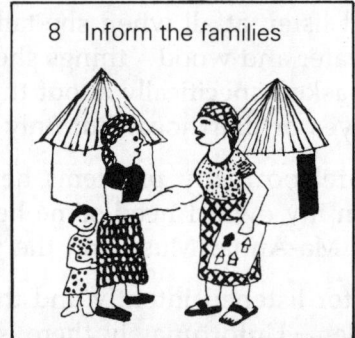

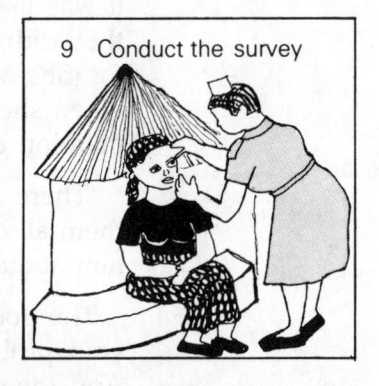

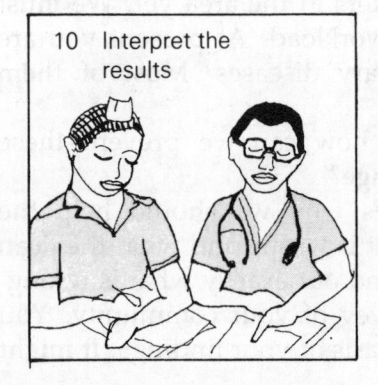

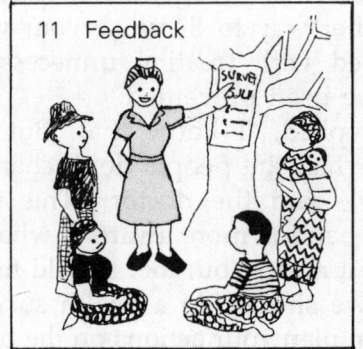

4. Discuss with important people
5. Inform and motivate the community
6. Draw a map
7. Draw a sample
8. Inform the families
9. Conduct the survey
10. Interpret the results
11. Feedback
12. Decide on Action

also help the community to become more interested. When they see you examine people in the village, they will see that you care.'

This was too much for Joyce. What she could see was that a survey meant more work for her, not less. It took a long time for the doctor to reassure her and make her agree to do a survey.

They decided to look at trachoma in Hanyane because they knew that people were concerned about this disease. The simplest method would be to see how many people over the age of 20 had entropion. This examination was quick and easy, so Joyce could do it with the help of one or two villagers. They planned the survey step by step.

QUESTIONS

1 What do you think about statistics?
   Why are they important?
   What are good ways of doing statistics?
2 What are the four most important diseases in the area where you work?
3 How can you find out about eye diseases and the health needs of the community in which you work? Discuss the advantages and limitations of the types of information you can obtain.
4 What do you think of the eye doctor? Is he typical of doctors you know?

DISCUSSION

Since Joyce met Musa some weeks ago she has learnt a great deal about him, his family and the village where he lives. It has taught her that:
1 Eye diseases are part of general health and are largely the result of the environment in which we live.
2 More poverty leads to more diseases.
3 It is more meaningful to fight disease where it starts, in the community, than to try and cure it later at the hospital.

Joyce's problem is that the more she knows the more she gets frustrated and discouraged. The doctor's advice is to step back and have a good look at the situation. In other words, he wants her to make a **community diagnosis**.

Steps in community diagnosis (see Survey, page 42)

If a doctor or health worker wants to treat a patient correctly, s/he will first make a clinical diagnosis. Exactly the same procedure must be followed in community health. As you see from the picture and Table 6.1 (adapted from C. H. Wood) the steps for both the individual and the community are similar:

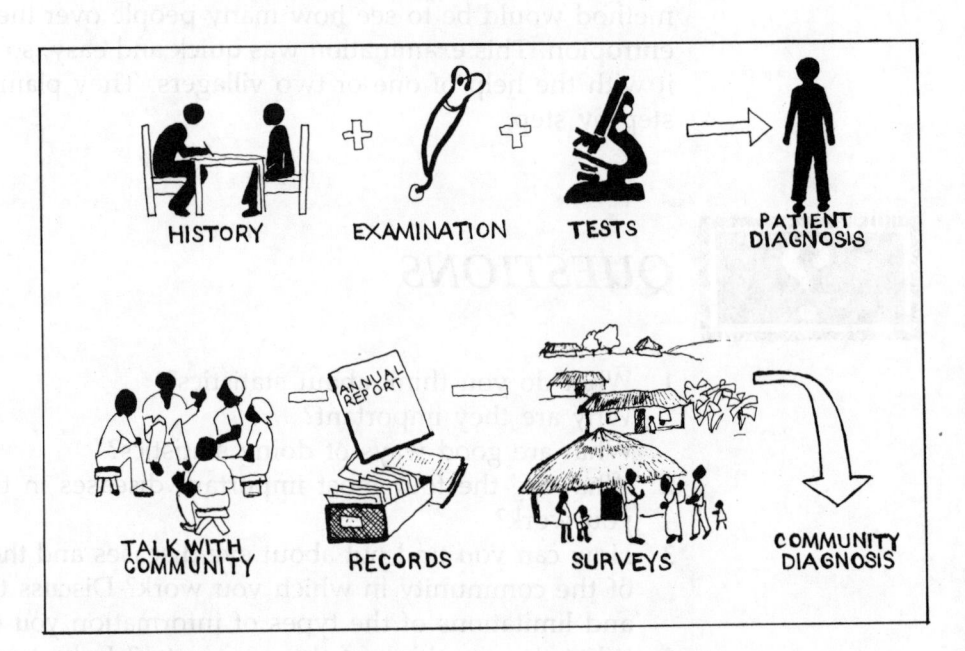

Individual and community diagnosis. From *Community Health* by C.H. Wood et al. AMREF 1981

Step 1: Talk with the people

This is time-consuming, but it is the most valuable step because we will discover:
- What people are worried about.
- The distribution of wealth and poverty within the community.
- Where people work.
- What people plant and eat.
- How people feel and what they think.

You will only get this information after you have developed a relationship of trust between you and the community. If people do not trust you, they will give answers to please you in order to get rid of you quickly.

Joyce has got her information from her visit to Ma-Anna's home, from Lerisa, from the chief, and from a community meeting. From them she learned that:
- The people are most worried about jobs, water and wood.

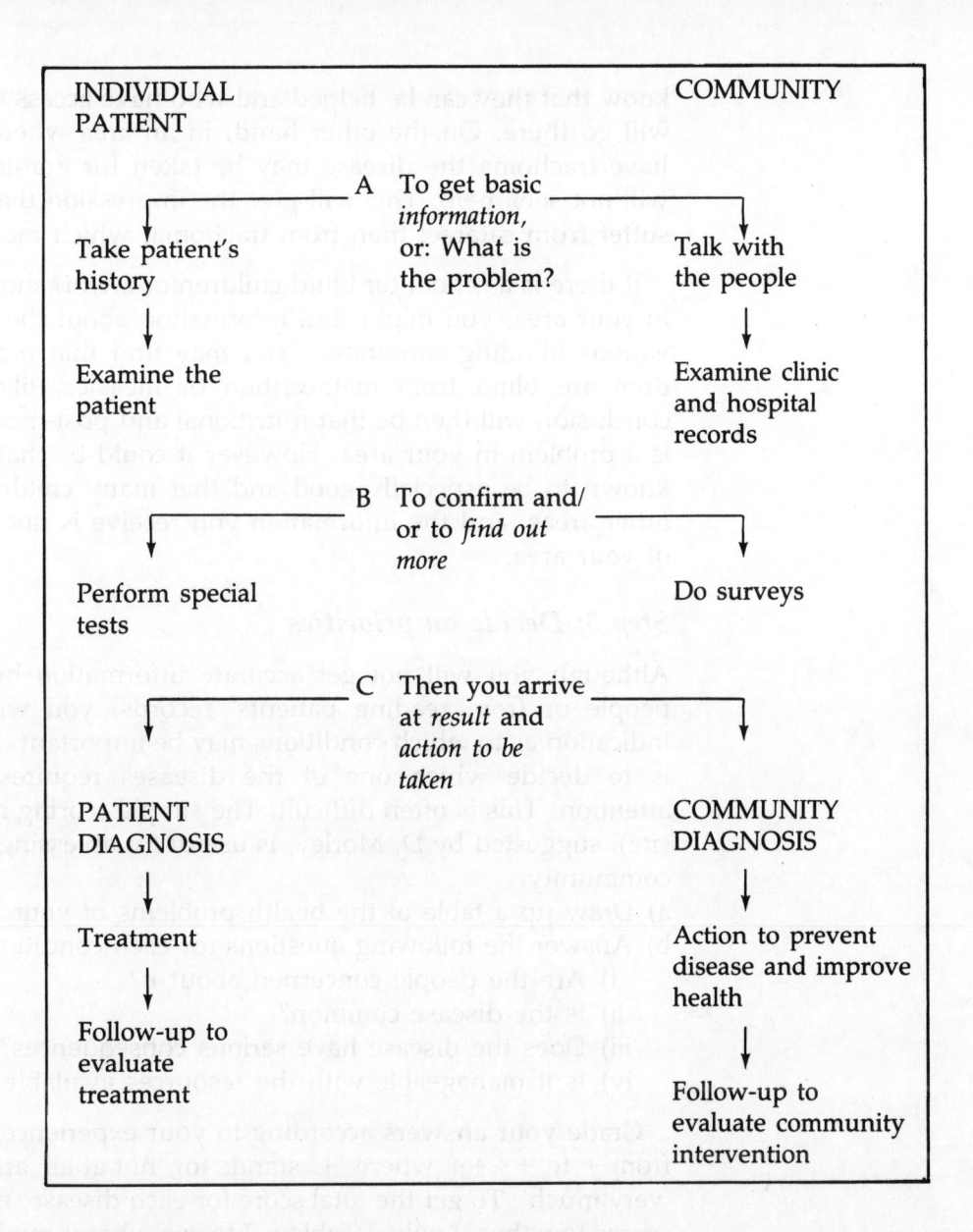

INDIVIDUAL PATIENT		COMMUNITY
↓	A To get basic *information*, or: What is the problem?	↓
Take patient's history		Talk with the people
↓		↓
Examine the patient		Examine clinic and hospital records
↓	B To confirm and/or to *find out more*	↓
Perform special tests		Do surveys
↓	C Then you arrive at *result* and *action to be taken*	↓
PATIENT DIAGNOSIS		**COMMUNITY DIAGNOSIS**
↓		↓
Treatment		Action to prevent disease and improve health
↓		↓
Follow-up to evaluate treatment		Follow-up to evaluate community intervention

Table 6.1

- Hygiene is poor, there is no safe water supply and wood must be collected far from the village.
- The main health worries at the moment are eye diseases and diarrhoea.
- People are poor and spend most of their time trying to survive. This leaves them with little energy to change anything.

Step 2: Information from clinic records

Clinic and hospital records show which conditions are seen most often. These are the diseases about which people are sufficiently concerned to seek help. But it does not mean that they are the most common. Other diseases may be more frequent, but people do not worry about them. For instance, most cataract patients who know that they can be helped and who have access to an eye clinic will go there. On the other hand, in an area where most people have trachoma the disease may be taken for granted and people will not seek help. This will give the impression that more people suffer from cataract than from trachoma, which may be wrong.

If there is a school for blind children or a workshop for the blind in your area, you might find information about the importance of various blinding conditions. You may find that most of the children are blind from malnutrition or measles, like Musa. Your conclusion will then be that nutritional and post-measles blindness is a problem in your area. However it could be that this school is known to be especially good and that many children come from other areas, and the information you receive is not representative of your area.

Step 3: Decide on priorities

Although you will not get accurate information by talking with people or from reading patients' records, you will get a good indication as to which conditions may be important. Your next step is to decide which one of the diseases requires your special attention. This is often difficult. The simple scoring method (opposite), suggested by D. Morley, is useful for assessing priorities in a community:
a) Draw up a table of the health problems of your community.
b) Answer the following questions for each condition on your list:
    i) Are the people concerned about it?
    ii) Is the disease common?
    iii) Does the disease have serious consequences?
    iv) Is it manageable with the resources available to you?

Grade your answers according to your experience, using a scale from + to ++++ where '+' stands for 'not at all' and '++++' for 'very much'. To get the total score for each disease, multiply all the scores together. Look at Table 6.2 to see what it might look like for Hanyane.

The highest score is for trachoma (96) and lowest for retinoblastoma (4). Although retinoblastoma is clinically extremely serious, the disease is so rare that people do not know about it and, by the time a patient is taken to the clinic, it is already beyond treatment. Joyce is therefore right to decide that she should do something about trachoma in her community.

Having taken a community history (Step 1), performed a community examination (Step 2) and decided on priorities (Step 3), Joyce is ready to find out more about her community. She will do a **survey**. This will provide a yardstick by which she can measure her success after taking action. This will be discussed in the following chapters.

Disease	Concern	Frequency	Seriousness	Manage-ability	Score
Diarrhoea	+++	+++	+++	+++	3 × 3 × 3 × 3 = 81
Scabies	++	++++	+	++	2 × 4 × 1 × 2 = 16
Measles	++	++	+++	+++	2 × 2 × 3 × 3 = 36
Trachoma	+++	++++	++	++++	3 × 4 × 2 × 4 = 96
Retino-blastoma	+	+	++++	+	1 × 1 × 4 × 1 = 4

Table 6.2

Exercise

Administrative work should be kept to a minimum in a busy rural clinic. The more cumbersome statistics are, the less likely it is for figures to be tabulated correctly. It is better to have a handful of easily understood, simple statistics than to have a lot of complex and confusing data.

You want to improve your clinic records. You want to retain the essential facts and discard unnecessary items. Therefore, for each item, you should ask yourself:
a) Is it important?
b) Is it necessary for deciding on strategies in your work?

Now draw up a format for your own clinic and discuss it with your teachers and colleagues.

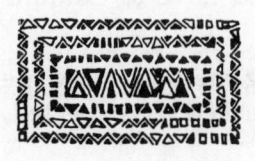

SUMMARY

The assessment of health problems in individual patients and in the community follows the same principles, listed below:
a) Listen to what people are worried about.
b) Examine records for common diseases.
c) Decide on priorities.
d) If necessary, do a survey.

References
Morley, D., *Paediatric Priorities in the Developing World* (Butterworth, Guildford, 1983)
Wood, C.H. et al., *Community Health* (African Medical Research Foundation, Nairobi, 1981)

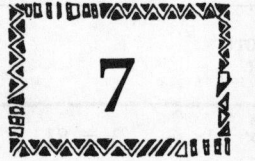

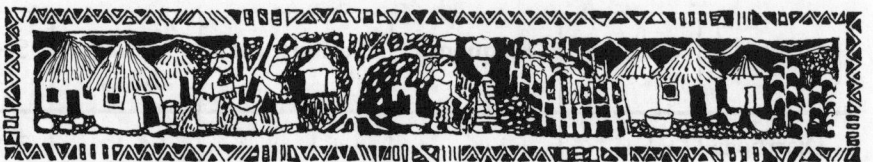

Why draw a map?
– Knowing your village

Joyce was preparing for the survey. She visited the chief and his councillors to introduce the idea. They were a bit reluctant, but when Joyce said that she would bring eye ointment along for those who had eye troubles, they became interested. They said they would arrange a village meeting the next day so that Joyce could inform them about it.

When she arrived in Hanyane the next afternoon about 60 people were waiting for her under the big tree in the centre of the village. The first thing Joyce wanted to know was whether they were still worried about eye diseases. Some mothers answered that this was so. Their children refused to go to school because of their sticky eyes.

Joyce went on to explain that she wanted to help them to get rid of these eye diseases. But to do so she needed to find out how bad it really was in Hanyane. Therefore, she would have to examine the eyes of many people.

'Would anyone here be interested in helping me – to show me the way and introduce me to the families?' she asked. As expected, it was Lerisa who offered her services.

The following day Joyce and Lerisa met to draw a map of the place. They walked up and down the many paths. It was hot and tiring. Lerisa started to complain. She couldn't see why they had to draw a map. Afterall, she knew most of the people, and the chief had a list of all the stands. Joyce suggested they have a rest under a tree.

She explained why a map was useful for them. She gave five reasons. What do you think these reasons were? Write your answers in the spaces below.

1 ....
2 ....

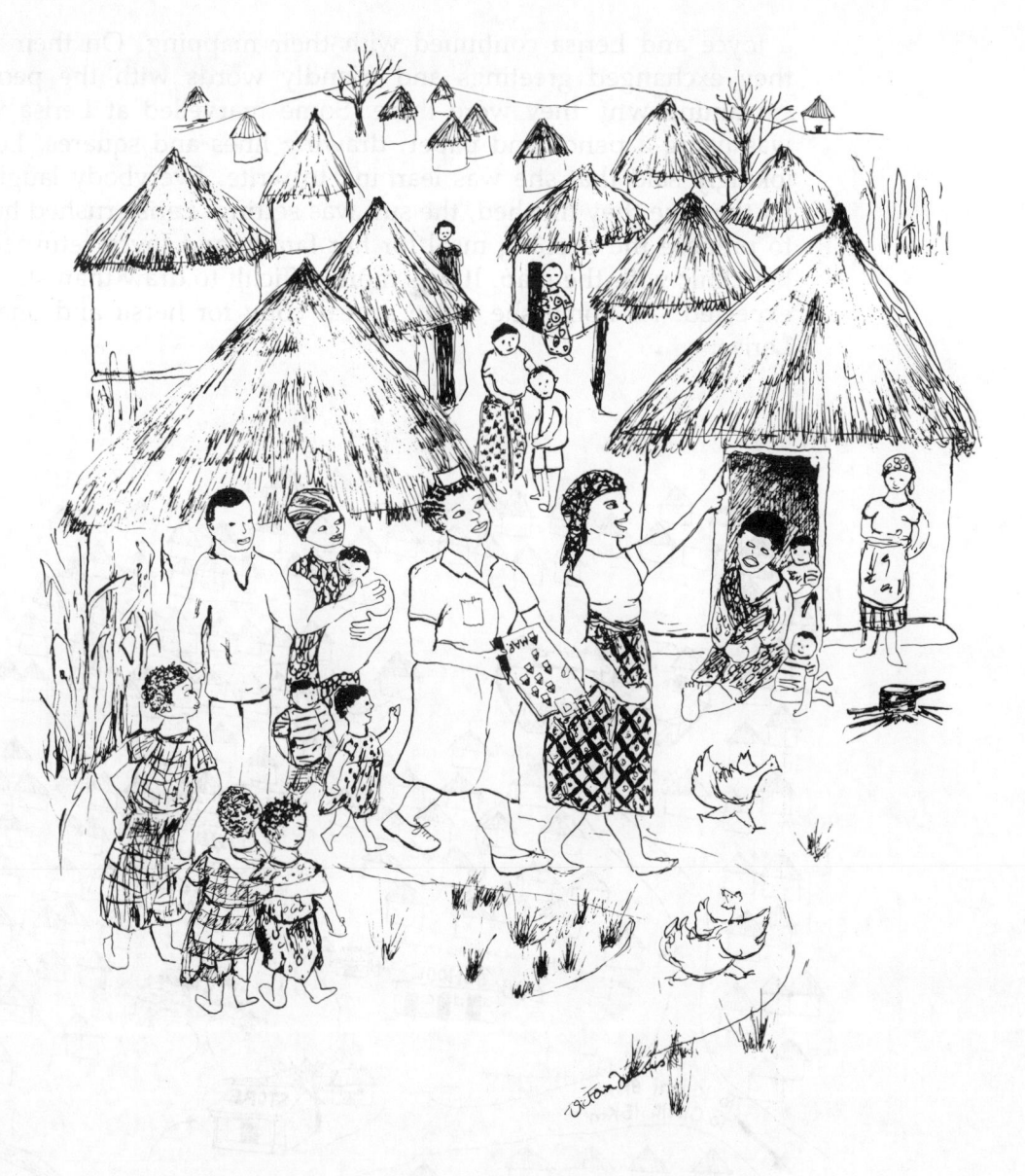

Joyce and Lerisa walked up many paths drawing the map

3 ....
4 ....
5 ....
(If you can think of more than five reasons, add them to the list.)

Lerisa added her own good reasons: 'Today, people will get to know you. Many people don't know what's happening because they haven't attended the meeting. Now we can tell them. That means they will then be less suspicious when you come to examine their eyes.'

Joyce and Lerisa continued with their mapping. On their way they exchanged greetings and friendly words with the people, explaining why they were there. Some marvelled at Lerisa who was using a pencil and paper, drawing lines and squares. Lerisa jokingly said that she was learning to write. Everybody laughed. By the time they finished, the sun was setting. Lerisa rushed home to prepare the evening meal for her family and Joyce returned to her clinic with the map. It was more difficult to draw than she had expected. At home she made a neat copy for herslf and one for Lerisa.

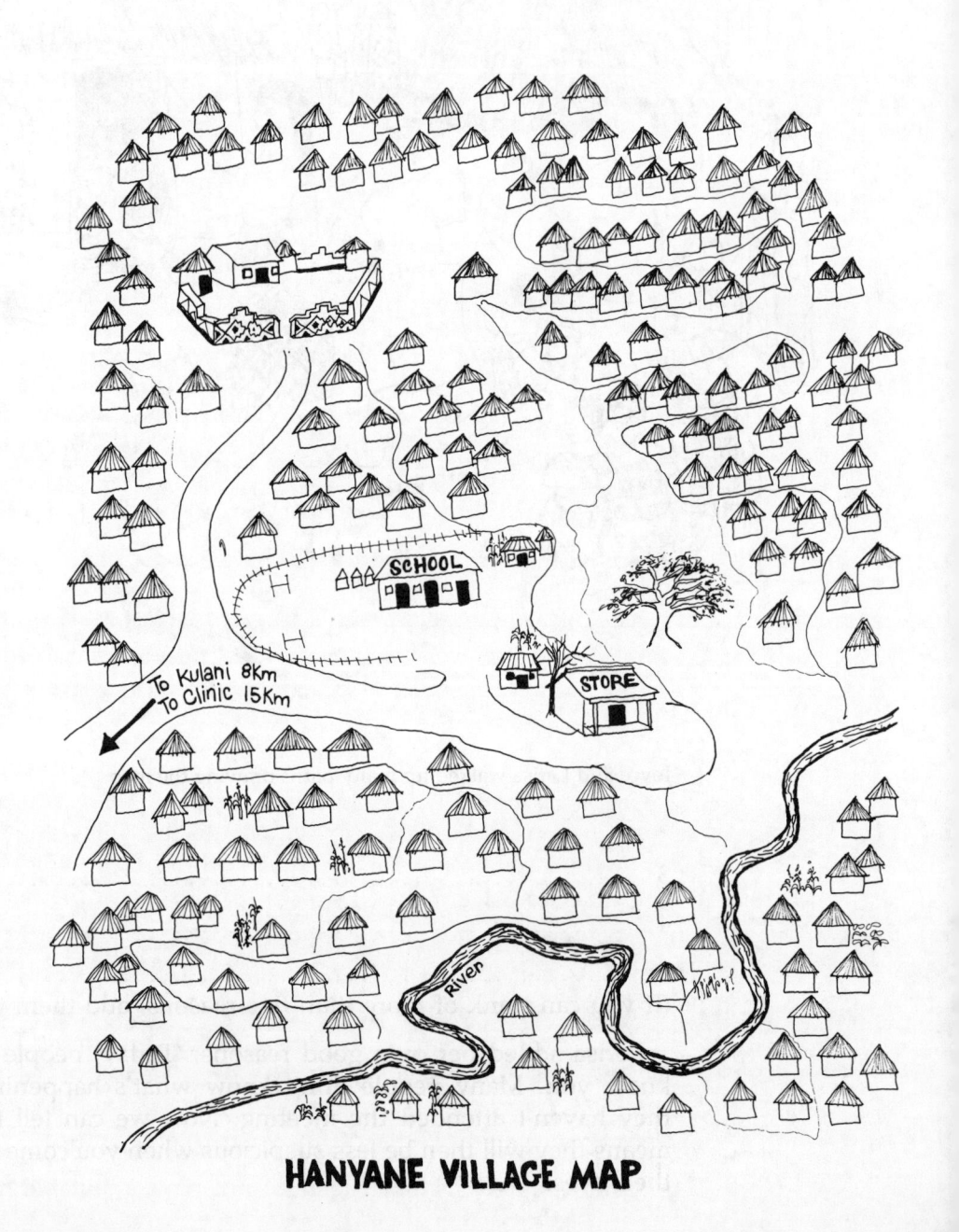

HANYANE VILLAGE MAP

QUESTIONS

1. Have you ever drawn a map of the place where you work?
   a) Was it easy?
   b) Where did you have problems?
   c) What methods do you know for making a map?
2. In addition to the houses, what would you like to enter on your map?
3. Using your experience from the area where you work, which houses on the map of Hanyane village would you allocate to:
   a) The better-off people?
   b) The poorest people?
   c) Ma-Anna?
   d) Lerisa?

DISCUSSION

We have seen how Joyce, in preparing for the survey, visited the chief (Step 4: Discuss with important people) and discussed it at a village meeting (Step 5: Inform and motivate the community).

Step 6: Draw a map (see 'Survey', page 42)

Maps are useful for finding your way in an unfamiliar area. They are usually made for tourists or business people who travel in a foreign country, or for government departments and the army. Such maps are very accurate. One needs special equipment to make them. Maps may also be made from photographs taken from an aeroplane.

Joyce and Lerisa do not have any special equipment. They had to rely on their own eyes, their legs and their imagination. For their purposes, walking up and down the village has been good enough to obtain a reliable record of all the dwellings and important objects in Hanyane.

The illustration on page 52, shows you how to draw a map.

You can also get a bird's eye view when the village you want to map out is situated at the foot of a mountain. You climb up the mountain slope until you have a good view of the layout of the village and draw your map. Smaller details can be filled in by walking through the village later on. This would be the most accurate map you could do by yourself.

Unfortunately most villages do not have a suitable mountain in

LEARNING HOW TO DRAW A MAP

1 Make a model village

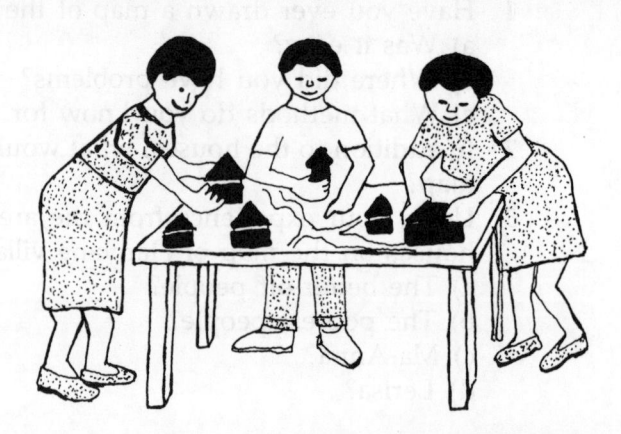

2 There are two ways of looking at the village:
   i) Eye level

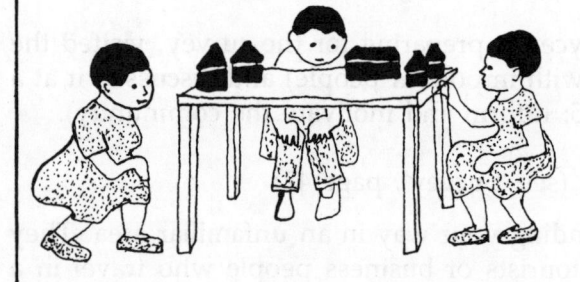

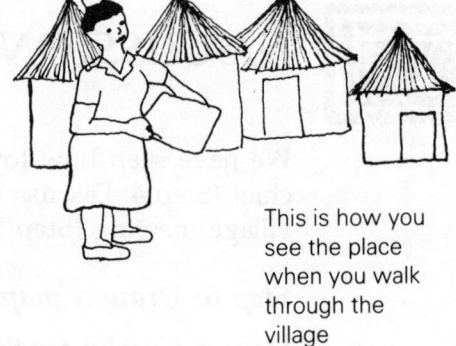

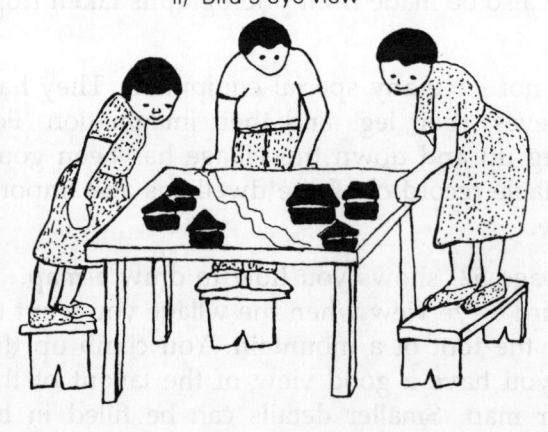

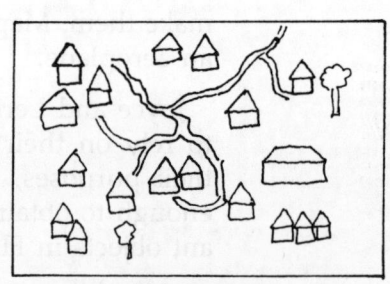

This is how you see the place when you walk through the village

   ii) Bird's eye view

This way you can see the whole layout of the village at once. This is the view used in mapping the vicinity. Then you have no choice but to walk up and down the village and draw the houses, roads, paths and other landmarks on your way. It will be time-consuming, and the measurements will not be accurate. But it is time well spent, because you get an overall picture of the place. For example, you see where and how people live, how their houses are built, and how far they have to go for water or to the shop. You will also meet people and be able to answer their questions.

Your map is also useful for monitoring progress in your village. When you have marked essential facilities on your map (water outlets, toilets, vegetable plots, shops, and anything else you think is important), you can make a note of any changes taking place over the years ahead. You can also indicate the households requiring special attention, e.g. families with severe trachoma, malnourished children, or the physically or mentally disabled.

The doctor told Joyce to draw a map in preparation for her survey (Step 6). She must know the exact number of households and estimate the number of people living in the village so that no one will be forgotten. She also needs the map to determine the population sample she is going to examine. This will be discussed in the next chapter.

The people of Hanyane would have been upset if Joyce had set about making her map without letting them know, in advance, what she was planning to do. This is why she introduced herself first. Whatever you do in a community, always remember that you are a guest. Do not assume that because you are a health worker you are always welcome! Introduce yourself politely, according to local custom, and ask the villagers for permission to work there. This avoids ill feelings and mistrust towards you and the health services.

SUMMARY

1. A simple map any health worker can draw is a useful tool to get to know the community you work with and to monitor changes taking place. It is also helpful for drawing a random sample when doing surveys and for subsequent follow-up.
2. Remember that you, the health worker, are a guest in the community.

8

Choosing a bag of beans
– A random sample

Joyce numbered the houses on the map and found that there were 204. The doctor calculated that she should choose 30-35 households randomly. This meant examining every sixth family, starting with a random number between 1 and 6. Joyce suggested that Lerisa should draw the first number, so that she could see for herself how it was done and that no one was cheating.

She took the map to Lerisa's home and showed it to her. She had to help her find her own house on it. It was number 123. Lerisa was surprised that there were so many families living in Hanyane.

'How long will it take you to examine all these people?' Lerisa asked.

'I will only see about 30 families,' said Joyce.

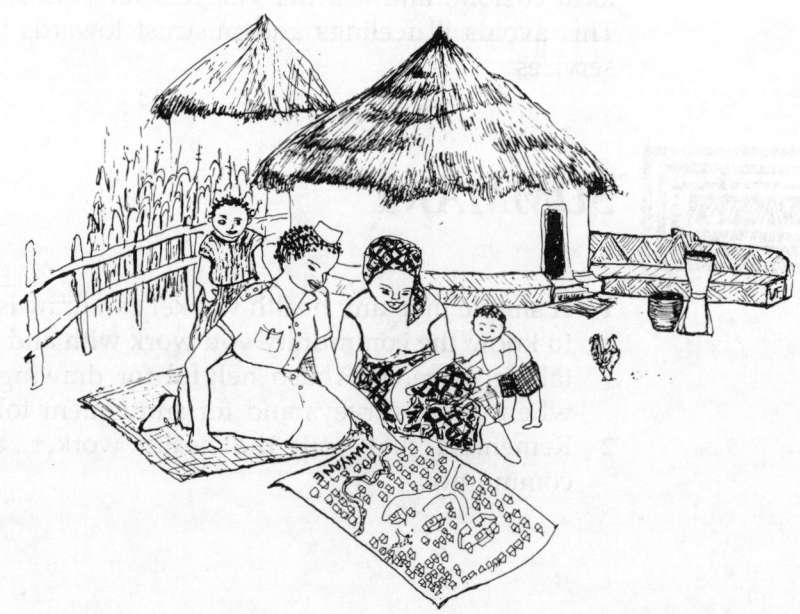

Joyce and Lerisa looked at the map. They had to select 34 of the 204 houses

Lerisa was worried. This would cause trouble. Most people were looking forward to a free eye examination. They would also blame Lerisa for being unfair. Joyce wondered how best she could explain the reasons for examining only a few. Then she asked Lerisa whether she had ever bought a 20 kg packet of beans. Of course she hadn't. She never had enough cash to buy such large quantities.

'Now imagine,' said Joyce, 'that you had enough money to buy a big bag of beans. You don't quite trust the dealer. He might have put a few good beans on top and rotten beans at the bottom. You want to be sure of what you are buying. So, you would empty the whole bag on the floor and test every bean, wouldn't you?'

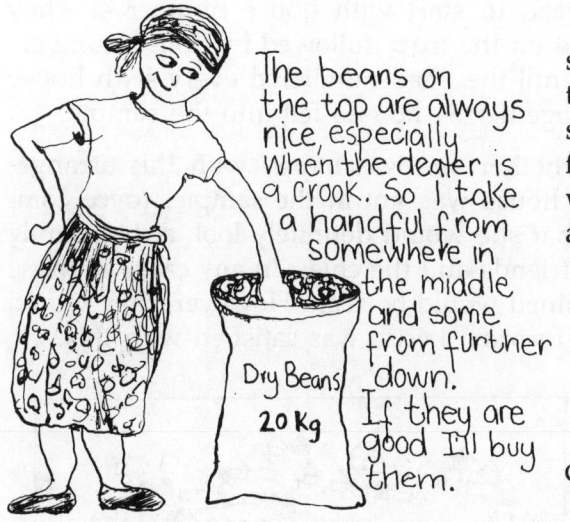

Lerisa objected. Did Joyce think she was stupid? She could do it much better than that. She would just take a handful from somewhere in the middle and another from the bottom. If all were good then she would know that the whole bag was good and she would buy them.

Choosing a bag of beans

Joyce explained that the same can apply to a survey. To know whether trachoma is a problem you don't need to see every family. Lerisa said, 'In that case, if we don't need to see everybody, at least we must see my mother's place, and my aunt down at the river, and of course my own family. We mustn't forget the teacher and the chief, because they are important people. And then there are my friends, Ma-Anna and Mavila. Let us go to all these people and examine their eyes.'

Joyce laughed and said, 'Oh, in that case *you* would be biased, if only your friends are seen and nobody else. The people in Hanyane would really have the right to say that this survey was only for your friends.'

After some arguing, Lerisa agreed to do it the way Joyce had suggested. This was to examine every sixth household in Hanyane. To do that Joyce prepared six tickets with the numbers 1 to 6 written on them, and folded them together so that the numbers couldn't be seen from outside. Then she put the six folded tickets into a pot and asked Lerisa to shake it. Then Lerisa had to draw out one ticket and see what number it was. It was number 4. She looked on the map to see which house this indicated.

'Oh, no, not this house! Old Kwatisa lives there. She is a horrible woman. She always chases children away and she is angry with everybody. I'm not going to see her. I suggest that I draw another number and then we start with another house.'

Joyce disagreed. It would no longer be a matter of chance, and the houses must be chosen strictly by chance. 'Don't you think it would be nice if we visited Kwatisa for the survey so that she feels that people care about her? Maybe she is grumpy because nobody cares about her. Perhaps she will be friendlier afterwards.'

Lerisa and Joyce agreed to start with house number 4. They marked house number 4 on the map, followed by house numbers 10, 16, 22, and so on, until they had numbered every sixth house on the whole map. Altogether 34 houses fell into the sample.

Joyce asked Lerisa whether she was happy with this arrangement. She wasn't. Her house was not in the sample. Joyce comforted her, promising that she would definitely look at her family and the families of her friends and the chief. In any case, all those who wished to be examined would be seen. However, they would not be counted for her records. Lerisa was satisfied with this.

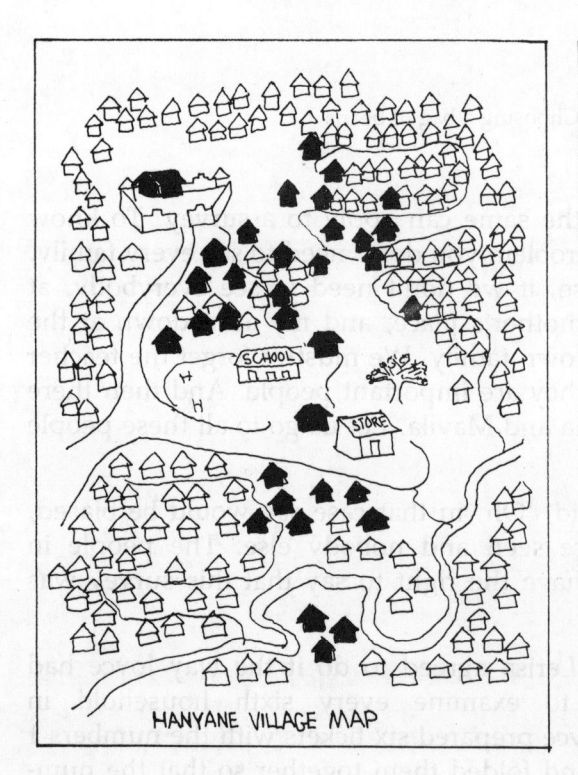

Lerisa's choice of 34 homes

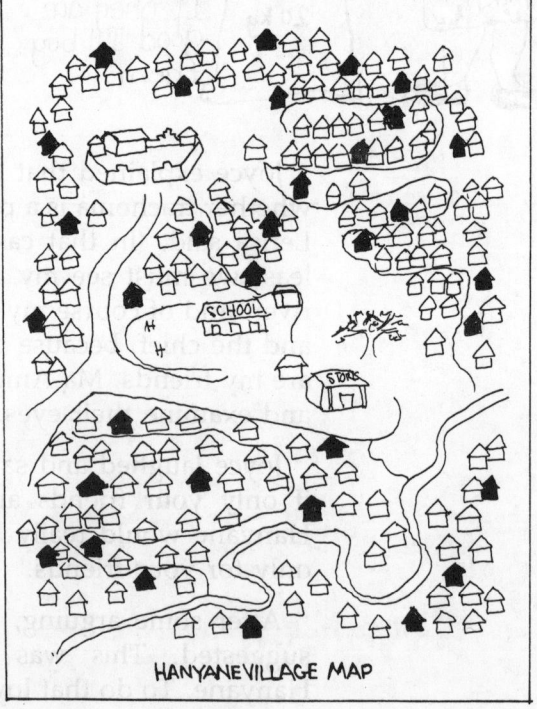

Random sample of 34 homes. Every sixth house was chosen, starting with No 4

QUESTIONS

1. Have you ever taken part in a survey?
   a) What did you learn?
   b) What were the difficulties you experienced?
   c) How did the people react?
2. a) What is a sample survey?
   b) What is a random sample?
   c) What is a biased sample?
   d) What is a representative sample?
   Give examples of each.
3. Why will Joyce only examine people *above* the age of 20 for entropion?

DISCUSSION

Joyce feels that trachoma is a problem in Hanyane. She has drawn the map and prepared for a survey. Now she is ready to begin. She wants to use a simple, yet reliable, method to find out how big the problem is. In order to save time, she will not examine every person in Hanyane. Instead, she draws a **sample**.

Surveys are always time-consuming. As an organiser of a survey, therefore, you might look for voluntary helpers or hire extra staff. If no suitable helpers can be found or there is no money to pay additional staff, you have to do the survey yourself. This may mean that you have to interrupt your normal duties. You may even have to close your clinic.

If you do not want to waste your time and energy you must decide first of all if you really want to do the survey. If the answer is 'yes' you must plan the survey well and carry it out correctly. This is not easy. Joyce had the eye doctor to guide her. You probably know an experienced field worker who can help you. There are also good books on survey techniques which are easy to read (e.g. M.T. Feuerstein's *Partners in Evaluation*). In Table 8.1 we can merely point to a few essentials you should know and consider.

Before starting a survey, answer the questions in Table 8.1:

Questions	Answers for Hanyane
1 Which disease will I investigate? (e.g. malnutrition, trachoma, xerophthalmia, etc.)	Trachoma
2 Why do I want to do the survey? (e.g. to take preventive measures, to set up a mobile clinic, to know whether any action is needed or not, etc.)	People are worried about trachoma and clinic records indicate that it is common. But Joyce does not know whether people in Hanyane are in real danger of going blind from trachoma and whether special action is required.
3 What do I want to *know* about the condition? (e.g. how many people suffer from it, what disabilities does it cause, what are people's beliefs about it, etc.)	How many people have entropion (the complication of trachoma which can lead to blindness)?
4 Who will be examined? (e.g. the whole nation, a certain village, children, mothers, etc.)	People over the age of 20 in Hanyane village. The reasons for looking only at the adult population is that entropion is a late complication in trachoma and is rarely seen in young people.
5 Is the survey *necessary* to decide on the action to be taken?	Yes.
6 Who will *benefit* from the survey? (e.g. doctors, pharmaceutical companies, politicians, the health services, the people, etc.)	The people of Hanyane and Joyce.
7 Which *survey method* will be most suitable?	Random sampling – examining every sixth household.
8 Who will do the survey? (e.g. medical students, nurses, teachers)	Examination for entropion is fast and does not require any equipment. Therefore the study can be done by Nurse Joyce alone or with one or two helpers from the village.

Table 8.1

If the answers to questions 5 and 6 mean that neither the health services nor the people will benefit, and that the outcome of the survey will not influence your actions, then *don't do the survey!* Once you have decided that the survey will be useful and should be done, then you must choose the best method (Question 7).

Should we, for instance, examine all people who come to the hospital (**hospital population**), or all children who come to the child health clinic? In both cases, we may find less people with trachoma than in the population at large. Those attending health facilities are more health conscious, live nearby, or have the money to travel. If, on the other hand, we examine the people in the poorest section of a village, where they lack the necessary facilities, we will probably find more disease than in the average population of that village. In both these examples, we deal with a **selected population** – we have a **biased sample** and our results are therefore biased. Lerisa's choice of families would have been a biased sample.

In order to get a true picture, we would have to examine every person in a population. This, however, is not practicable, even if we had enough finances and staff. Fortunately, there are other, simpler ways to get a fairly true picture of the problem: using the principle of Lerisa's bag of beans in a population survey, we obtain what is called a **representative sample** of the population. In order for a sample to be truly representative, make sure that:
- Every person or unit (e.g. family) of the population has an *equal chance* of falling into the sample. This is called a random selection (random meaning 'chosen by chance').
- The *size* of the sample is adequate for the accuracy required.

Only then can you confidently generalise and predict for the whole population.

Samples

Here are two methods for obtaining a representative sample:

Step 7: Draw a sample (see 'Sample', page 42)

a) Random sample
The doctor had calculated that the size of the sample would be adequate if one sixth of the adult population were examined. So Joyce examined every sixth house. In your sample, to ensure that every house has an equal chance of being included in the sample, the starting point must be chosen completely by chance. That is why Joyce asked Lerisa to randomly draw one of the numbers between 1 and 6. The number drawn will be the first house from which to start.

Should you decide to examine 10% of the population in a settlement, you would use the same method but going to every tenth house. Or, if you want to examine 10% of all school children, you would number the children and examine every tenth child, starting with a random number between 1 and 10.

b) Random cluster sample
Alternatively, you can divide the area to be surveyed into sections of approximately equal size, say about ten families. Draw the dividing lines on your map. Number the sections and, again, make

tickets with all the section numbers. Draw the required number of tickets after having mixed them in a bowl. The numbers drawn will be the sections where you will examine *all* households within the boundary of that section. This method is less accurate, but more convenient, because it means less walking from one house to the next.

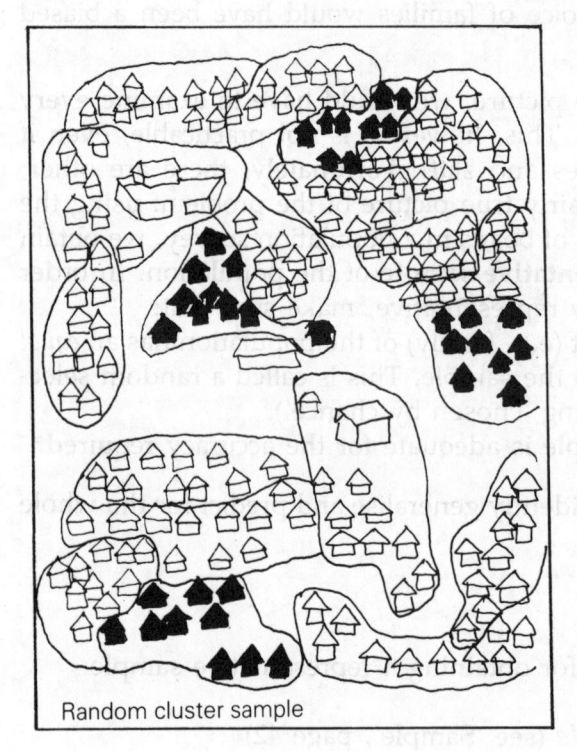

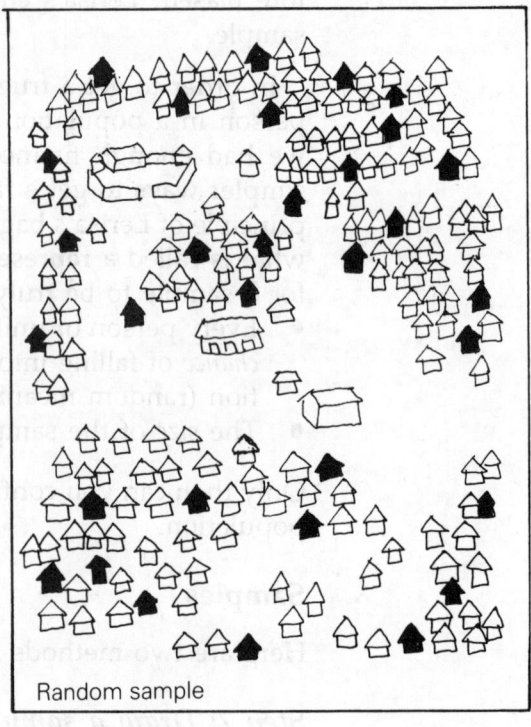

Two methods of choosing a random sample

Exercise

Plan a survey for the area you are working in. Answer questions 1–8 in Table 8.1 for your own area.

SUMMARY

1 If neither the people nor the health services benefit from a survey, then don't do the survey.
2 When doing a survey, take care that your sample is not biased. Random sampling methods, if done well, give a fairly accurate picture of the health problem you want to investigate.

Reference
Feuerstein, M.T., *Partners in Evaluation* (Macmillan, London, 1986)

9

Ten people with entropion – Interpreting the survey results

Preparations for the survey were completed as planned. Joyce explained the procedure once more at a village meeting. Lerisa asked two of her friends to help. They visited all 34 homes the day before the survey and asked all adults to stay at home for Joyce's visit. This long and tedious preparation turned out to be very worthwhile.

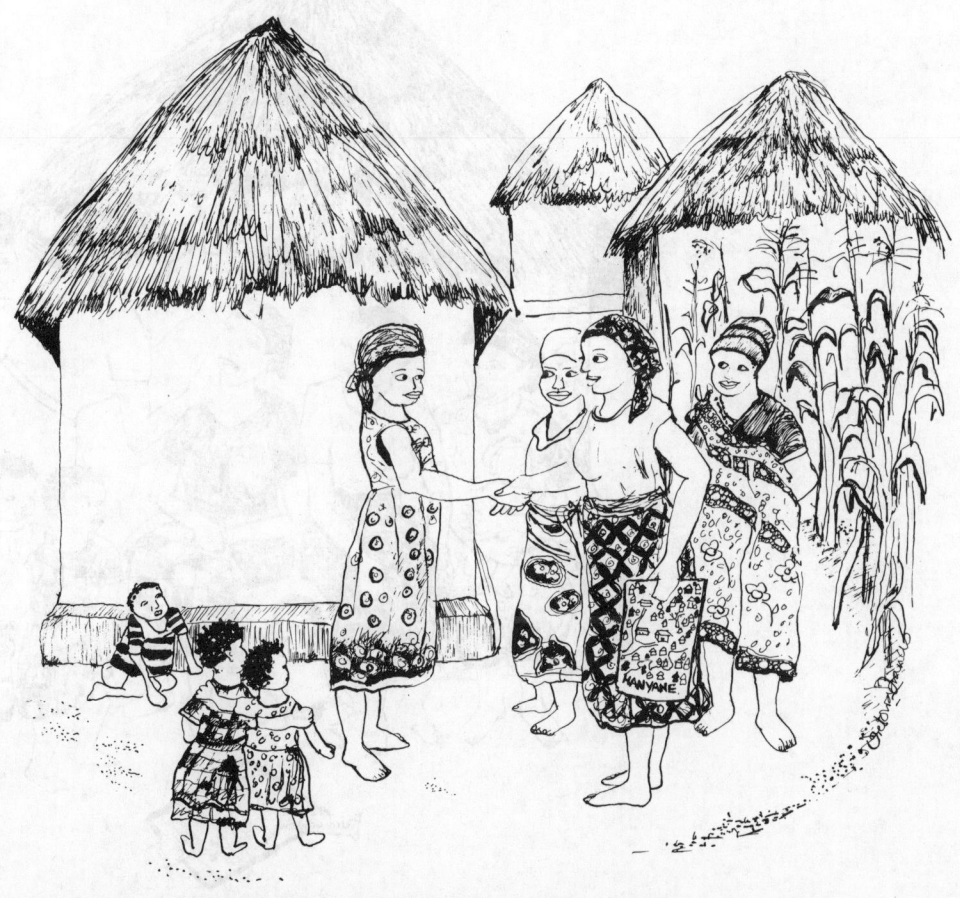

Lerisa and her friends visited all 34 homes before the survey

The survey went smoothly – people were ready for the nurse and willing to be examined. The only person who refused was Vho-Mudau. One hundred adults were present in the 34 homes of the sample. But many people who were not part of the sample wanted to have their eyes examined. Mothers came with their children. These examinations took a long time because children's upper eyelids need to be turned inside out. The children cried and some mothers had to run after the older ones who tried to escape. In many of the little ones the inside of the upper lid was red, swollen and rough. This is what trachoma looks like. Fortunately, Joyce had enough tetracycline eye ointment with her to treat the children who needed it. Examination for entropion was easy – she just had to look at people, without even touching their eyes.

While going from home to home, Joyce noticed that the more affluent people lived near the shop and the school, their homes were well-built and clean, and the people looked healthy. There was no entropion and only one child had mild trachoma. In other

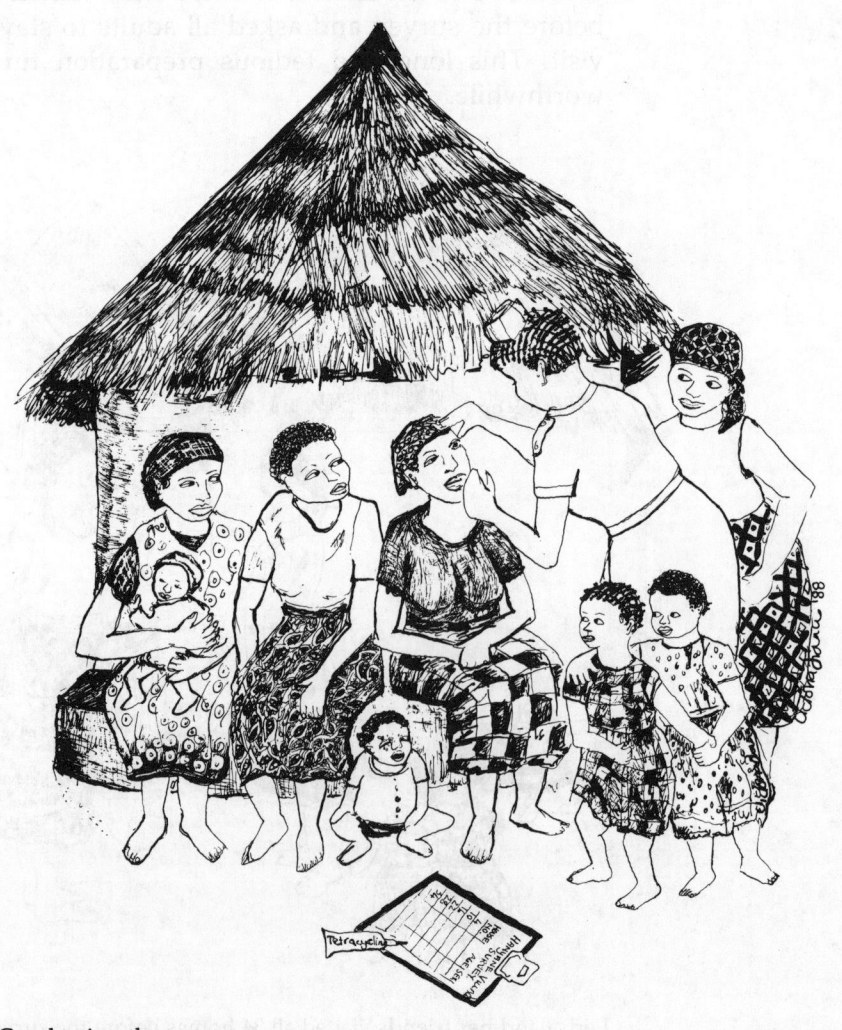

Conducting the survey

areas, especially where Ma-Anna lived, the people were extremely poor – there were no gardens and the women looked tired and their homesteads were untidy. The number of children, goats and fowl in the yards made it even worse. Flies settled on the children's faces, around discharging eyes and noses – the children didn't even swat them away. In these households she found most of the cases of entropion. One of them was Kokwana. Her house was number 58, and was one of the sample. It was also striking to find many young children with severe trachoma, while older children and adults seemed less affected. Most people had some scars on the inside of the upper eyelid which showed that they must have had trachoma in the past.

The outcome of the survey is shown in Table 9.1 below.

	Men	Women	Total
Persons over 20	30	70	100
Entropion cases	1	9	10
% entropion	3%	13%	10%

Table 9.1

These figures indicated that, of all the adults in this village, about one in ten had entropion and was at risk of going blind from trachoma. Joyce wondered if this meant trachoma was a serious problem. She decided to discuss the results with the doctor before reporting back to the villagers.

What should she tell the people?

QUESTIONS

1 Why were the children not counted in the sample? Why are there more women in the sample than men?
2 What are the signs of active trachoma?
What are the signs of old (inactive) trachoma?
3 Joyce found that some groups of people in Hanyane were more affected by trachoma than others. How do you explain this?
Where do you find most cases of trachoma in your own area?
Where is trachoma uncommon in your area?
4 Can you help Joyce in the interpretation of her results?
a) Is trachoma a problem in Hanyane?
b) Who is most at risk of going blind from trachoma? Why?

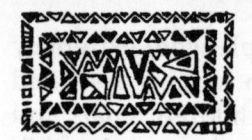

DISCUSSION

Before reading on, refresh your knowledge of trachoma (Part 3, Section C, page 225), in order to understand the following discussion notes.

We have now reached Steps 8–10 in our community diagnosis (see 'Survey' page 42):

Step 8: Inform the families

The families in the random sample have been informed and asked to be present on the day of the survey. If this information is not given to the people, they may leave home for visiting, fetching wood or working in the fields. The sample is then incomplete and of little value.

Step 9: Conduct the survey

Joyce has examined all the families in the sample. To make people happy, she also examined those additional people who wanted to be seen. However, these were not included in the final count as this would make the sample selective and therefore biased.

Step 10: Interpret the results

The results of the survey have been calculated.

1 Joyce's observations on trachoma

a) 10 people out of the sample of 100 had entropion, i.e. 10%. This is very high and confirms the impression that *trachoma is a serious problem*, and an important cause of potential blindness.

b) Entropion was most frequently found in the areas of Hanyane where *hygiene was poorest*. The disease was less common in the central section of the village where the well-to-do people live, and also in those families living near the river.

c) Entropion was seen in *women* more often than in men: 13% of all women and only 3% of all men had entropion. This may have been because there were more women in the poor section of Hanyane than in the centre of the village. The women may also have been much older than the men. But, on checking the records, Joyce found that this was not the case. If the sample's findings are a true reflection of what is happening in the village, then *women aged 40–60 years are at greater risk of blindness from trachoma than are men of the same age.* How do you explain this?

d) Although children were not counted in the survey, Joyce noted that active trachoma was more common in *pre-school children* than in older children and adults.

2 Risk factors and high risk groups

The survey has shown that trachoma is more common in some areas in Hanyane, and also in some groups of people. Hence, although anybody can catch trachoma, people living under certain conditions or people belonging to a certain group are more at risk of getting the disease than others.

Factors which increase the **risk** of illness are called **risk factors**. Poor hygiene and lack of water are risk factors for trachoma, but also for other diseases common in Hanyane, such as gastro-enteritis and scabies. **Groups** of people who are at greater risk than others are **high risk groups**. For example, women are a high risk group for entropion and young children are a high risk group for severe active trachoma. Surveys help health workers to find these factors and groups and to plan appropriate action. In Hanyane one would therefore try to improve hygiene and pay particular attention to women and young children.

Exercise

For each of the diseases listed in Table 9.2 below, name an important risk factor and a high risk group for the area where you work:

Disease	Risk factor	High risk group
Xerophthalmia		
Glaucoma		
Ocular trauma		
Measles		
Epidemic conjunctivitis		
River blindness		

Table 9.2

SUMMARY

1 Surveys are only of value if well planned and carefully conducted.
2 Surveys are useful for identifying risk factors and high risk groups. Armed with this information, appropriate action can be taken.

10

Disappointment with the survey – Where is the action?

The chief sent an urgent message to Joyce to attend a village meeting. He told her that the villagers were unhappy about the survey. They had had to stay at home all day instead of going to the fields. They felt that Joyce had used them for her own gains and hadn't kept her promise to come back with medicines.

Joyce was upset. She still had not seen the doctor to discuss the survey results and all the eye ointment had been used up. But she could not delay the report-back any longer. Next day she went to Hanyane. She was very nervous. Would people still respect her? She took her place next to the chief uneasily. The chief opened the meeting as usual and then it was Joyce's turn to speak.

Joyce thanked the gathering for their good cooperation during the survey and apologised for being late with the report. 'Do you still remember what I was looking for?' she asked.

When the people said that she had been looking for 'shinyeku', Joyce was puzzled. She had not heard that word before. However, she learned that shinyeku was the popular name for 'in-turning eyelashes'. She was also told that there was a certain old lady of Hanyane who pulled eyelashes out for a fee. It usually helped for a while. Joyce was glad that people knew so much already. This made it easier for her to explain more about the disease. The old lady's treatment was nearly the same as what Joyce did at the clinic. The people liked to hear her say that. It was the first time that a nurse had respected their old traditions.

Joyce went on to explain how these eyelashes can cause blindness if nothing is done about them. The many children she had seen with trachoma would get shinyeku later in their lives, because trachoma in childhood was the beginning of it. Therefore, she had given eye ointment to these children on the day of the survey. They could get more medicine at the clinic later on when fresh supplies arrived.

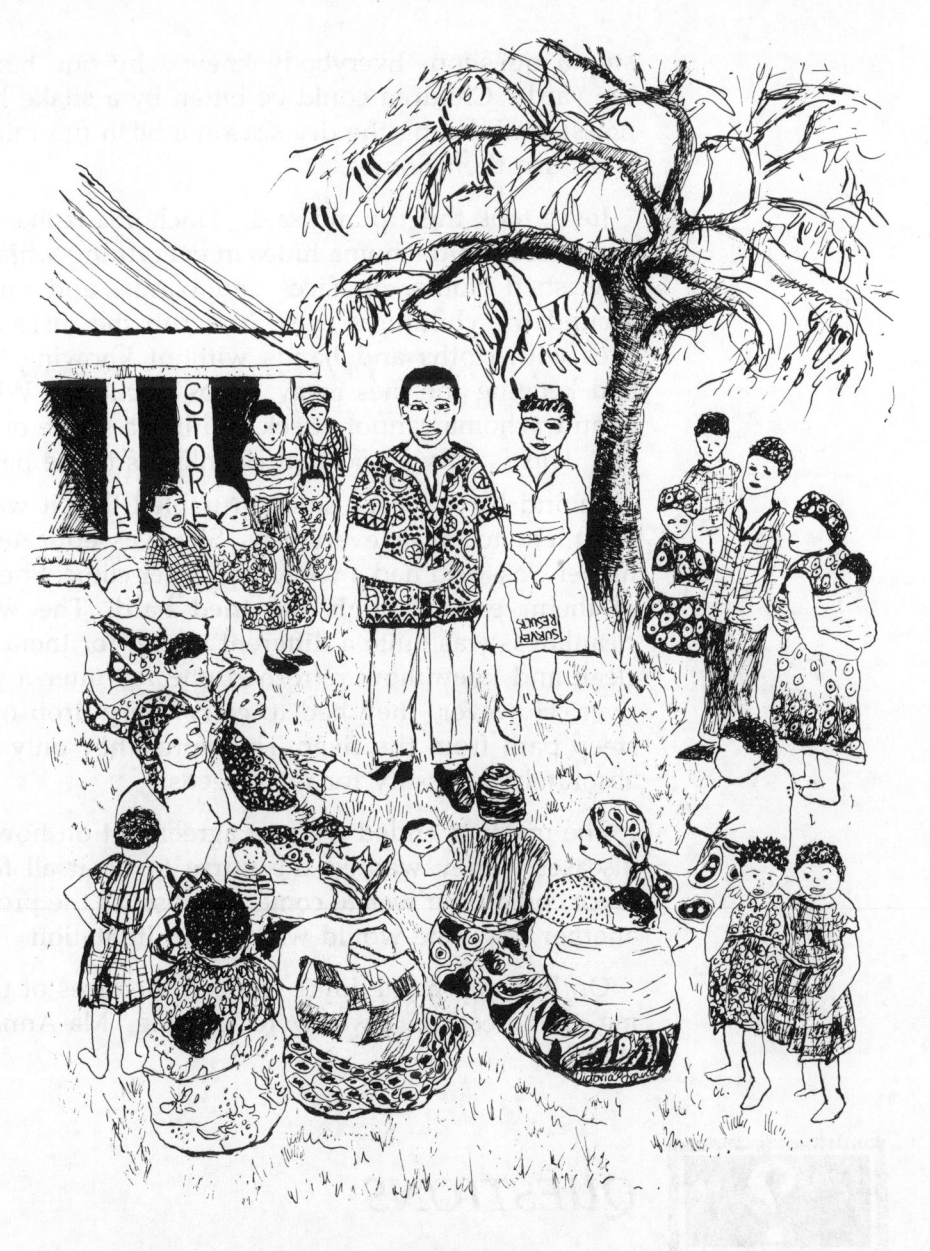

The people were very disappointed. They wanted medicine immediately. Hadn't Joyce promised she would cure their eye diseases after the survey?

'There is another medicine which is much better. You can even do it yourself,' Joyce said.

'What is it?' the villagers asked.

'This medicine is called "wash face and hands every day"'.

'That's not a medicine,' they shouted.

Joyce pointed towards the next homestead and asked why they kept the grass so short around the yard. The old ladies shook their heads. This nurse was really strange. First, she talked about washing the face being a medicine and now she asked such a

67

stupid question. Everybody knew why one had to clear around the yards. Children could be bitten by a snake hiding in the high grass. And during the dry season a bush fire might come too near and burn their homes.

Joyce took this up and said, 'Trachoma is like a snake hiding in the grass. But trachoma hides in everything which is dirty. It is on unwashed cloths, on faces and hands, and on the legs of flies around the children's eyes. You rub the disease right into your eyes with cloths and hands without knowing it. So cleanliness, and keeping the flies away, stops trachoma. When everything is clean trachoma cannot attack you like a snake or scorch you like a fire. This is why I said that cleanliness is the best medicine.'

Behind Joyce's back some grumbled that it was easy for her to ask them to wash every day. She was educated, belonged to a higher class and had a water tap at her clinic. She wasn't really one of them, even though she tried hard. The whole business of cleanliness was quite a different matter for them. They liked to be clean and knew how refreshed one felt after a good wash in the river. However, they had to carry every drop of water along the steep path from the river. Therefore, they only carried what was absolutely necessary for their needs.

The meeting ended without agreement on how to get rid of eye diseases – they wanted the nurse to do it all for them. All that Joyce could offer was to come and discuss the problem of trachoma another day. She would wait for an invitation.

On her way home Joyce recalled the faces of the people attending the meeting. Two were missing: Ma-Anna and Kokwana. Why?

QUESTIONS

1 Have people in the area where you work got a popular name for entropion/trichiasis?
   a) Is it useful to know popular names of diseases? Why?
   b) Have you met any local practices for treating entropion?
2 What do you think about Joyce's health education?
   a) Contents?
   b) Presentation?
   c) Credibility? (Can you believe it?)
   d) Feasibility? (Is it possible?)
3 Are you satisfied with the outcome of the meeting? What are your own experiences with village meetings?
   a) List five things that can go wrong with village meetings.

b) List five advantages of village meetings.
4 How do people in your area react to surveys? Is it good to inform people about the survey results?

DISCUSSION

Step 11: Feedback (see 'Survey', page 42)

Hanyane's experience is not unusual. Surveyors rarely deem it necessary to report back. The same people would not treat an individual patient like that. They would inform him about the results of any special tests done. Why are whole communities treated so carelessly? They have as much right to know as the individual person has.

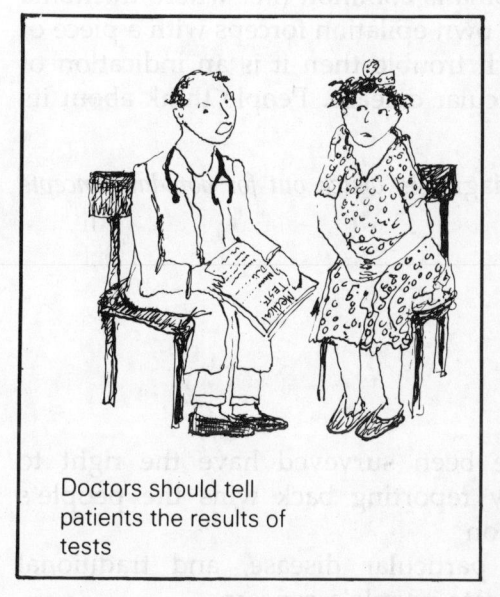

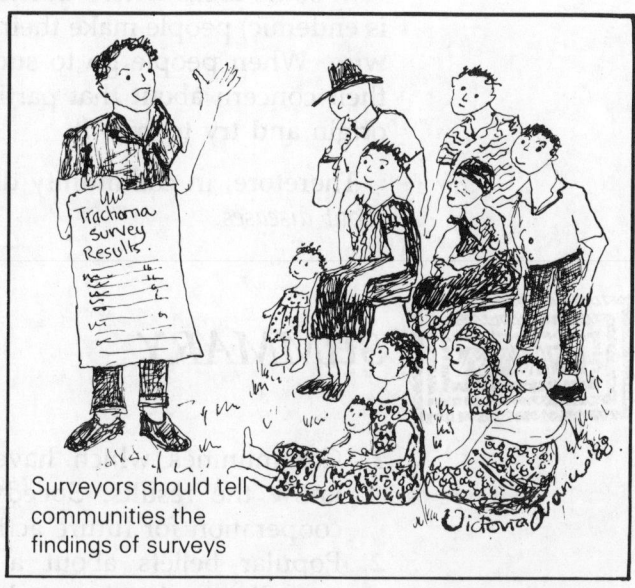

| Doctors should tell patients the results of tests | Surveyors should tell communities the findings of surveys |

The failure to report back is not always due to carelessness. Joyce had the best intentions but did not know what to tell the people.

Evaluating a survey involves laborious and time-consuming work. For health workers, time is a rare commodity. So, all those record sheets, compiled during the survey, get left in a heap on the shelf until the day comes when the health worker can work on them. That day may never come and the survey, as well as the people it was meant to serve, are forgotten. It is much better to do a rough estimate of the results to convey to the community as soon as possible and attend to the details later. The people will appreciate your courtesy and concern. They may even offer their own

69

ideas on how to solve the problem, and you will have won their support.

Another reason for the failure to report back is the belief that people do not understand anyway. Doctors need to learn the art of telling their patients what is wrong with them; surveyors need to find ways of presenting their findings to communities. If this is done well, people will understand and will want to act.

> REPORTING BACK IS AS IMPORTANT AS GIVING MEDICINE

Why is 'shinyeku' important?

People knew exactly what Joyce was looking for when she examined them. They had a word for it in their own language ('shinyeku' – in-turning eyelashes) and even a method to treat it (epilation).

In some areas where trachoma is common (i.e. where trachoma is endemic) people make their own epilation forceps with a piece of wire. When people go to such trouble then it is an indication of their concern about that particular disease. People think about its origin and try to cure it.

Therefore, in community diagnosis *watch out for popular concepts about diseases*.

SUMMARY

1 Communities which have been surveyed have the right to know the results. Speedy reporting back wins the people's cooperation for future action.
2 Popular beliefs about a particular disease, and traditional remedies for its cure, indicate people's concern.

PART 1   SECTION B
Action towards eye health

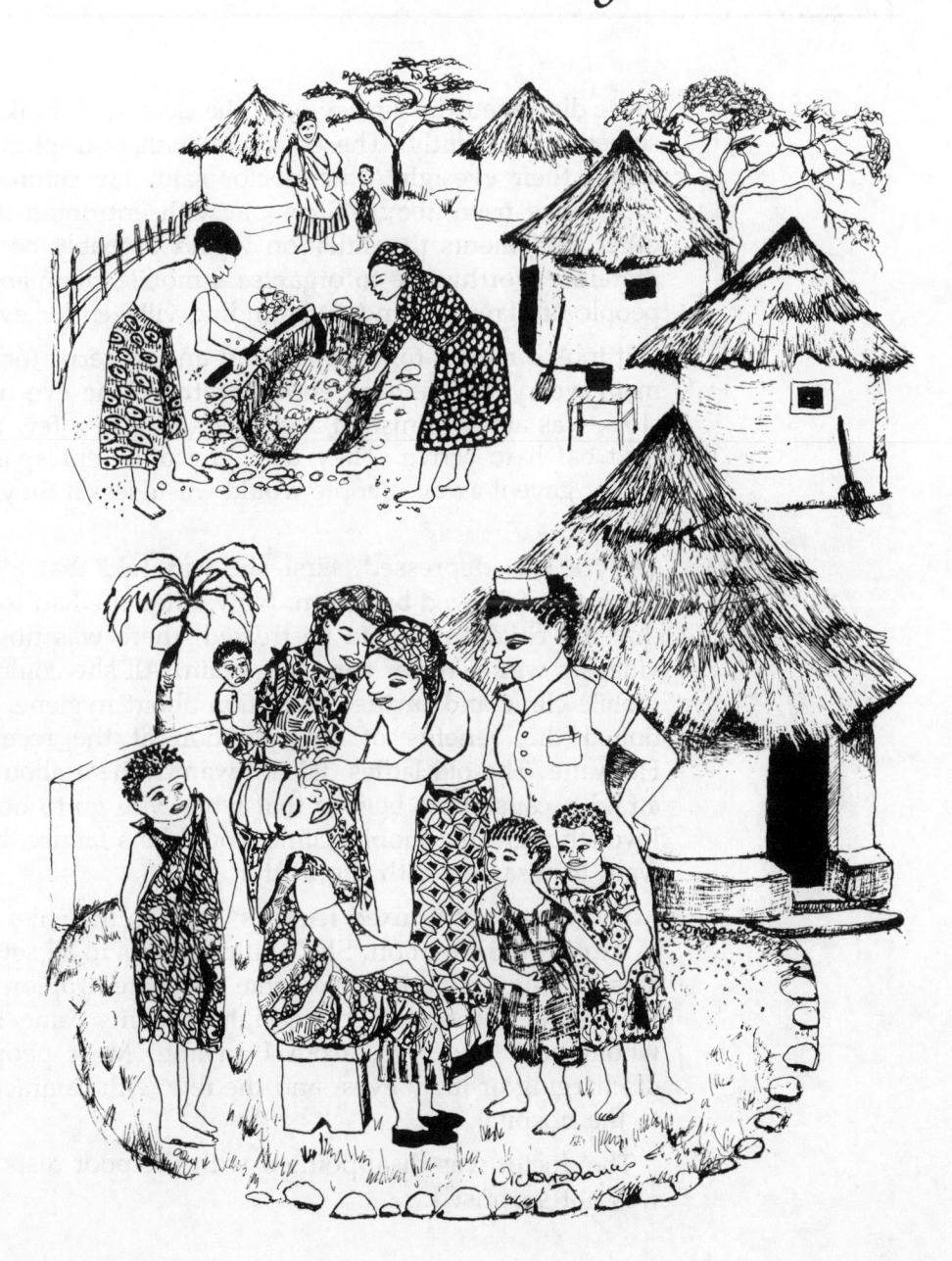

11

Operation? No thank you – Inappropriate action

Joyce discussed the survey with the doctor. 'I think we have to do something urgently. These people with entropion are at risk of losing their eyesight,' the doctor said. He estimated that there must have been about 40 people with entropion in Hanyane. In other settlements the situation would probably be similar. It was therefore worthwhile to organise a mobile clinic and to invite the people of Hanyane and surrounding villages for eyelid surgery.

It took a month to organise staff and material for the clinic. The main worry was finding enough tetracycline eye ointment. Their stock was almost finished and it would take a few months for the next batch to arrive. They used the ointment sparingly, and no longer gave it away. People would waste less if they had to pay for it.

Joyce was depressed. First she was told that a survey should always be followed by action. Now, after she had told the villagers that the children had to be treated, there was no ointment. The villagers would never trust her again. All she could offer was the mobile clinic and further education about hygiene. She had mentioned the benefits of an operation at the recent meeting in Hanyane. The old ladies did not want to hear about it. They were afraid because they believe that when you go to hospital you die. Joyce thought the mobile clinic would be a failure, but she did not want to disagree with the doctor.

She went, with mixed feelings, back to the chief and the elders to explain the situation. She sent messages to all settlements in the area, asking for patients to come for the entropion operation. On the day of the mobile clinic eight patients came for surgery, of whom only two were from Hanyane. Most people came with discharging or itchy eyes, and the few with cataract were referred to the hospital.

The doctor was disappointed with the poor response, but Joyce was not surprised.

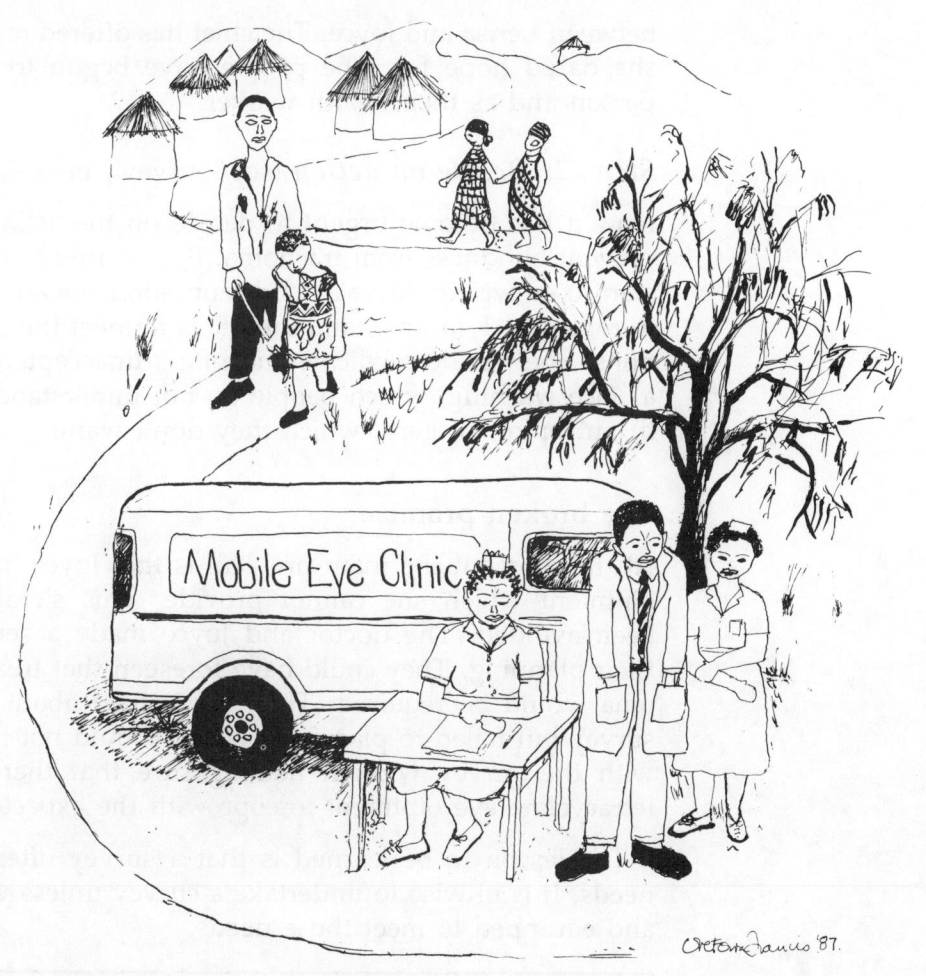

The mobile clinic was a disappointment

❓ QUESTIONS

1. Why do you think so few people came for the entropion operation?
2. What would help people to agree to the operation?
3. The shortage of eye ointment has further damaged Joyce's credibility. How could it have been avoided?

DISCUSSION

Joyce has started off well with her community diagnosis. She has learned much about the community she is serving from her visits to Ma-Anna and the chief. A relationship of trust is developing

73

between Lerisa and Joyce. The chief has offered more support than she dared hope for. The people have begun to accept her as a person and as their health worker.

Step 12: Decide on action (see 'Survey', page 42)

Now it has become urgent to decide on the action to be taken to prevent blindness from trachoma. But, at this crucial point, things start to go wrong. Joyce's good reputation is waning. First she fails to report back in time, and then fails to meet the people's expectations. She has no medicine and offers unacceptable alternatives:
a) face washing, which people do not understand, and
b) entropion surgery, which they don't want.

1 The broken promise

At the moment the main problem is that Joyce has promised eye ointment which she cannot provide. This situation could have been avoided. The doctor and Joyce made a serious mistake in their planning. They could have foreseen that treatment for trachoma would be required. They had talked about action after the survey but failed to plan for it. They should not have gone ahead with the survey without making sure that there was sufficient tetracycline eye ointment to cope with the expected demand.

The lesson to be learned is that a survey often reveals urgent needs. It is unwise to undertake a survey unless you are prepared and equipped to meet those needs.

> IF YOU FAIL TO PLAN, YOU PLAN TO FAIL

2 The wrong action

For a doctor or a nurse, health has top priority. It is frustrating for them to see that, for most rural people, health is very low on the list of priorities. People are more worried about the essentials of daily life such as income, wood, water and food.

The eye doctor in the story is convinced that, by organising the mobile clinic, he is doing the best for the people. He has observed that many adults required entropion surgery. In community health language this is called **observed needs**. He believes that it is only lack of knowledge which prevents the people from using the health services properly. All that the people of Hanyane need is to know about trachoma. The doctor assumes that, when people *know* then they will be eager to go for the operation. He is under the illusion that knowledge leads to action.

What he has not thought about is how people feel about their needs. Entropion has been with them for a long time – they even have their own way of treating it. Why should they take time off from their everyday life-sustaining duties and submit themselves to an unknown operation?

Health workers are usually outsiders to the communities they serve. Therefore, they are in danger of taking the wrong (i.e. inappropriate) action. They make their plans as they see it and expect the people to comply. Think about the meaning of the word 'compliance' – it means to act according to someone's command, leaving no freedom of choice. Is this the best way to solve a problem?

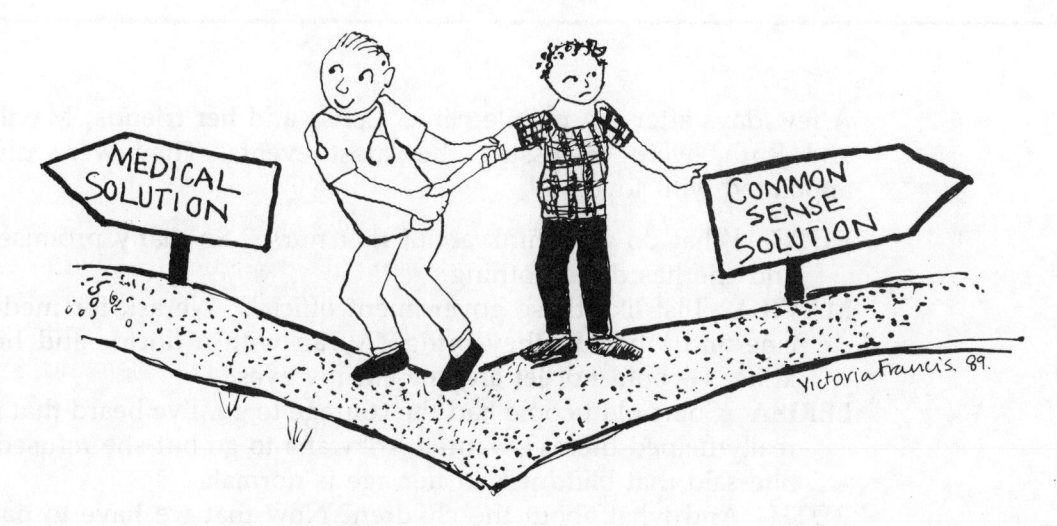

Compliance

SUMMARY

1. If you know a survey cannot be followed by appropriate action, don't do the survey.
2. Knowledge does not always lead to action.
3. Action *for* the community instead of *with* the community is often inappropriate action.

12

Where is the medicine?
– Health at a price

A few days after the mobile clinic, Lerisa and her friends, Mavila and Ruth, were discussing the latest events. They were disappointed with Joyce.

RUTH What do you think about that nurse? So many promises and she has done nothing.

MAVILA Just like these government officials. We ask for medicine and what do they bring? A van with a doctor and his knife. I would not let anyone cut my eyes.

LERISA Some old people had the courage to go. I've heard that it really helped them. I wanted Kokwana to go but she refused. She said that blindness at her age is normal.

RUTH And what about the children? Now that we have to pay for the eye ointment, many will not be able to treat their own children. Are you on the nurse's side for this also?

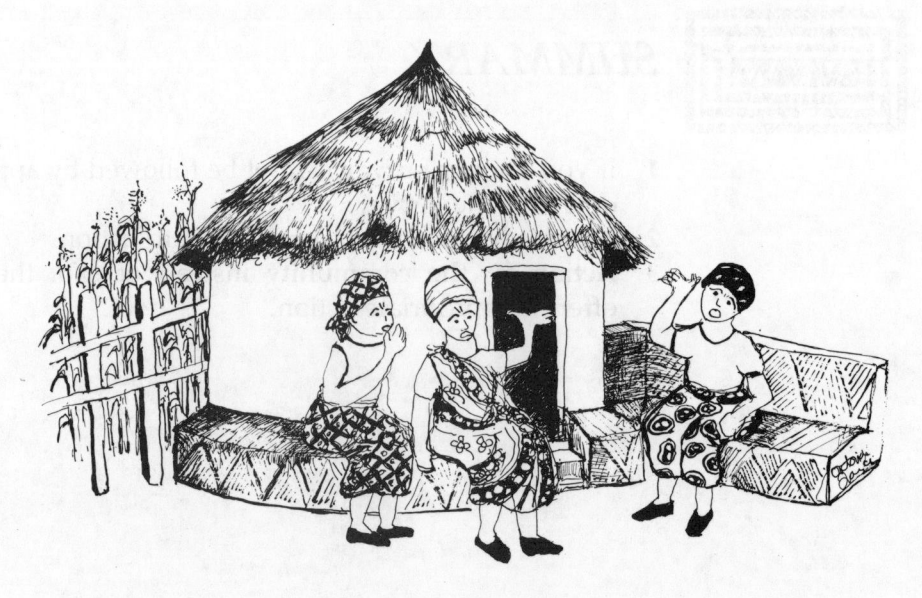

'What do you think of that nurse? She promises help, then we don't see her'

Lerisa had to admit that she could not understand this either. During the survey she saw that the poorest people had most of the trachoma in the village. They couldn't pay for medicine while the rich people who needed it less could afford it. There were rumours in the village that the teacher and the shopkeeper bought the medicine for their whole family. People were upset about this. Was health only for the rich?

Now that they were aware that something had to be done about trachoma, and were willing to treat their children, there was no medicine.

Lerisa was getting worried about the way her friends were talking. She felt responsible. She had encouraged Joyce to come to Hanyane to help them solve their health problems. In spite of her own disappointment, Lerisa thought there was still a chance of working with the nurse. 'We must go to the nurse,' she said. 'Why should we always wait for someone to come here and help us? Let us pay her a visit.'

When the three friends arrived at the clinic the next day Joyce was busy with the child health clinic. They couldn't talk with her right away because it was too noisy with the children crying at the tops of their voices. Joyce invited the three friends to watch her while she weighed and examined the children. She explained what she was doing and showed them the children suffering from trachoma.

After Joyce finished the clinic they sat down with a cup of tea. At last they could talk undisturbed. Joyce was glad they had come. She had been worried about the failure of all her previous efforts and feared that people had turned away from her. She knew it had been her own fault. She had promised more than she could do. One should think before speaking, especially in front of those who might believe every word one says. Happily things seemed to be getting sorted out again. It was wonderful how quickly people could forgive.

'We are unhappy in Hanyane,' the three told Joyce. 'We are especially worried about Ma-Anna. As you know Musa is already blind. Must the other children also lose their eyesight because Ma-Anna can't afford to buy eye ointment?

Joyce understood their worries. She herself was unhappy about the situation. She had a few tubes of ointment she could give free of charge to those of the poor who needed it most.

'How can we know who needs it?' asked Lerisa. 'We are not nurses. You once promised that you would teach us more. Would you do it now?'

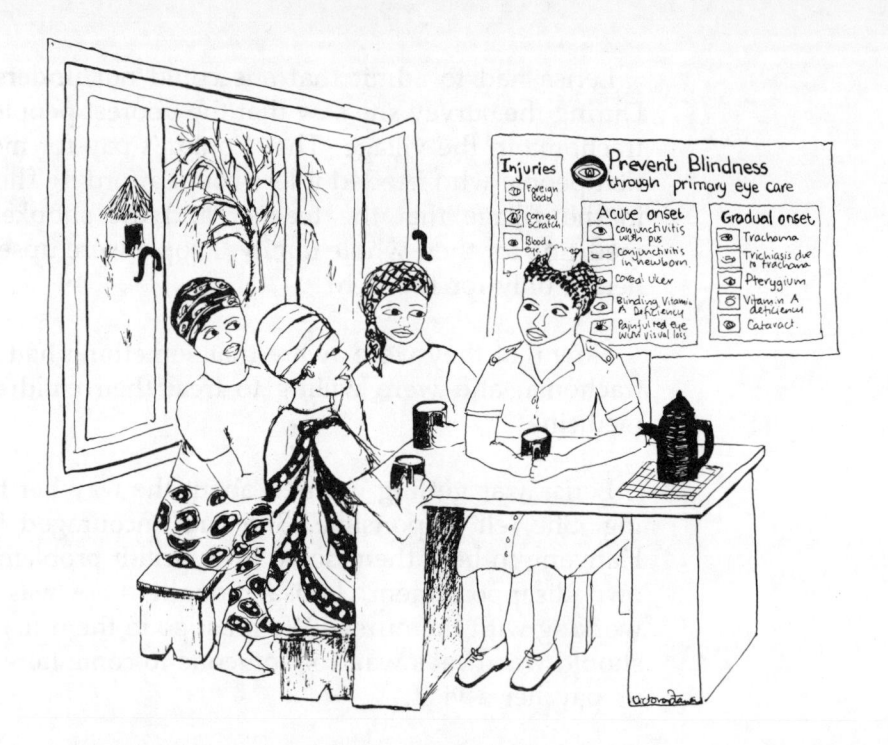

Joyce was a bit surprised and thought to herself, 'When do I have time?' But she had offered to teach them. Her journey towards community health had begun. Now that people were truly interested she could not turn them away.

'Of course I will,' said Joyce. 'If you gather some more of your friends who would be interested then I will come to Hanyane.' They made a date for Thursday afternoon the following week and promised to have a group ready.

'Will Ma-Anna be there?' asked Joyce.

Lerisa explained that Ma-Anna was too depressed about Musa. She was not interested in trachoma because she was told that Musa became blind from measles, not trachoma.

QUESTIONS

1. What are the advantages of providing medicine free? What are the disadvantages?
2. Who has easiest access to health services where you work? Why do some people find it difficult to utilise the health services?
3. What do you feel about sharing your knowledge with village people?
4. Are the people in the area where you work passive receivers of health care or active doers? Why?

DISCUSSION

1 The costs of health

Health care is an expensive commodity. One of the principles of primary health care is to provide basic health services for all. But when it comes to sharing available resources, this principle is often overlooked. The specialised health care units in the cities get the greatest share, while remote areas are neglected and left without the necessary services. You are a frontline fighter for health and you should use your position to fight on behalf of your deprived community for a more just distribution of health facilities.

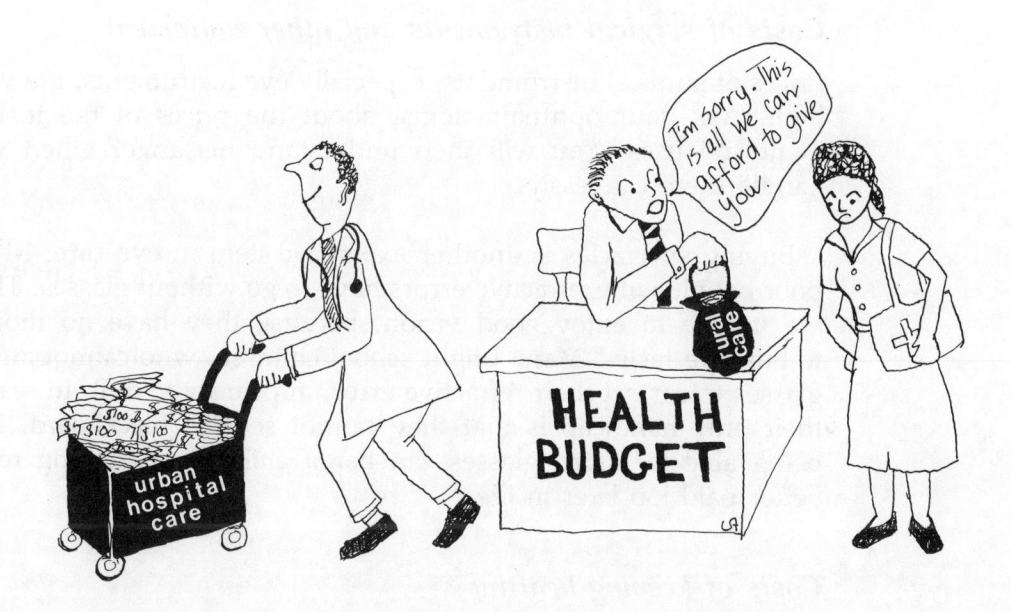

Why is health care so expensive?

Costs of personnel

Do you know how much has been spent on your training? Try to find out. Bryant calculated that the money spent for the training of one doctor would be sufficient to train four nurses or 26 nursing auxiliaries. Once trained and in their job, more money is spent on the salaries of a few doctors than on the other health workers. Because money means power, those earning most have the greatest say about how health care facilities should be organised. This is one of the reasons why health facilities are concentrated in urban areas, and provide the best equipment and care for the wealthy.

Costs of medicines

Most medicines are produced by the multinational pharmaceutical companies. The primary concern of business is to make profits, hence essential medicines are often very expensive. Some developing countries have tried to produce the most important drugs themselves. A few have succeeded, but most find it very difficult. It therefore happens that health departments have no funds to purchase the most essential drugs. It also happens that drugs destined for rural clinics are sold in the cities to make money. This means that the clinics have no medicines and people may die as a result. We do not know why there was no eye ointment in Hanyane. From your own experiences with similar situations, you can probably come up with several possible explanations.

Costs of surgical instruments and other equipment

Prices of surgical instruments, especially eye instruments, are very high. Ask your ophthalmologist about the prices of the instruments he uses. You will then understand his anger when you handle them carelessly.

Buying spectacles is another expensive item in eye care. Many poor people with refractive errors have to go without glasses. They are unable to enjoy good vision, because they have no money to buy spectacles. Many bright school children, who cannot afford glasses to correct their refractive error, appear to be dull. In reality their only handicap is that they cannot see the blackboard. Not being able to afford glasses can bar a child from training for a better paid job later in life.

Costs of keeping healthy

In Chapter 4, we discussed why poverty is the greatest obstacle to health. People with money, who have access to food, good sanitation and clean water, and who have a safe job, are healthier than the poor who may lack these essentials. To fight poverty, a lot of capital is required which poor countries simply do not have. There are many reasons why poor countries remain poor. One is that rich countries exploit cheap labour in developing areas making the rich richer and the poor poorer and more sick.

Preventable disease is not confined to the poor. It also occurs amongst the wealthy when they indulge in unhealthy junk food, tobacco and alcohol, or overeat and avoid taking exercise. These are the people who run to the pharmacist or doctor with the slightest discomfort and spend a lot of money on medicines. They believe health can be bought in the chemist shop or at the hospital.

2 Wise use of available resources

Let us assume that Musa had one eye totally destroyed and on the other eye he had a dense central corneal scar. This eye would be suitable for a corneal graft which would help him see again. This operation is very expensive and requires costly equipment. For the money spent on a corneal graft, about 3,000 children could be vaccinated against measles and given a dose of Vitamin A, which protects them from nutritional or post-measles corneal ulceration.

> PREVENTION IS NOT ONLY **BETTER** BUT ALSO **CHEAPER** THAN A CURE

Prevention does not only save money. It spares innumerable years of suffering for those children whose blindness could have been prevented.

Do you know of any other blinding eye conditions where prevention is cheap and easy?

SUMMARY

1 The costs of health care include money spent on training and salaries of health workers, medicines, equipment and buildings.
2 Usually, most available resources are spent on curative care in the cities.
3 Unless preventive care is accompanied by effective elimination of poverty, unnecessary disease will not disappear. However, material and political costs involved in removing poverty are tremendous. Hence keeping healthy is more costly than we like to believe.

Reference
Bryant, J., *Health and the Developing World* (Cornell University Press, 1969)

13

The best medicine
– Keeping snakes away

A group of women gathered at Lerisa's home. They were all young mothers, most with babies tied on their backs. Some toddlers were playing. Lerisa's mother and another old lady sat at a distance, keeping a watchful eye on these young women. They wanted to know what was going on. They wouldn't allow them to learn any nonsense from that nurse.

Joyce was pleased to see the little group of mothers and the grandmothers as well. Could this be the beginning of better health in Hanyane?

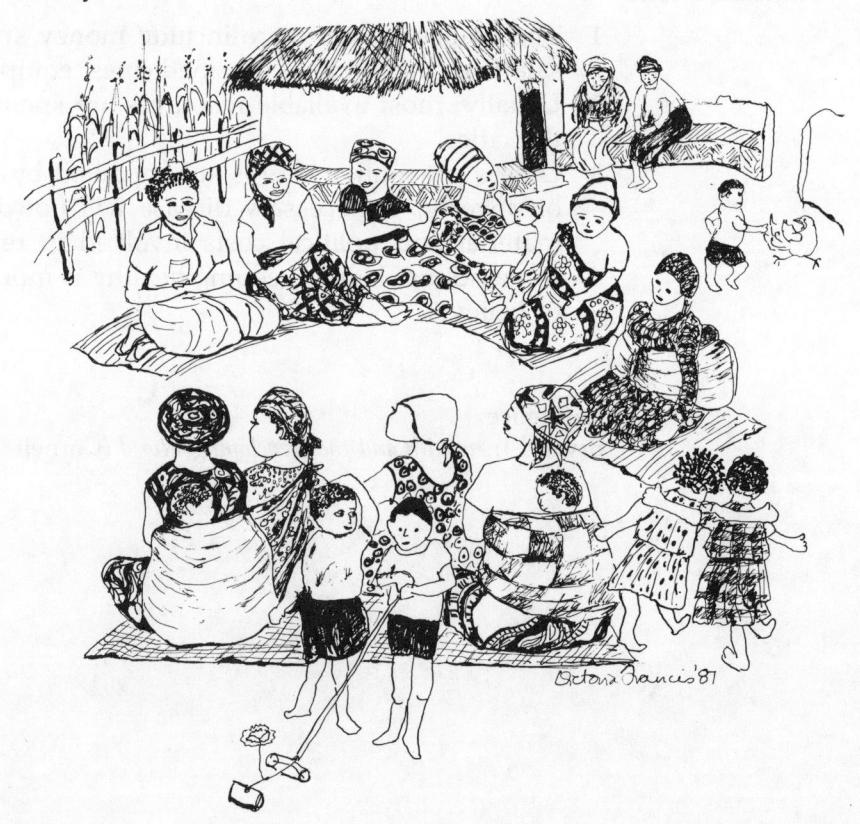

They began by complaining about the lack of eye ointment. They wanted Joyce to examine all the children and tell them who should get ointment. Joyce could not promise that. She was too busy at her clinic. The best method was still to improve hygiene. But how could she convince them? Maybe a better understanding of the disease could make face washing more acceptable. She explained in simple terms the clinical course of trachoma.

'Do you still remember the village meeting when we spoke about the reasons for cutting the grass around the houses?' Joyce asked.

'Yes, you told us that trachoma is a snake hiding in the grass.'

Joyce was shocked. She had not expected people to take it literally. So she had to find another way. She noticed a mother wiping her baby's face and then her own face with the cloth she was wearing. This is a better illustration, Joyce thought. She asked for a volunteer to help her demonstrate. The lady would act as her 'baby'. Joyce then crushed a piece of yellow chalk into a fine powder and put some of it below the 'baby's' eyes.

'Imagine the baby has trachoma,' Joyce said. 'I've put this chalk below the baby's eyes to show that trachoma is hiding in the pus.' Then Joyce asked the woman playing baby to pretend to cry. 'My baby is crying. What must I do?'

'You must comfort it. You must wipe its tears,' they all said.

Joyce wiped her 'baby's' face with a cloth. Everyone could see the yellow powder on the cloth. Trachoma was now hiding in the cloth. Then she said she had itchy eyes and rubbed them with the stained cloth. The powder was now on her face.

The group agreed that this was exactly what they used to do. Sometimes they didn't use a cloth but used their fingers instead. Would this also carry trachoma from person to person? 'Of course it does', said Joyce. 'And the flies do the same. They are attracted by all the dust on the children's faces. They sit around the children's eyes and fly, with trachoma sticking to their feet, to the eyes of other children.'

The group got quite excited. Now they began to understand better. What Joyce had explained was very familiar to them. Ruth added her own story: 'We have a traditional belief in our village: Every woman who has children and is pregnant again must notify her mother-in-law about her new pregnancy. If she doesn't, then after the baby is born her mother-in-law gets shinyeku (entropion) and later goes blind.'

Joyce was delighted to hear this. 'You are so clever. You already know that many children can be the cause of shinyeku and later blindness. The fact is that when you catch trachoma very often during your life, the disease can make you blind. You get it from the young children in the way I showed you with the chalk.'

The mothers and grannies all talked at once:
'Now we understand what you meant when you said that washing face and hands is a medicine.'
'Does it also mean to wash the cloths more often?'
'What about the flies?'
'Cattle and goats near the house bring lots of flies.'
'When our children have diarrhoea flies swarm onto the stools.'
'You must cover the stools with soil. We do the same when we go to the bush.'
'Or build a toilet.'
'Flies also sit on our children's runny noses and skin sores.'
'They are wherever food and rubbish are left uncovered.'

The group carried on talking for a long time. It was very exciting to learn so much in one afternoon. Water was the biggest problem for them. A tap in the village would help. Joyce let them talk, careful not to provide them with ready-made answers. It was hard for her not to interfere. It would have saved her a lot of time to tell them immediately what to do. With a guiding remark here and there from her, the group finally decided that they could make a start with cleanliness in their own homes. This way there would be nowhere for trachoma to hide.

HOW TRACHOMA SPREADS

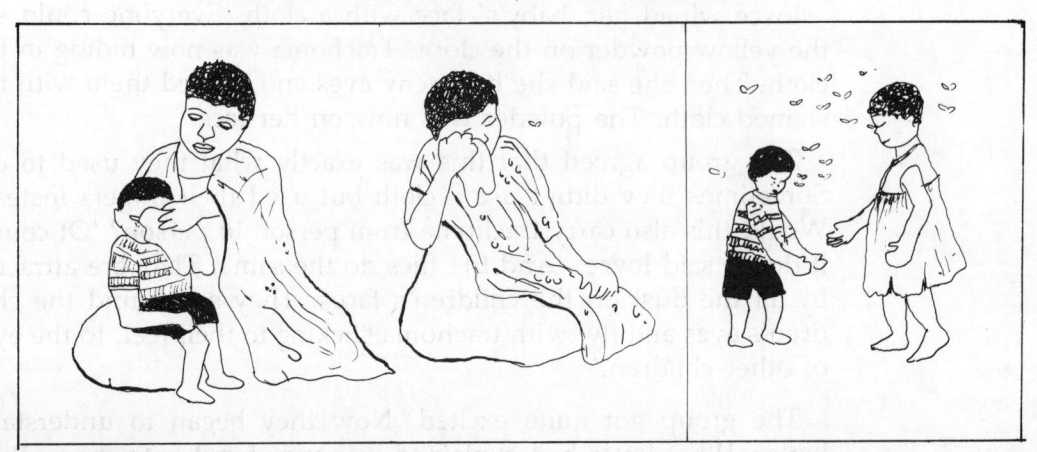

QUESTIONS

1. Describe the classification of trachoma (see Part 3, Section C).
2. What are the popular beliefs about trachoma in your area?
3. What are the most important methods of trachoma transmission in your area?
4. Think of a way in which you could explain trachoma transmission.

DISCUSSION

Trachoma, the most important cause of *preventable* blindness in the world, is commonly found in arid areas in Africa and Asia. This eye disease is the one most commonly seen by rural health workers and is one where community health care is far more effective than hospital treatment.

You, the rural health worker, are the person best able to deal with this problem. Therefore, you will want to have a good understanding of the nature of trachoma.

1 How much do you know about trachoma?

You have already learned a lot about the disease from reading Chapters 9 to 11 and the notes in Part 3. Check your understanding of these sections before reading any further.

Exercise
a) What has the story taught you about trachoma in Hanyane?
b) How would you answer the same questions for the area you work in (see Table 13.1)?

Question	Answer for Hanyane	Answer for your own area
1 Is trachoma a community problem?		
2 What complication of trachoma may lead to blindness?		
3 What is the traditional method for treating trachoma and/or entropion?		
4 Are men and women equally affected?		
5 In which section of the village is trachoma most common?		
6 In which age group is active trachoma most severe?		
7 How does trachoma spread within the family?		
8 What is the treatment for trachoma?		
9 How can people prevent the spread of trachoma?		

Table 13.1

2 How does trachoma cause blindness?

If you catch trachoma only once, or if it is very mild, you need not be afraid of going blind. One single spell of the disease, especially when it is mild, heals spontaneously without disabling complications. Such cases do not even require treatment.

Trachoma is only a danger to eyesight when a person contracts the disease many times over a period of months and years. Every new infection with *Chlamydia* triggers off another tissue reaction. This results in the scarring of the conjunctiva, trichiasis and entropion. Blood vessels grow into the cornea, and the cornea can develop an ulcer, especially in the presence of bacterial conjunctivitis. The additional trauma of eyelashes rubbing on the cornea (entropion) leads to dense scarring and finally blindness. It is therefore essential that people should be protected from frequent reinfection.

In Part 3, Section C, environmental factors favouring reinfection are listed under the **four Ds** (**D**ry, **D**irty, **D**usty, with **D**ischarge) and the **four Fs** of transmission (**F**lies, **F**omites, **F**ingers and **F**amily). Instead of discussing them in isolation, let us look at how they might have contributed to Kokwana's blindness. Try, yourself, to find the four Ds and four Fs in her life story.

When Kokwana was born, living conditions and the climate in Hanyane were much the same as they are now. Cattle were kept near her family's homestead; water was scarce and seldom used for washing. When she was a toddler, Kokwana was left with the other children to play in the dusty yard. Like most children, she always had a runny nose and sores on her skin. Her little hands were dirty with mucus from her nose, which often contains *Chlamydia*. Filth and bad smells attracted swarms of flies. During the seasons of epidemic conjunctivitis, flies were especially abundant around the children's discharging eyes. This was when Kokwana was infected with trachoma for the first time. She was then one year old. Nobody worried about it. Slightly discharging eyes were considered to be normal in young children.

Kokwana slept with all the other girls in the girls' hut where they huddled together on one mat and shared one blanket between them. Such close physical contact, day and night, made it easy for the *Chlamydia* to spread amongst the children, causing repeated infections.

By the time she was eight years old she had had trachoma many many times. Like most children, she could see well and had few complaints apart from slight discomfort and an intermittent discharge from her eyes. Kokwana was then old enough to be in charge of her little brothers and sisters. Most of them also had trachoma. Kokwana carried the youngest child on her back. When he cried she wiped his face with the same cloth that she used to dry the sweat from her own face. In this way, she caught the disease again.

When Kokwana became a young woman she worked in the fields where the wind often blew dust and sand into her face and eyes. When she had her own children she wiped their faces with the same cloth she used on her own face, or she used her fingers. In this way she became infected again and again, this time from her own children. The repeated infections with trachoma began to damage her eyes – the eyelashes started to turn in. This made her rub her eyes even more. Kokwana had many children. Each one of them had trachoma and they kept reinfecting each other and Kokwana.

Kokwana is now a grandmother and looks after Ma-Anna's children. She wipes the noses and eyes of her little grandchildren with her own cloth, getting herself infected again. The scarring has now led to entropion and the cornea has turned cloudy. Now her vision is failing. If nothing is done for her entropion soon, she will be totally blind.

Kokwana's brother also had trachoma as a child, but his eyes are still good. His job was to herd the cattle, so he had little close contact with his younger brothers and sisters. Later he found work in the city and did not see much of his own children who remained in Hanyane. Even if he had stayed at home, it would not have been his business to nurse the children. So he was less at risk of getting repeated infections.

Now you can see why far more women than men have entropion and are blind with trachoma (Chapter 9).

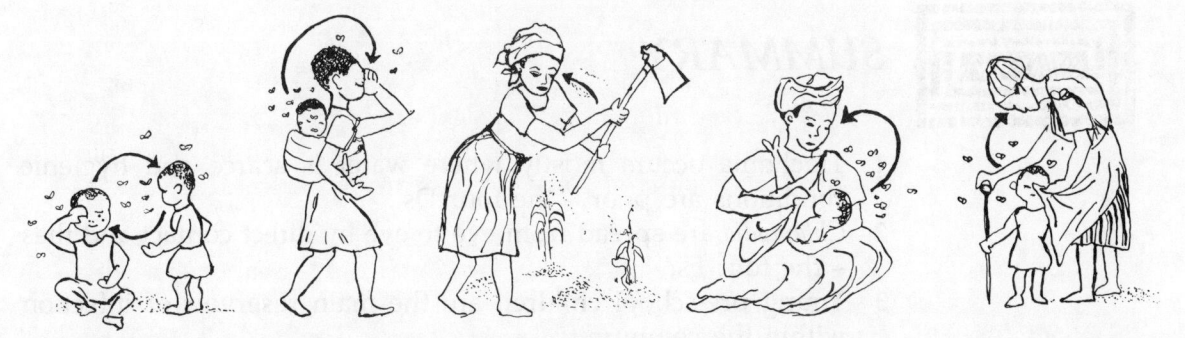

Kokwana's life story: women are frequently reinfected with Chlamydia and exposed to dust.

3 How can trachoma be prevented?

The epidemiology of trachoma can be summarised in the cycle illustrated on page 88. Poverty leads to poor hygiene. Where there

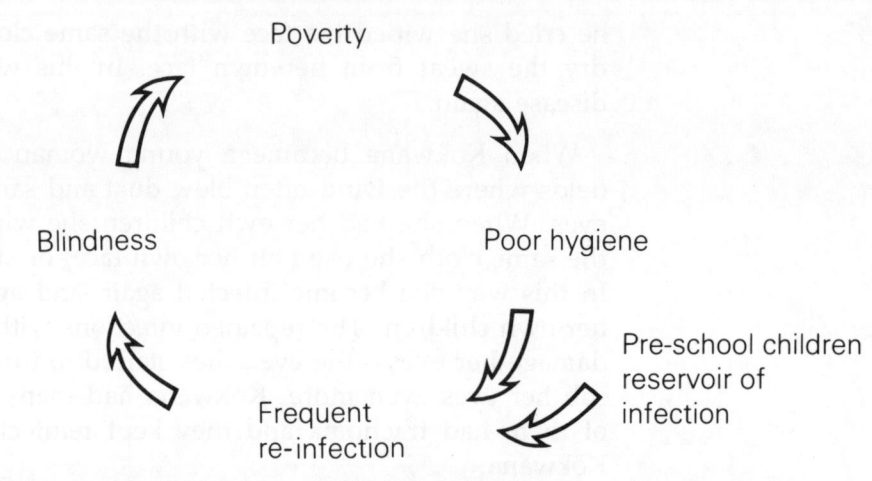

Poverty → Poor hygiene → Pre-school children reservoir of infection → Frequent re-infection → Blindness → Poverty

Essential components in the cycle of blinding trachoma

is dirt, the disease spreads easily from the young children and frequent reinfections take place. These lead to blinding complications and blindness. Blindness makes poverty worse because blind people do not earn money. So hygiene will not improve and trachoma will go on and on.

To prevent blindness from trachoma we must break this vicious cycle so that reinfections are avoided. The most effective, but also the most difficult, intervention would be to remove poverty. This, however, takes far too long. So, we have to act where we can to:
- Improve hygiene
- Reduce the *Chlamydia* by treating young children.

The story of Hanyane will tell you more about this.

SUMMARY

1. Trachoma occurs mostly where water is scarce and hygienic conditions are poor – the four Ds.
2. *Chlamydia* are spread from eye to eye by direct contact and flies – the four Fs.
3. Young pre-school children are the main reservoir of infection within the community.
4. Blindness occurs as a result of repeated infection.
5. Those most at risk of going blind from trachoma are mothers and grandmothers.
6. Trachoma is a family and neighbourhood disease.
7. To prevent blindness reinfection must be avoided. This can be achieved by improving hygiene (particularly daily face washing), and treating all young children.

14

The Tidy Ladies – Self-praisers or Health Carers?

After the first meeting, the group met a few times with Joyce, sometimes at the clinic, sometimes in Hanyane. The eleven ladies were proud of their new knowledge and Joyce was pleased to have such keen students. They formed a little club called the 'Tidy Ladies'. They discussed among themselves how to keep their homes clean and how much time they spent washing. They visited each other and admired their beautifully kept and well ornamented yards. Most of the Tidy Ladies belonged to Hanyane's middle class families – neither the very poor nor the well-to-do ones.

One day the chief's wife and the teacher's wife joined the group. These two ladies were well educated and good at needlework. Soon the group was concentrating on embroidery and crocheting table mats to decorate their homes. The homes were by now very well kept. On Joyce's advice they had dug refuse pits and built pit toilets. They also made sure that each member of their family had their own face cloth and towel. If what they had been told about trachoma and cleanliness were true, they should now be safe.

They were all very content, except for Lerisa. She was worried that Ma-Anna had refused to join the group. She had tried to convince her to join them, but to no avail. She decided to try again and went to see her.

When Lerisa arrived at Ma-Anna's home, she found Musa tucked into a corner inside the house. Kokwana didn't want to have him outside. It was shameful to have a blind child. People should not see him. They were also afraid that he might hurt himself if they left him to toddle around. Lerisa again encouraged Ma-Anna to join the Tidy Ladies. She could learn much. It was all about eyes. In addition, they had a good time together, crocheting, embroidering, and drinking tea.

Ma-Anna turned her back to Lerisa. 'Leave me alone,' she said angrily. 'Don't you see that I don't fit into your club? I'm too poor

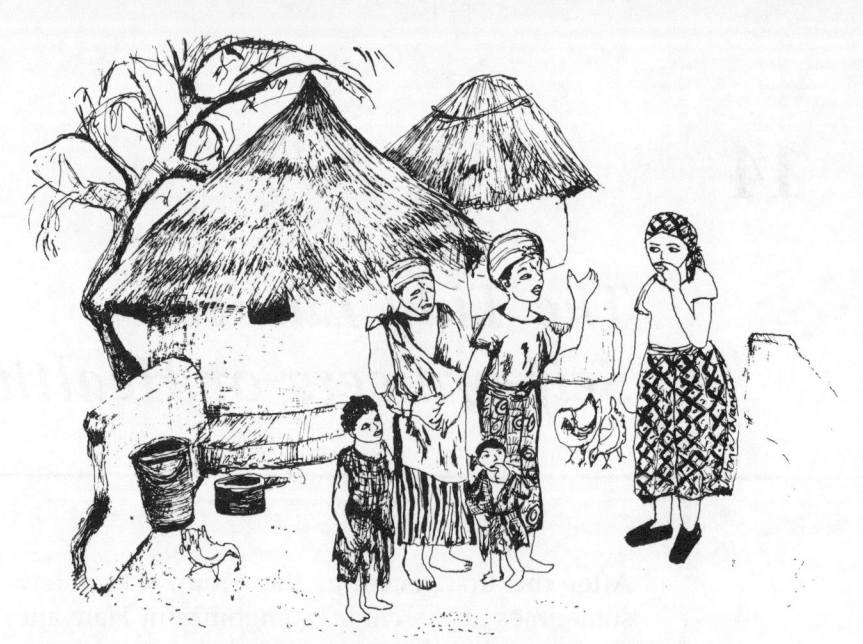

'Don't you realise that I don't fit into your Tidy Ladies club? The others will despise me because I'm poorly dressed'

for those snobs. You, too, are not the same any more. You look down on me since you started mixing with the "educated".'

Lerisa was hurt. Her friend just didn't believe her when she said nothing had changed between them.

Lerisa returned home, tears in her eyes. Why must she lose a good friend? Had her association with the 'better-offs' of Hanyane really changed her so much? Had she become aloof to other people's struggles? Was her club of Tidy Ladies really so snobbish? She felt responsible for it. It was she who started it all. She decided that on the following Thursday the Tidy Ladies must discuss how they wanted to continue, and what the aim of the club should be.

QUESTIONS

1 What is the attitude towards blind children in the area where you work?
2 If you were living at Hanyane, would you think it worthwhile to join the Tidy Ladies?
   Should Ma-Anna join?
3 Why have none of the poor mothers of Hanyane joined the Tidy Ladies?
   Why are there no men in the club?
4 What do you understand by the term 'community'?

DISCUSSION

You may have heard of the Declaration of Alma Ata on primary health care. There, paragraph IV reads: 'The people have the right and duty to participate individually and collectively in the planning and implementation of their health care.' Joyce is delighted to see that the theory she once learned is becoming reality in Hanyane: Lerisa and her two friends have taken the initiative. They have managed to get a group of interested mothers together to learn about trachoma. A good start has been made towards true community participation in health. She dreams of the time when everyone in Hanyane will work together to make the whole village spotlessly clean so that trachoma and other diseases of dirt will disappear.

Have you had similar dreams about your community? Have they come true or have you been disappointed? You will probably want to warn Joyce to look more critically at her Tidy Ladies, and to find out why Lerisa is suddenly so unhappy. Some of the questions Joyce will have to answer are:
- Is everyone in the community the same?
- Are particular interest groups exclusive?
- Does community participation in health care guarantee that the poorest in the community are reached?

1 Concepts of 'community' in primary health care

The word 'community' is used widely amongst health workers, rural developers, agriculturalists and politicians. They talk of community health care, community eye care, community participation, community involvement, community needs, community decisions, and so on. Most people who use these terms would have difficulty defining exactly what they mean. But they imagine that communities are homogenous, with a strong sense of belonging together. They have the illusion that communities are eagerly waiting for them to initiate concerted community action. Then they believe all community members will act as one body.

In reality, every village is composed of *individuals* and various groups of people, all with different interests. Village elders may share, or quarrel over, issues of power. Church groups share their faith, but may exclude those with different beliefs. Women's groups share their interests in home crafts. The wealthy and poor have different interests. Each of these individuals and groups react to project initiatives according to their own interests.

There are differing groups in Hanyane also. The wealthier ones, like the shopkeeper, the teacher and the chief, live in the village centre while the very poor, like Ma-Anna, live on the outskirts of the village. The shopkeeper is interested in selling his goods at a high price in order to make money. Ma-Anna wants the opposite – sufficient land to subsist on so that she is no longer forced to buy food at a price she cannot afford. The Tidy Ladies are interested in good housekeeping and nice needlework. They have become the 'better educated' group in the village.

2 Elitism

The Tidy Ladies have learnt how to prevent trachoma through cleanliness. They apply their learning in their own homes. They feel superior and regard themselves as the elite of Hanyane. An attitude of 'insiders' and 'outsiders', 'them' and 'us', has developed creating tensions in Hanyane. The Tidy Ladies think the outsiders are ignorant, untidy and lazy. The 'outsiders' despise the Tidy Ladies for their snobbish attitude.

Not being part of either group, Joyce believes that the Tidy Ladies are the beginning of good community participation in Hanyane. She sees herself moving towards the goal of primary health care available to all, including the very poor. She is not yet aware that the Tidy Ladies' elitism is a serious obstacle on her road and that the poor are even more excluded than before. She still has to learn to look critically at what appears to be community participation. It is seldom a guarantee of good health for all.

SUMMARY

1 'Community participation' is no guarantee that the poorest are reached with primary health care.
2 Village organisations easily become exclusive. They are then unsuitable vehicles for the spread of health awareness in the community.
3 Those most likely to 'participate' are the better-off in a community.

Reference

World Health Organization and United Nations Children's Fund, '*Alma Ata 1978, Primary Health Care.*' Report of the International Conference on Primary Health Care, Alma Ata, USSR, 6–12 September 1978. (World Health Organization, Geneva, 1978)

Why has my child got trachoma? – A community problem affects everybody

Joyce and the Tidy Ladies gathered for another meeting, this time at Mavila's place. One of them brought a cake for their tea. She had sold some of her table mats and bought ingredients for the cake with the money. The ladies sat together, chatting, drinking tea, embroidering and crocheting. 'Our houses look much better now,' remarked Ruth.

'It just required a bit of effort. Now we can enjoy our needle-work,' Mavila added.

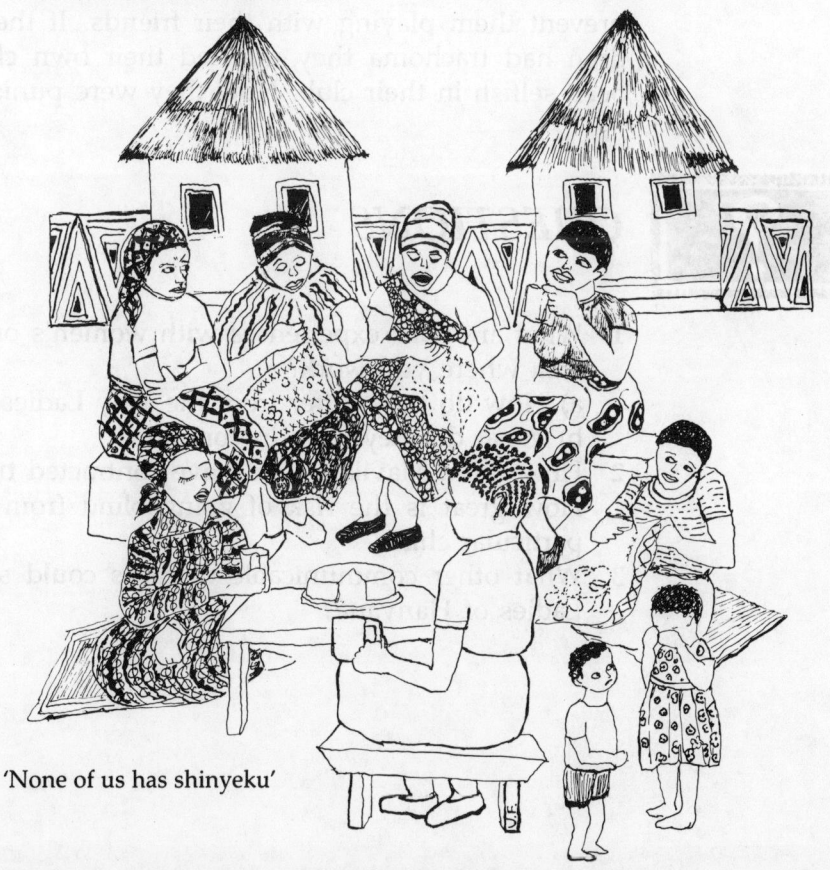

'None of us has shinyeku'

The teacher's wife, Leah, boasted that it was she who taught them needlework. Thanks to her the club had become respectable. Lerisa said nothing. She was wondering how she could introduce her problem. Eventually she said, 'We've been together for six months now and we've learned a lot about trachoma and cleanliness. We help each other, but what about those who are not in the club? Ma-Anna, for instance.'

The other women objected. 'We can't tolerate a slut like Ma-Anna. It would spoil our good name. Other people should just do as we have done and keep their homes clean.'

Mavila's little girl watched with big, envious eyes as the ladies gossiped and enjoyed their cake. She slowly came nearer, too shy to ask for a piece. There she stood, rubbing her eyes. One of the group noticed her. 'Is she rubbing her eyes?'

The others looked. 'Surely not! Mavila's home is spotless. It can't be trachoma.' Joyce turned out the child's upper eyelid. There it was: all red with lots of little bumps: trachoma.

'Impossible,' everyone shouted. 'Then everything you told us is not true. We've worked hard for nothing.'

Joyce had to explain once again the mode of transmission. While there was still trachoma in Hanyane no one was safe. After lengthy arguments they agreed that it was not enough just to look after themselves. They could not lock the children inside their houses to prevent them playing with their friends. If the neighbour's children had trachoma they infected their own children. They had been selfish in their club. Now they were punished for it.

QUESTIONS

1. What are your experiences with women's organisations in the area where you work?
   a) How do they differ from the Tidy Ladies?
   b) What do they have in common?
2. How could Mavila's child have contracted trachoma?
   How great is the risk of going blind from trachoma for this particular child?
3. What other communicable diseases could spread to the Tidy Ladies of Hanyane?

DISCUSSION

The Tidy Ladies had wanted to keep themselves separate. 'Others' should not disturb them. They thought that would guarantee their good health. The discovery of the child's trachoma has shattered their illusions.

The problems of the Tidy Ladies are that:
1 They have become alienated from their community.
2 They have forgotten the aims of their club.

1 Alienation

The Tidy Ladies have become strangers in their own community. They have lost touch with the reality of living in Hanyane and no longer feel part of their community and its problems.

Although there are now some beautifully clean individual houses, overall living conditions have not changed in Hanyane. There is a lack of jobs, and men seek work elsewhere. People still cannot produce enough food. There is still no good water supply. Cattle, who attract flies, are still kept near the houses. Most children still have unwashed faces and trachoma continues to be transmitted. As long as all this continues, no child is safe from being infected with trachoma.

A small exclusive club which makes things better for members only does not help. Until a majority of the community join together to tackle communal problems, nothing will really change.

2 The purpose of the club

When someone gets excited about something, he or she will find other people who share the same interest. They may then form a club or association to pursue that interest. After a while, the initial excitement wanes and the original purpose of the group is forgotten. The group may then dissolve quietly or just plod along without any purpose other than to enjoy each other's company at more or less regular intervals. This is what happened with the Tidy Ladies. They lost sight of their original plans to fight trachoma in Hanyane and became a tea party club.

One way to avoid this pitfall is to clearly formulate the group's aims and objectives at the beginning and write it down. Such notes serve as a reminder later on, at times when there is a danger of the group going astray. A good plan helps us to proceed towards an objective and it can be used to monitor progress.

SUMMARY

1 Community organisations may become exclusive and isolate themselves from the rest of their community, serving only their own interests.
2 Such groups do not help to improve the health and quality of life in the community at large. They remain, therefore, vulnerable to the common communicable diseases and other community problems.
3 When initiating a community group, the members should clearly define their aims and plan for appropriate action.

16

Becoming a Health Carer
– Being alone is difficult

The experience with Mavila's little girl taught the Tidy Ladies that they would never be free of trachoma while others in Hanyane still had the infection. Lerisa suggested that, instead of keeping their newly acquired knowledge for themselves, they should teach the others. Joyce encouraged this idea. She suggested that each of the ladies should choose about ten homes in their neighbourhood and advise people on better hygiene.

Over the next few weeks the club members tried to follow Joyce's advice. It was far from a success. Whenever one of the ladies knocked at a door she was not welcome at all. People said they were busy and had no time, or they accused them of meddling in their private affairs. Not being a relative, the visitor had no business to interfere.

At the next meeting, they shared their experiences. They all had the same story to tell. The refusals also made them feel more and more uncomfortable when doing visits. One lady confessed that she was now so scared that she didn't want to go on her own any more. Maybe going as a group of two or three would help her.

The rest of the group agreed. They would all feel happier and more confident if they went in groups. It might also help them to be accepted – it would not be so easy to close the door on a group.

From then on the Tidy Ladies went visiting in groups. They were singing and dancing on their way to make their presence known. People came out of their houses to see what was going on. But there were still many problems. For one, people wanted medicine, not words. For another, some resented being told what to do by neighbours instead of by nurses.

QUESTIONS

1 Is it acceptable in the area where you work to visit and advise neighbours who are not relatives?
2 What type of person would be most acceptable for home visits: man, woman, married, unmarried, elderly, young, etc.?
3 Do you think the Health Carers at Hanyane should be given medicines to treat minor troubles?
How are village health workers equipped in your area?

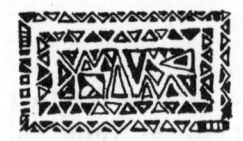

DISCUSSION

We have arrived at an important turning point in our story: the Tidy Ladies have made their first steps in a new direction, back to their own community. Sometimes a traumatic experience is needed to open our eyes. The trauma for the Tidy Ladies has been the discovery of trachoma in Mavila's child's eyes. This has made them think again. Instead of crocheting, they now go out to the people and share their knowledge. But it is not as easy as they imagined it would be.

1 The problem of visiting homes

Joyce learned in her training that health education is best done by visiting the people in their homes. Now she feels that she is extremely lucky to have as many as eleven health educators to do this job. It should be easy for the group to cover the whole settlement of Hanyane if each one cared for a sufficient number of families.

This has been Joyce's theory – the theory of an outsider. The reality has been different – the Tidy Ladies were not accepted. People were suspicious. They knew these ladies – they had grown up together. They were no better than the rest of the village. How dare they enter their homes and talk about cleanliness. Advice on domestic matters is only acceptable from one's own relatives, not from neighbours. In addition, the Tidy Ladies felt very insecure. Their training had been short, and they were afraid that they would not have the right answers to questions.

Traditionally the main task of a community health worker is to do home visits. His or her efficiency is usually assessed by the number of home visits done in a given period of time. But are home visits always a good thing? Before introducing home visiting

as the main ingredient of a primary health care programme, we should ask ourselves:
a) How do people feel when they are visited by a health worker?
b) How do you feel when you get an unexpected visitor?
c) How does the health worker feel when entering a home?

People's reaction to a visit (a) and b) above)

Health workers are often regarded as unwelcome intruders into private affairs. When Joyce visited Ma-Anna's home for the first time, all the family were apprehensive. They felt uneasy because their home was untidy and they had no time to prepare themselves to receive a visitor. Advice on health which interfered with their old traditions was also not very welcome.

This sort of reaction is quite common. But because most people are polite, they receive their visitors with the customary friendliness. In particular, they do not want to offend someone whose help they may require at some other time. Thus health workers are led to believe that they are always welcome and that people are keen to hear the 'gospel' of disease prevention.

The health worker's apprehension (c) above)

A health worker, too, feels uneasy when entering a home. S/he does not know what situation s/he is going to meet and whether s/he will be able to approach it correctly. S/he feels threatened when confronted with problems for which s/he has no answer. His or her reputation as health worker is at stake. The Tidy Ladies feel insecure, and even Joyce felt uncomfortable at Ma-Anna's home. The health worker feels most secure in his or her office. There s/he is on familiar ground and patients come to him or her because they trust him or her to provide the help they need.

Being aware of the uncomfortable feelings of both parties involved in a health visit does not mean that home visits should be abolished. It should encourage us to be more sensitive in our approach.

2 Improved methods of sharing knowledge

The group of Tidy Ladies found their own solution to their problem: to go visiting in small groups. This had several advantages:
a) The Health Carers could support each other, giving courage to the shy. They also helped each other to get the message across. What one of them had forgotten, another remembered. Holding hands made them feel secure.
b) People found it easier to accept them in a group. It was no longer a case of an individual poking his/her nose into another's private affairs.

c) As a group, they were able to use different, more attractive, methods of education like singing, dancing and play acting. This was fun and attracted people's attention.

3 Flexibility

Joyce suggested a method which did not work but both she and the group were flexible enough to change the method and attempt new, hitherto untried, ways.

This is important when working with communities. It can be dangerous to stick stubbornly to old, traditional methods simply because they have always been used. It is to Joyce's credit that she has not been offended by the failure of her own method and that she has been able to accept the initiatives of others.

SUMMARY

1 Both the visitor(s) and the visited feel uncomfortable during home visits. Consideration and imagination needs to be used to benefit from this potentially useful teaching situation.
2 In certain circumstances, visiting in groups may be easier and more acceptable than visiting as individuals.
3 Working in and with communities requires much flexibility on the part of the health worker.

17

You must! – Health Carers: police or friends?

The women were now confident when visiting as a group. Three members of the health club – Ruth, Mavila and Sarah – visited Ma-Anna's home to deliver their talk on hygiene. Ma-Anna and Kokwana told them, in no uncertain terms, that they were not welcome. Their problem was blindness from measles, not trachoma. In any case, if they had any worries, they would go to the clinic. They trusted the nurse.

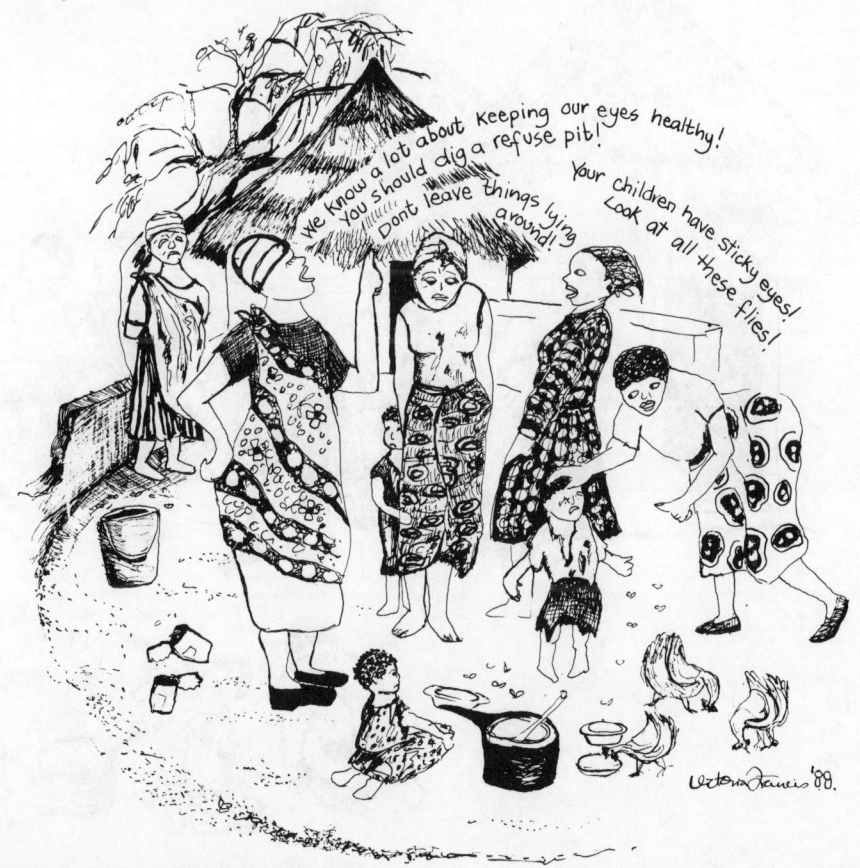

Three Tidy Ladies with Ma-Anna

The three ladies were undeterred. They insisted that they knew a lot about eyes and that they came on orders from Joyce. Although they were not invited, they started to look around the house and yard. They then heaped their admonitions on the two startled women:

'Your children have sticky eyes. They must have trachoma. Look at all the flies! You must keep your children clean – they're awful.'

'You must also keep your house clean. Don't leave things lying around like this – it attracts flies. Sweep the yard every day.'

'You mustn't leave the pots unwashed after meals. Flies sit on the food and then your children eat it.'

'You must dig a refuse pit.'

'You mustn't use your cloth for wiping everyone's faces without washing it.'

'You must wash the children's faces every day and their hands many times a day.'

'We don't see a toilet. You must build one.'

'Do what we tell you. We'll come and see you again in three weeks time. By then you should have a refuse pit, or we will tell the chief.'

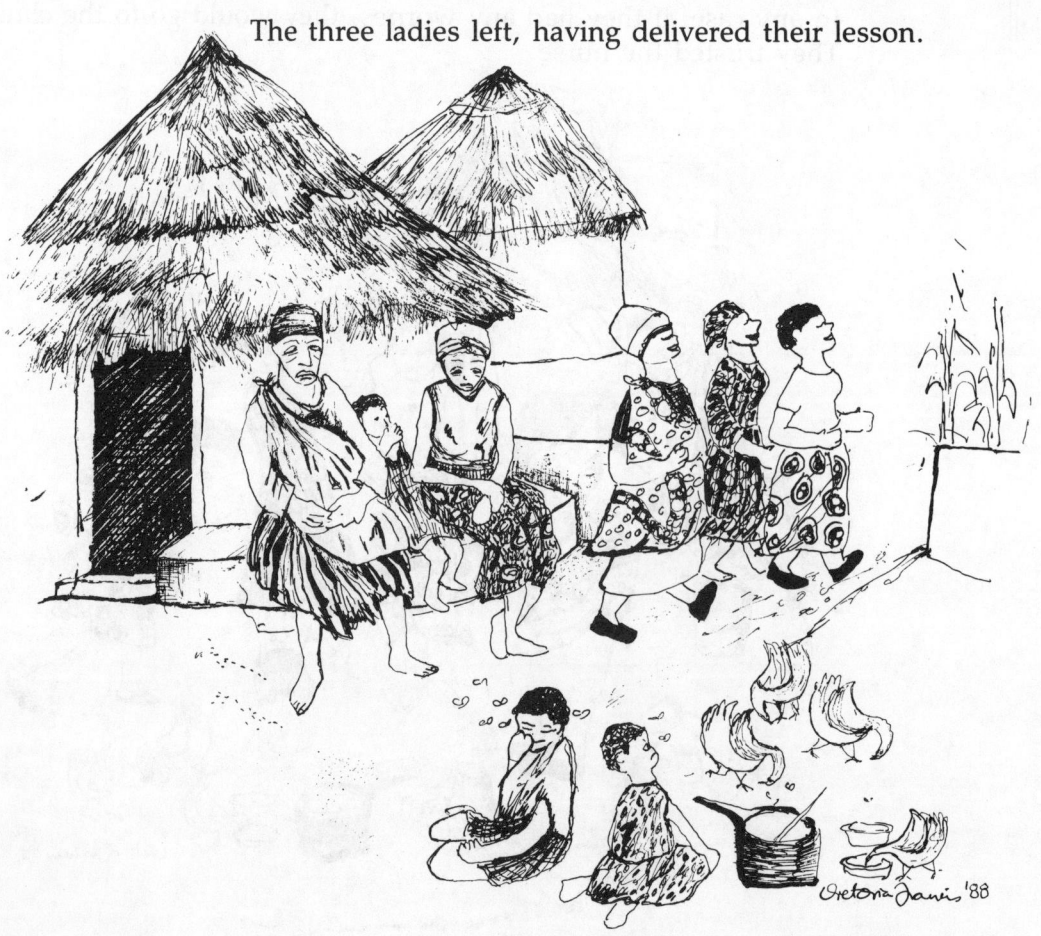

The three ladies left, having delivered their lesson.

'You must, you must, you must. Who do you think you are – the police?'

Kokwana and Ma-Anna were glad to see them go. They were angry. These ladies treated them like children, playing nurse and policeman at the same time. They objected to being ordered around like that. How could they dig a refuse pit in this hard and stony soil? They didn't have any suitable tools or sufficient strength to do it. A toilet was out of the question. There was no money to pay a builder. And all that talk about cleanliness. One got tired of hearing the same thing over and over. Their home was a long way from the river. They could not carry more water than they did already.

They wondered why Lerisa wasn't with these ladies. They were sure that, with her, the others would have behaved differently. Kokwana suspected that Ma-Anna had angered her friend. The old lady was very fond of Lerisa. She told Ma-Anna to go and see her about this incident.

QUESTIONS

1 What were the feelings of Ma-Anna and Kokwana at the beginning and at the end of the visit by the Health Carers?
2 Make a list of the mistakes made by the Health Carers. How would you have approached Ma-Anna?
3 Make a list of the correct messages they tried to put across.

DISCUSSION

The three ladies really 'had a go' at poor Ma-Anna. True, they overdid it. Health workers are seldom as insensitive as this. But we all make similar mistakes and have to learn the art of sharing knowledge.

1 **'Teaching' the 'ignorant'**

Teaching is often seen as a one-way process:
a) The teacher possesses knowledge.
b) The teacher decides what part of his/her knowledge to impart.
c) The teacher lectures.
d) The student accepts and memorises the lecture without any question.
This approach is that of an adult to a child.

Many health workers believe that ignorance makes the poor sick more often than the rich. If people had sufficient knowledge, they could avoid falling ill. The story of Hanyane shows that the poor are the victims of a social order which maintains their poverty and disease.

2 Education to change habits and attitudes

Some ignorant health educators believe that what people do and think is wrong and has to be changed and that a change in behaviour will automatically lead to good health. Do you remember the Tidy Ladies? Their change in behaviour did not prevent trachoma in their own children, because the social and economic situation in Hanyane has not changed.

Many of us health workers believe that it is our job to *change the poor*. For example, we have learned that trachoma is associated with dirt. Therefore, we assume that, if we change hygiene habits, we have solved the problem. We know that xerophthalmia results from a lack of vitamin A in the diet. Therefore, we assume that we only need to change eating habits to prevent xerophthalmia.

This is unrealistic. When water has to be carried over long distances and when there is no land to plough, it is hardly possible to improve practice. A hostile environment often makes it impossible for people to respond to new ideas.

To achieve health for all, rich and poor, the 'have-nots' should educate the 'haves' to change *their* habits and attitudes.

3 Good health education

So far we have discussed inappropriate health education. As the story unfolds, you will learn more about alternative methods of improving health.

Good health education should help people become aware of the root causes of their poor health. It respects the good things people do and enhances their self-confidence. It is built upon the people's own experience and treats them as adults and equals. Thus it can help them to effect changes in their environment, making health more attainable.

If you want to know more about health education, read Werner, *Helping Health Workers Learn*.

SUMMARY

1. Health education does not automatically lead to better health.
2. It is not ignorance that makes poor people sick, but poverty and a hostile environment.
3. People are experienced adults and want to be treated as such.

Reference
Werner, D. and Bower, B., *Helping Health Workers Learn* (Hesperian Foundation, 1982)

18

Refuse pits prevent trachoma – Working together

Rumours reached the clinic that some of the Health Carers were bossy on their home visits. Joyce saw that she had to do something about this as soon as possible, before too much damage was done. Her Hanyane women had progressed so well. They were so enthusiastic that Joyce had to handle the situation carefully. The group had recovered from 'elitism'. They were no longer the Tidy Ladies but had become Health Carers. She mustn't allow 'authoritarianism' to take over now. The question was how to go about it. She vaguely remembered some of the methods she learned long ago at a workshop on community health. Now that the time had come to use it, she wished she had taken better notes. She had forgotten many of the details. The only thing she remembered was an exciting exercise called role play. In this exercise people take on different roles so that they can see how people react and how others feel in a difficult situation. Maybe Joyce could try that.

At the next group meeting Joyce organised a role playing exercise on home visits. Mavila was to play mother of a problem family. Two others were asked to visit her and instruct her about hygiene for the prevention of trachoma. The two shouted down at poor Mavila, just as she had done at Ma-Anna's home with Ruth and Sarah.

Mavila felt humiliated. She was almost in tears when she burst out, 'You can't do this to me. It's awful.'

After the play, the actors and spectators talked about the scene and how everybody felt. They recognised their own behaviour during health visits. They realised now how hurtful bossiness can be.

Through discussions and more role playing, the group arrived at new ways of giving health education. Instead of talking *down* to a person, as if to a child, they must talk *with* people as friends and

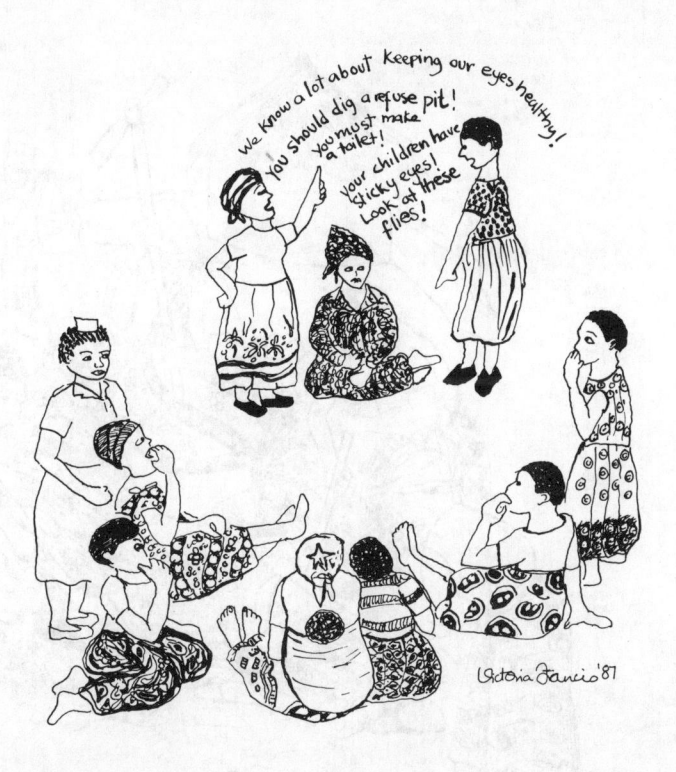

In the role play they experienced how it feels to be humiliated by those who have knowledge and status

equals. Afterall, in Hanyane they *were* friends and equals. The only difference was that they had had the chance to be taught about trachoma and hygiene. Before they met Joyce, their ways of living were neither better nor worse than those of the people they were now advising. So, why not share what they had learned informally, at the river for instance, or at the shop or through a friendly visit at a neighbour's home?

Back home, the Health Carers put their new ideas into practice. It was so much easier now. They invited people into their homes to see what a refuse pit looked like and how it was used. But most of the Hanyane people were still sceptical. First they wanted to see how the Health Carers had changed. Then, slowly, they began to accept the Carers. They invited them into their homes to get advice on hygiene, or to proudly show them their finished pits.

Lerisa saw that Ma-Anna and Kokwana could not manage to dig a pit on their own. The soil where Ma-Anna lived was especially hard and stony. She asked two friends to come with her and help dig a pit at Ma-Anna's home. Ma-Anna was surprised – she hadn't expected this. Happily she joined in as, to the rhythm of their song, they swung their picks and hoes.

Many followed this example and helped the old and frail to dig their refuse pits. The mothers taught their children how to use the

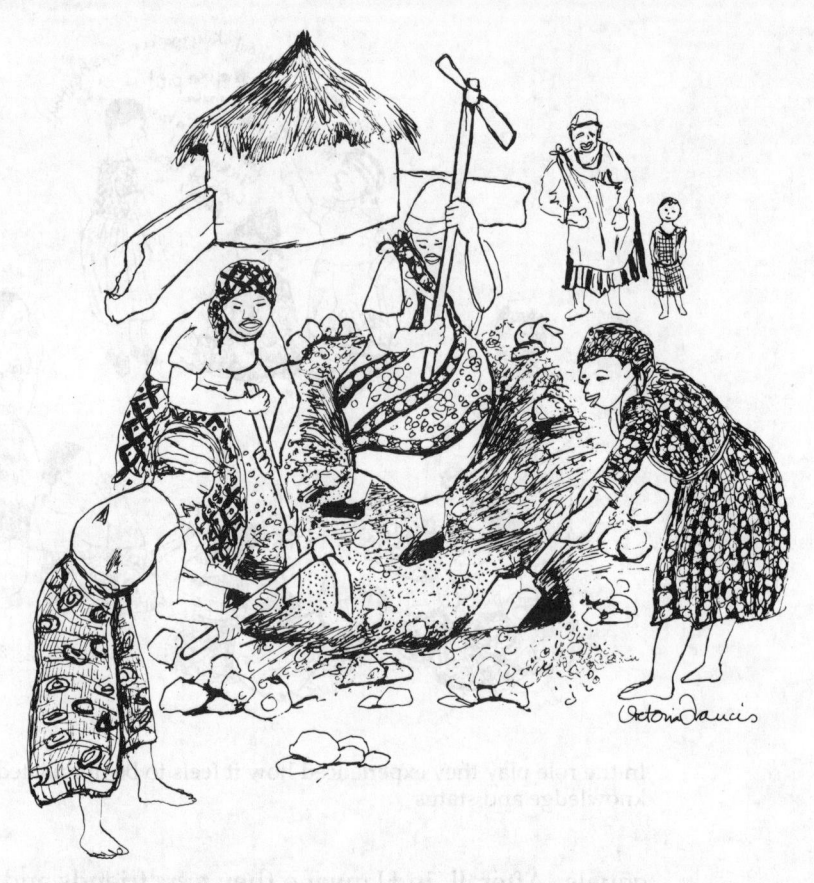

Lerisa and her friends helped Ma-Anna dig her refuse pit

pits and the teachers reinforced the message at school. Regularly the refuse had to be covered with soil or burned to prevent flies breeding there. As it was something new, the children took great delight in collecting rubbish and throwing it into the pit. In due course, the pits became full. One old man had a good idea: he planted a pawpaw tree in it. Two years later this tree was bearing bigger and juicier fruit than all the other pawpaw trees in Hanyane.

QUESTIONS

1 What is the point of good refuse disposal?
   What methods do you know?
2 How do refuse pits or other good methods of refuse disposal prevent trachoma?
3 Have you ever used role playing or popular theatre? What is their advantage?

DISCUSSION

1 The value of role playing

Seeing the other side

The three ladies who visited Ma-Anna belong to the better off in the Hanyane community. They did not intend to hurt Ma-Anna. They have learnt that good hygiene prevents trachoma and are keen to deliver their lesson. Their problem is that they have never experienced extreme poverty in life as Ma-Anna has. They do not know about the struggles she faces in caring for her family. Ignorance of the other person's situation can give rise to much unnecessary hurt. Role playing can help us to understand another person's situation. When you act out the role of another person you feel like that person and see how you appear in their eyes. The role play worked very well with the Health Carers. It made them think about their own attitudes and helped them to find better ways of working with their community.

Approaching sensitive community issues

Role playing and popular theatre can be a way to solve problems in a community. There are situations where open discussion would be offensive and could polarise the various parties involved. For example, Joyce could not tell the chief of Hanyane to his face that it was unfair to fine people for not having a toilet when he had not built one for himself. However, if a group can present an amusing play about a similar situation, everyone will feel free to discuss it without fear of causing offence.

2 Working together

The Tidy Ladies have now become Health Carers. Whilst they were the Tidy Ladies they cared only about themselves and kept others out. Since becoming Health Carers they have begun working with the people, helping each other.

There are several reasons why health workers may find it difficult to work together with their communities as equals. First, they have knowledge others lack. Second, some demand respect and teach down to the people, usually sitting on a chair overlooking the listeners who sit on the ground. Third, others who want to work with the people may be thwarted in their efforts by the people themselves. Health workers are considered special and the people want to keep it that way.

Customs vary with countries and regions. As a health worker, you must be sensitive to local customs and find the correct way to work with your communities.

Joyce usually sits at the same level as the people with whom she is talking. In her area, this is the acceptable way to show that you feel at one with the people.

Look at all the pictures in this book where Joyce is with the Hanyane people. Where does she sit or stand, and why?

There are many games which are helpful for group work. You will find lots of ideas in: Hope and Timmel, *Training for Transformation* and Johnston and Rifkin, *Health Care Together*.

SUMMARY

1 Role play helps us to understand the feelings of another person. It is also a useful tool for approaching and solving sensitive issues.
2 Working with the people, instead of talking down to them, wins their hearts and their respect.

References
Hope, A. and Timmel, S., *Training for Transformation* (Mambo Press, 1984)
Johnston, M.P. and Rifkin, S.B., *Health Care Together* (Macmillan Publishers, 1987)

19

Treating trachoma – Medicine wins more community acceptance

As time went on, the Health Carers became more popular. Several women from the community asked to join them. This time everyone was welcome, even the very poor. Thus all levels of Hanyane society were now represented in the group.

As the chief's wife was also a member, they had all the support they needed from the chief. This made things easier. (They discovered the disadvantage later. What do you think it was?)

One problem was still not solved. The community continued to ask for eye ointment. At one of their meetings at the clinic, the Health Carers complained again about it. It was time that Joyce did something about the medicine issue. She should examine the children and say which ones must get ointment. They knew a limited amount of eye ointment had arrived.

Joyce pointed to the crowd of patients waiting outside. 'You see how busy I am. We are going to have to stop our meeting now, so that I can attend to them.'

The Carers looked on as Joyce flipped the children's upper eyelids over to examine them for trachoma. She took the opportunity to show the group once more what trachoma looked like. Ruth thought that this looked easy enough. Couldn't the Health Carers try to turn the eyelids themselves?

Joyce was a little reluctant. Should she allow them to touch and turn the eyelids? But the ladies insisted until finally Joyce gave in. They washed their hands thoroughly before and after examining each person's eyes with soap and water. Then she showed them how it is done and allowed them to try on each other. She couldn't believe it: within half an hour they all managed so well that she allowed the better ones to try with a patient. They were all very excited. Now they were like nurses. Joyce made them promise to practice on each other and not to examine any one in the village before she was convinced that their practice was safe. Then she would show them how to apply ointment.

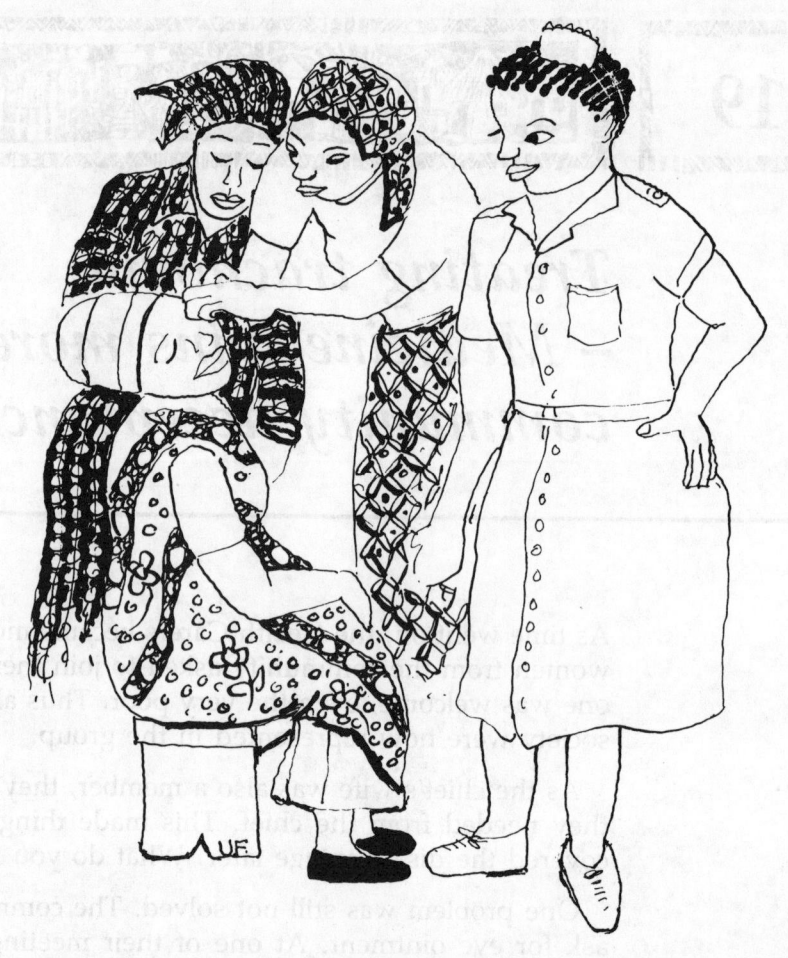

After some weeks, Joyce decided they were competent enough to examine their neighbours. She went with them on the first occasion and gave her blessing for them to examine the village people on their own.

Joyce provided the Carers with notebooks so that they could keep records on the people they examined. They had to write down who had trachoma and make notes on the presence or absence of refuse pits and toilets. Most of those who could not write had children at school who could help them.

At first, the Hanyane people were surprised and also suspicious. After all, the Carers were not nurses. How could they examine for trachoma and give out ointment? However, suspicion slowly gave way to respect. They could see for themselves that the children got better with the eye ointment. From now on people called the Health Carers the 'mothers of trachoma'.

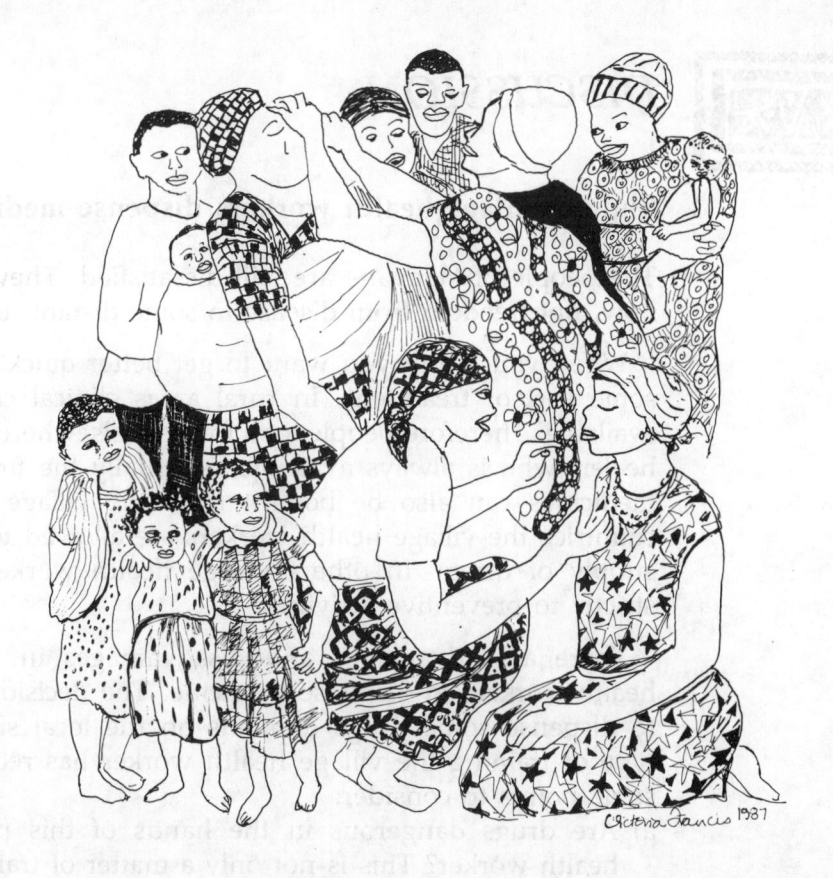

The people of Hanyane began to respect the Health Carers and called them 'mothers of trachoma'

QUESTIONS

1. Do you think it is safe to let the Carers examine people's eyes?
2. Should health carers /village health workers only do preventive work? Give reasons for your answer.
3. Should people have access to tetracycline eye ointment without having to see trained medical personnel (e.g. to buy it in the shop or be given it by health carers)?
   What is the practice where you work?
   What do you think about it?

DISCUSSION

1 Should village health workers dispense medicines?

The people of Hanyane are still dissatisfied. They want medicine now, not freedom from disease in some distant, uncertain future.

When you are ill you want to get better quickly. This requires some sort of treatment. In rural areas clinical care is often not available. Therefore people look for help elsewhere. The traditional healer, who is always available, is usually the first choice. Some medicines can also be bought from the village shop. In some countries the village health workers are allowed to have a limited supply of drugs. In others village health workers are confined strictly to preventive activities.

There are advantages and disadvantages in allowing village health workers to dispense medicine. The decision to allow them to dispense some drugs depends on the local situation and the type of training the village health worker has received. Here are some points to consider:

a) Are drugs dangerous in the hands of this particular village health worker? This is not only a matter of training but also of the intelligence and reliability of the village health worker.
b) What happens in an emergency, e.g. broncho-pneumonia in a child where one penicillin injection would be life saving? What is more dangerous: penicillin and injection needles in the hands of a community health worker (risk of AIDS, wrong use, etc.), or not being able to save the lives of children?
c) When people are sick they want medicine. If the village health worker is not allowed to give drugs, people may buy them at the shop and use them dangerously.

2 Balance between prevention and cure

The Carers first had to prove that they had acquired enough skills to treat trachoma. Once the effects of treatment were evident, the people trusted and respected them.

People were more satisfied once eye ointment was available for them. It also helped them to accept advice about preventive measures.

For the Carers, being able to examine and treat people increased their self-confidence. They felt important and more useful.

Disease prevention and health promotion alone lack credibility. Their benefits are not immediately visible. The better future they promise is too distant to be appreciated. It is therefore important to combine prevention with cure.

It is essential both to attend to the immediate needs of the sick and to prepare for better health in the future.

In certain instances, such as in the control of endemic trachoma, simultaneous preventive and curative action is necessary to achieve a speedy result. As long as there are a great number of children spreading *Chlamydia* in the community, the effects of improved hygiene will be delayed. Older people will continue to become reinfected over a prolonged period of time. This makes it difficult for the people to understand why they should wash their faces. They will soon be disillusioned. If you look again at the diagram on page 88, you will understand how important it is both to treat the young children with tetracycline eye ointment *and* improve hygiene.

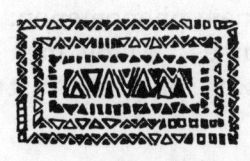

SUMMARY

1 The decision to allow village health workers to dispense medicines depends on local circumstances and the reliability of the individual worker. Advantages and disadvantages should be weighed carefully.
2 Disease prevention and health promotion not accompanied by curative care lacks credibility. People who are sick want to be helped now. Health in the distant future is meaningless to many people.

20

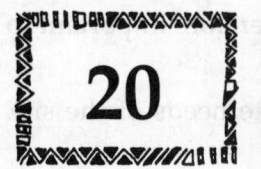

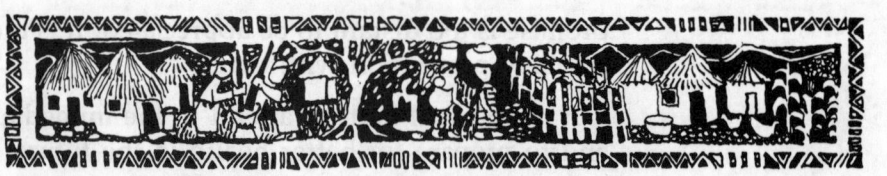

Counting the beans
– Self evaluation

Six months had passed. The Tidy Ladies had become known as the Health Carers. The fight against trachoma was under way and people in Hanyane were talking about this new phenomenon: 'Women so organised? Housewives turned nurses?' Many men were still sceptical about it and thought it was probably just another social activity.

The teacher was especially interested. 'Can all this teaching in the village really be effective?' he asked his wife, Leah, one day when she was sorting dry beans.

Leah showed him her record book. She had recorded the particulars of each of the ten families she cared for showing the name, age and sex of each person, and the dates on which she examined them. Those having trachoma were marked with a cross against their names, those without with a zero.

The records were impressive. In the first column, showing her first examination, there were many crosses. In the last column, six months later, most crosses had been replaced by a zero. These people no longer had trachoma.

'This really looks great,' he admitted. 'But, don't you think your results are good because you are my wife? People are more likely to listen to a teacher's wife.'

This argument angered Leah. 'You men always want to take the credit for what we women are doing.'

'I just want to make sure that you don't deceive yourself. Sometimes I think I have taught my pupils well. But, when I mark their tests, I discover that they have understood nothing.'

'How could we do such a test with our group?' Leah asked.

The teacher wanted to know whether all the Carers kept records, even those who could not write. They did. The illiterates were helped by their school-going children.

	Age	Sex	1.8.85	1.9.85	1.10.85	1.11.85	1.12.85	1.1.86	
♡ Mjaji	70	F	+	+	+	+	+	+	♡
Wilson	65	M	o	o	o	o	o	o	
Alinah	40	F	o	o	o	o	o	o	
♡ Moris	28	M	+	+	o	o	o	o	
Maria	12	F	o	o	o	o	o	o	
♡ Beauty	10	F	+	+	+	o	o	o	
♡ Moses	6	M	+	+	+	+	+	+	♡
♡ Nkhesani	4	F	+	o	o	o	o	o	
Njakanjaka	3	F	o	o	o	o	o	o	
Chipo	2	F	o	o	o	o	o	o	

A page from the Health Carers' record book

'Then it's easy,' the teacher said. 'You bring me all the records and I will make the calculations. We will compare the number of cases of trachoma before your group started work with the number of cases now. Then you will know what you have achieved.'

'Calculations? How are we supposed to understand complicated sums?'

The teacher looked at the beans Leah had been sorting and had an idea. He took her record book and put a bean in one dish for every case of trachoma she had seen on her first visit. In another dish he did the same for her last visit. It looked impressive. There were many beans in the first dish and only a few in the second.

At the next Carers' meeting Leah arrived with a big tin full of beans and two dishes. She showed the group what she had done with her records to see how much she had achieved with her ten families. Of course, all the other members were keen to see their own results. They all got busy with the beans. All of them found less trachoma cases at their last count. They took a goat skin. They piled all the beans of the first count into one heap, and those of the last count into a second heap. The first, showing the number of trachoma cases in Hanyane when the group began, was much bigger than the heap showing the remaining cases of trachoma in the village at the present time.

This was very exciting. They could see with their own eyes and feel with their hands the results of their labour. It had been worthwhile. All were very happy. They danced around the goat skin, singing and clapping their hands.

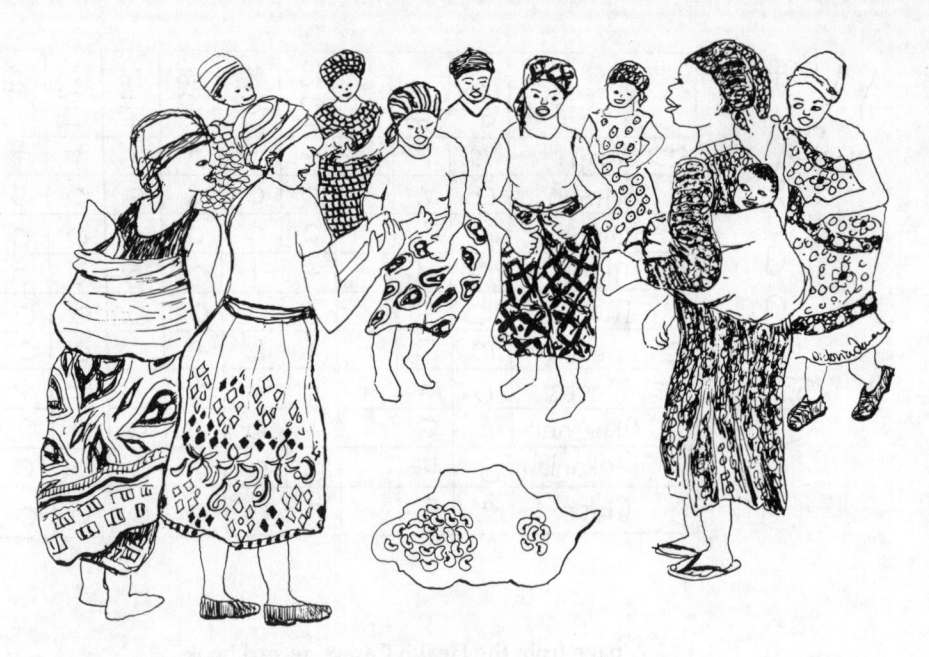

The Health Carers celebrate their success

Before going home, Lerisa looked for a long time at the heaps of beans. Why didn't they manage to completely wipe out trachoma? Ma-Anna's Rose still had the disease, she had seen it the previous day. Why?

QUESTIONS

1 What is evaluation and why is it important?
  Who should participate in evaluating community action?
2 How often should a project be evaluated?
3 Why is there still trachoma in Hanyane six months after the Carers started work?

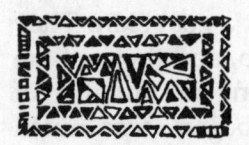

DISCUSSION

1 Why evaluate?

Over the last few months Joyce and the Carers have learned how to plan their action. They have implemented their plans. Joyce has done her survey. The Carers have taught their community about cleanliness and have treated the trachoma cases they encountered.

Now the time has come to see whether they have planned correctly and whether their activities have been successful. They are going to **evaluate** what they have done so far. Many things may have gone wrong. For example it could be that the Carers had given eye ointment to people who did not have trachoma, or that people did not understand their teaching about hygiene. It could also be that everything was done correctly but that, for some reason, it had no effect on the severity of trachoma.

If the Carers did not check for such mistakes, they would continue on the wrong track. Time and ointment would then have been wasted. Therefore evaluation is important.

2 What to do after evaluation

a) Evaluation may show that the *desired result has been achieved*. You will then decide either to stop the activity, or to continue as before to maintain the good result.
b) Evaluation may show that you are on the *right track*, but that there are *problems* that need to be remedied. You will then adapt your methods to overcome those problems.
c) Evaluation may show that *no progress* has been made. You then have to investigate why the applied method has failed. Having found the reasons, you will rethink your plan of action; for example if, after all your teaching, children's faces are still not being washed, you have to question why. If it is because of lack of water, you will first try to improve the water supply.

3 Self-evaluation

The Carers used an evaluation technique which is easy for everyone to understand. They could see with their own eyes that their efforts were bearing fruit. This is important. They have learned to monitor their own work. This new skill will make them more independent. From now on they would not forget to include regular evaluation exercises in their future programmes.

But the Carers must be careful not to unwittingly overrate their successes or underestimate their failures.

4 Evaluation from outside

Self evaluation with methods like those used by the Carers is not accurate enough for official use. Health services, organisers or donor organisations providing funds for special projects demand accurate figures on progress made.

Evaluators from outside are therefore requested to investigate a project. They make new sample surveys and questionnaires, which require a lot of time and effort. This is often very disruptive because the normal activities of a project come to a standstill while the survey is being conducted. Evaluation of this kind should therefore be scheduled carefully so that the work being surveyed can continue without too much interruption.

There is more to evaluation than what we have outlined here. If you wish to know more, read M.T. Feuerstein's, *Partners in Evaluation*. It is available from TALC.

Exercise

1 Evaluate your own project using Table 20.1 below.
2 Devise some methods for self-evaluation suitable for the people you work with.

Evaluation form				
Name of project or group	What were the objectives?	Did you reach the objectives?	Why or why not? (Reasons for success or failure)	What must be changed for the next time?

Table 20.1

SUMMARY

1 Projects should be evaluated at regular intervals to see whether the activities have been suitable to reach the set goal.
2 Depending on the outcome of evaluation, decisions on further action can be taken: either to find out the reasons for failure and change methods, or, if satisfied, to continue as before.
3 Self-evaluation may not be very accurate, but it promotes self reliance and gives satisfaction.
4 Evaluation from outside is usually more accurate but may be disruptive for the project.

Reference
Feuerstein, M.T., *Partners in Evaluation* (Macmillan, London, 1986)

21

Don't wait until you are blind – Cataract and glaucoma

The chief had some business at the neighbouring village, Kulani. He was relaxing at the cafe, sipping his beer when he overheard two old men at the next table talking about hospital and eyes. He listened to their conversation. He gathered that the name of the man with spectacles was Chauke. His friend's name was Baloyi. Their conversation went like this:

MR BALOYI Hello, my friend Chauke! It's a long time since I've seen you. I nearly didn't recognise you! You look so different with those funny thick spectacles. Your grandchild usually guides you to the cafe. Where have you left him?

MR CHAUKE I don't need him any longer. I had an eye operation at the hospital and now I can see again if I wear these glasses. I can see you clearly now, even the wrinkles in your face. Hey, I still can't believe that I can see again.

MR BALOYI Well, that's good news. Perhaps I also should go to the hospital. I don't see well at night. Even during the day it is becoming a bit difficult. Because I have no pain I never thought of going to the doctor.

MR CHAUKE Don't waste your time. As long as you can see, they do nothing. They only operate once you are almost blind. I went there almost a year ago because my eyes were getting weak. I had no pain either. The doctor told me: 'You have 'papa' (cataract) which will make you slowly blind. We can remove it once it is ripe. Come back when you can just see your hand in front of you. Then we will operate.'

MR BALOYI I'm glad you told me. I would have wasted time and money by going to the hospital. In this case I will just wait until I'm almost blind.

A few months later the chief met the two men again at the same cafe. Mr Baloyi was now completely blind and was led to the table by his little grandson. It appeared that Mr Baloyi was very angry with Mr Chauke.

MR CHAUKE I thought you went to hospital yesterday for the operation?

MR BALOYI I did. You gave me the wrong advice, you liar! You wished me to lose my eyesight!

MR CHAUKE No, no, Baloyi! Believe me, I meant it well. I told you exactly what the doctor told me. What happened?

MR BALOYI They told me it was too late. I should have come while I could still see well.

MR CHAUKE I can't understand. They sent me back home and operated only once I was blind.

MR BALOYI The doctor said I haven't got the same as you had. He said my disease is called glaucoma. It has to be treated early. My eyes are dead now and it's your fault.

MR CHAUKE I don't understand. We both felt the same: no pain, only slowly going blind. I really wanted to help you with my advice.

MR BALOYI You're a liar. You'll be cursed with blindness – I'll make sure of that!

At this stage the chief felt he had to intervene. He tried to calm the men down. There was surely a misunderstanding somewhere. He told them about the Carers in Hanyane who knew much about eyes. Maybe they could explain.

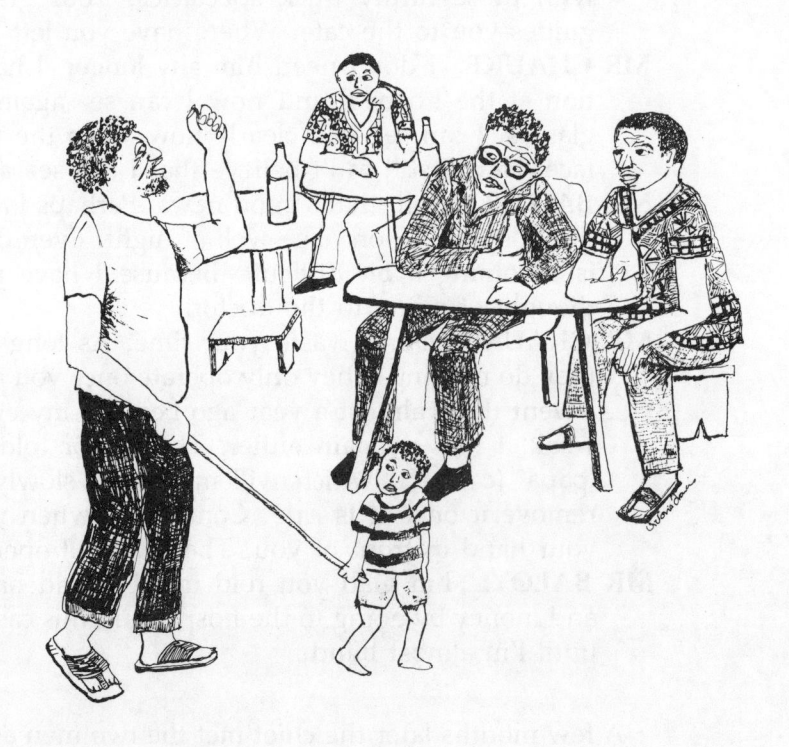

'My eyes are dead now and it is your fault'

Back home the chief asked his wife. She did not know and nobody in the group knew what to make of the story. They asked Joyce at their next group meeting.

'It is difficult for a person not specially trained in eye care to tell the difference between the two diseases, cataract and glaucoma. Both occur in the elderly and both are painless. But cataract can be cured with an operation while glaucoma must be treated long before the patient realises that there is something wrong.'

The Carers wanted to know what they could do about it. 'Everybody should learn to read and write,' Joyce said, 'and go on reading books and newspapers later in life.' The Carers laughed. This was another of Joyce's crazy ideas. How could reading prevent eye trouble? They thought the opposite was true.

Joyce explained about reading glasses and glaucoma. In the space provided, write down what you think Joyce told them.

....
....
....
....

Even if a literacy training programme for adults were started immediately, it would still take years before the old people were reading a lot. Something else had to be done in the meantime. The group could encourage the elderly of the village to have their eyes tested by the nurse. They could tell them the story of the two old friends at Kulani to persuade them.

'What about turning the story into a theatre play?' Lerisa suggested. 'People love theatre. They will talk about it afterwards and the message will spread.'

'We could organise a feast for the old folk,' Ruth added. 'We will bake some cakes.'

On the day of the party a large crowd had gathered. Nobody wanted to miss it. Joyce was there as well. She had to answer many questions, and reassured those who were afraid of an eye test or an operation.

A day at the clinic for the elderly was then arranged. The shopkeeper offered to provide transport for those who couldn't walk the distance. A great number of elderly people gathered at the shop. Even Kokwana was there. There were so many that the shopkeeper had to make two journeys with his van to ferry them all to the clinic.

Many elderly people now went for eye tests

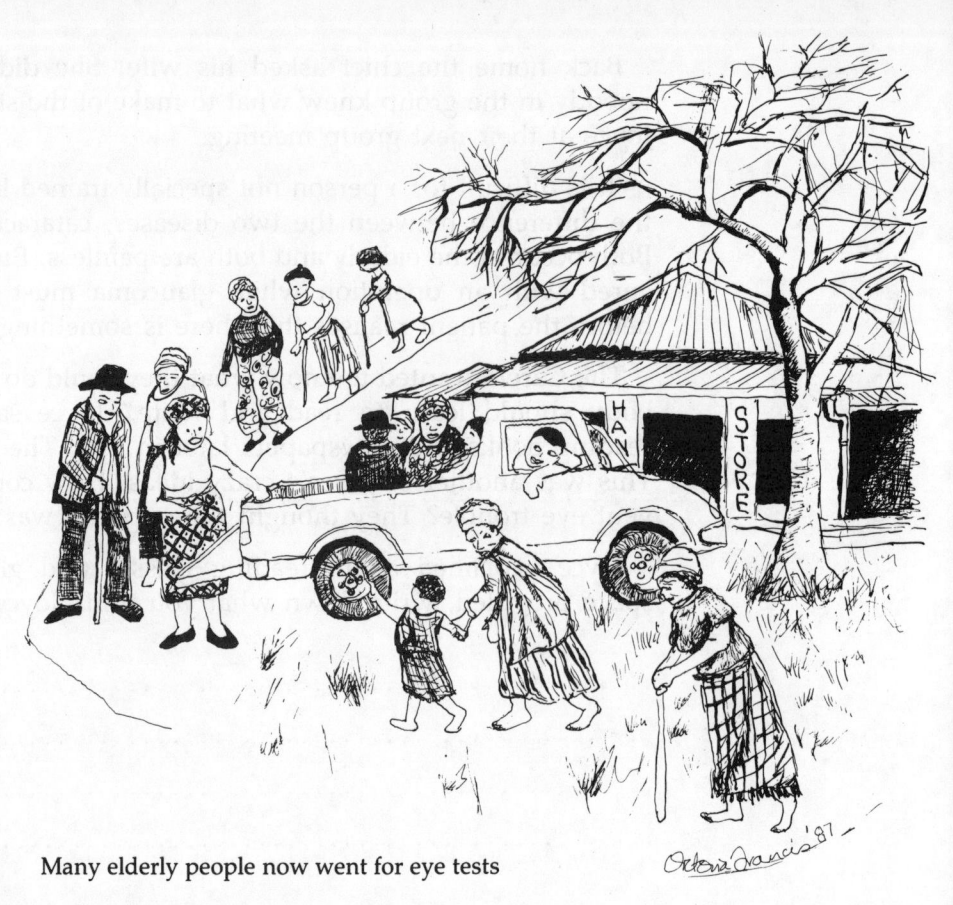

QUESTIONS

1. What is your experience with glaucoma patients in your area? At what stage of the disease do they present for the first time at the clinic or hospital. Why?
2. What could you do to motivate people to come for regular eye checks?
3. What has poverty and illiteracy to do with blindness from cataract and glaucoma?
4. What eye diseases cause blindness in the elderly? Can all of them be prevented?
   Which ones are most common your area?

DISCUSSION

Old people play an important role in their families. Usually grandmothers look after the little ones while the mothers work. In this way, the elderly contribute indirectly to the family income. Blindness in the elderly is not only a matter of discomfort. It might force a mother to stop work and remain with her children. This can mean hunger for the family. It is therefore important for health workers to help the old preserve their eyesight.

In the story, one of the two friends had his eyesight recovered while the other one lost it. This was because of his friend's unfortunate advice, which confused glaucoma with cataract.

Sadly, in rural areas, many **glaucoma** patients come too late for treatment, even in places where eye care facilities are available. There are three main reasons for this:
1 By the time a patient notices decreasing vision, irreparable damage has already been done to the eye. (Read the section on glaucoma and cataract in Part 3, Sections C and D.)
2 The usual age when glaucoma starts is between 40 and 60 years old. This is also the age when most people require glasses for near vision. A good doctor or nurse prescribing reading glasses always measures, at the time, the intra-ocular tension to detect early glaucoma. In populations where the majority of adults are illiterate or are not used to reading books or newspapers, people have no reason to ask for glasses. They therefore miss a good opportunity for early diagnosis. Now you will understand why Joyce suggested adult education classes at Hanyane.
Therefore:
Good education can lead to early diagnosis of glaucoma.
3 Patients with early **cataract** are told that they should wait until they cannot see enough to walk before coming for surgery. Thus news spreads that doctors do not want to treat elderly patients unless they are blind. This misunderstanding arises because, for ordinary people, cataract and simple open-angle glaucoma are almost the same:
- Both are eye diseases
- Both are common in people over 50 years of age and older
- Both are painless
- Both cause blindness which arises only slowly.

Neither cataract nor glaucoma are preventable. What, then, have these diseases got to do with poverty?

Surgery, the treatment for cataract, is almost always successful; and early treatment for glaucoma can arrest the disease. Yet millions of people in the world are blind from cataract and glaucoma. Some of the reasons are:
1 Poor countries cannot afford to provide enough facilities for cataract surgery.
2 Existing facilities are mostly in the big centres, out of reach to the people who cannot afford travel expenses and hospital fees.

3 We said that illiteracy may be responsible for late diagnosis of glaucoma. In poor countries the standard of education is often low and many people cannot afford to send their children to school.
Therefore:
Blindness from glaucoma and cataract is much more common in poor countries than in affluent countries.

Exercise

Fill in Table 21.1 below. This will help you to teach village health workers the differences between cataract and glaucoma.

	Cataract	Glaucoma
1 What is the damage to the eye?		
2 How do you recognise the disease?		
3 How is it treated?		
4 What will happen to the vision after treatment?		

Table 21.1

SUMMARY

1 For ordinary people, cataract and glaucoma are the same.
2 Adults who are literate and use reading glasses have a greater chance of early diagnosis of glaucoma.
3 Cataract and glaucoma are not preventable, but they can be cured and managed, provided people have sufficient and easy access to ophthalmic surgery. In poor countries, eye services are usually inadequate.

PART 1   SECTION C
Village development leads to health

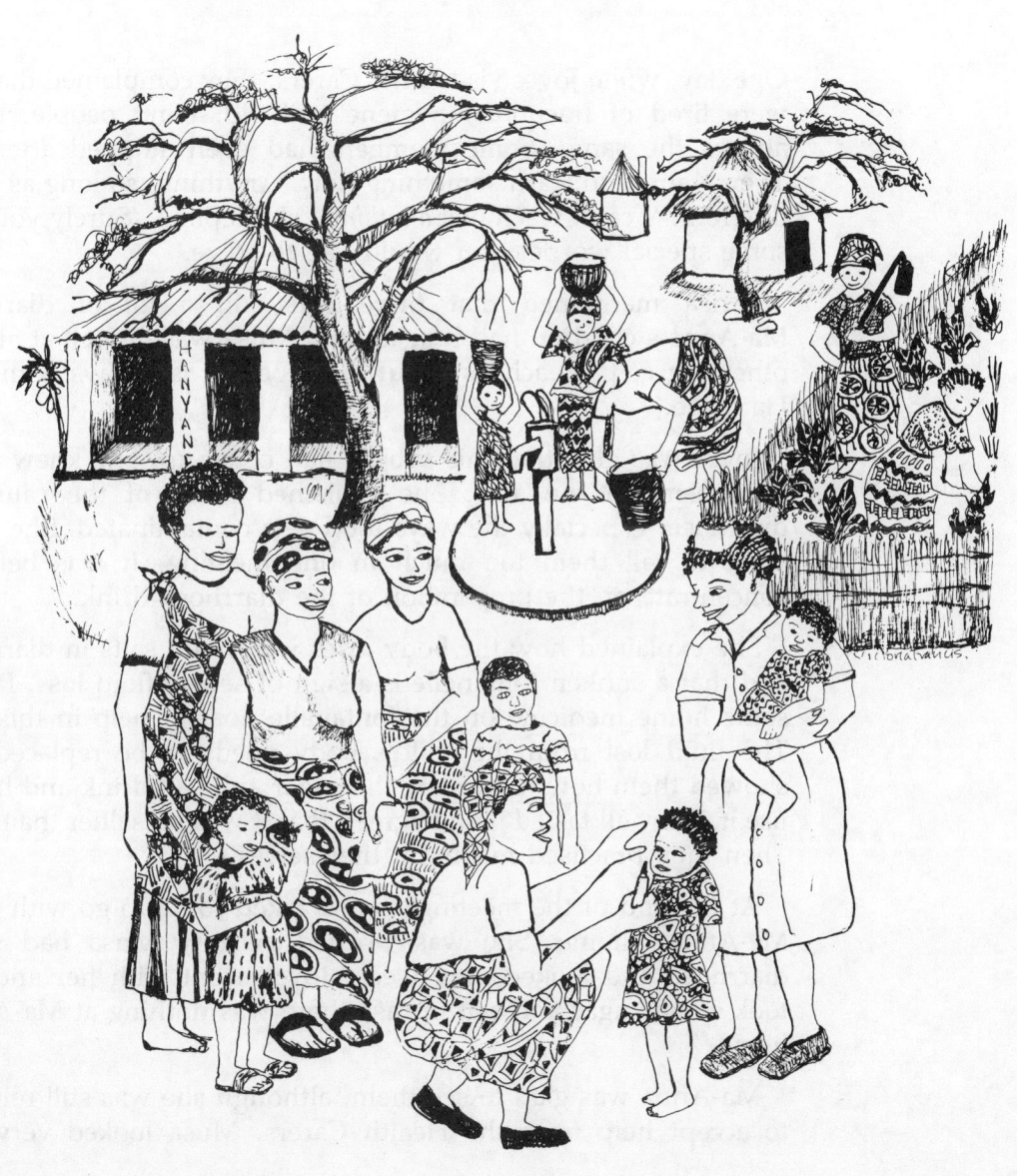

Musa is dying of diarrhoea – Ma-Anna becomes a Health Carer

One day, when Joyce visited her Carers, they complained that they were tired of trachoma, hygiene and old, blind people. It was always the same. Some members had even stopped attending. They wanted to learn something new. Anything, so long as it was different. 'I can't teach just *anything*,' she replied. 'Surely you have some special worries you would like to solve.'

Lerisa mentioned that there was still a lot of diarrhoea. Ma-Anna's children had it again and Musa wasn't well at all. The others agreed. 'Teach us about diarrhoea. It is always with us in Hanyane.'

Joyce was glad that this subject had come up. She knew it was a problem in the area. She explained some of the causes of diarrhoea, especially the ways food gets contaminated. She didn't want to tell them too much in one meeting. It was better to concentrate on the preparation of the diarrhoea drink.

She explained how the body loses water and salts in diarrhoea, and that a sunken fontanelle is a sign of severe fluid loss. Putting some home medicine on the fontanelle doesn't help in this case. The fluid lost from the child's body needs to be replaced. She showed them how to prepare the sugar and salt drink and how to use it. They all tasted it and agreed that it was no saltier than tears. Then they practised making it themselves.

At the end of the meeting, Lerisa asked Joyce to go with her to Ma-Anna's home. She was worried because Musa had severe diarrhoea and looked very weak. Joyce went with her and they took some sugar and salt in case there was nothing at Ma-Anna's home.

Ma-Anna was glad to see them, although she was still reluctant to accept help from the Health Carers. Musa looked very sick.

Joyce lifted a fold of skin on his tummy. The fold remained standing for a while and then slowly receded. Joyce explained that this was a sign that Musa's body had lost a lot of fluid.

'Let me try myself,' said Lerisa. She then compared it with her own skin: the difference was clear. Her skin snapped back immediately when she let go. Lerisa was happy to have learned something important.

Lerisa then told Ma-Anna what she had learned about diarrhoea and taught her how to make the diarrhoea drink. She explained carefully how to use it – for every stool a cupful. Musa sipped the drink, spoonful by spoonful.

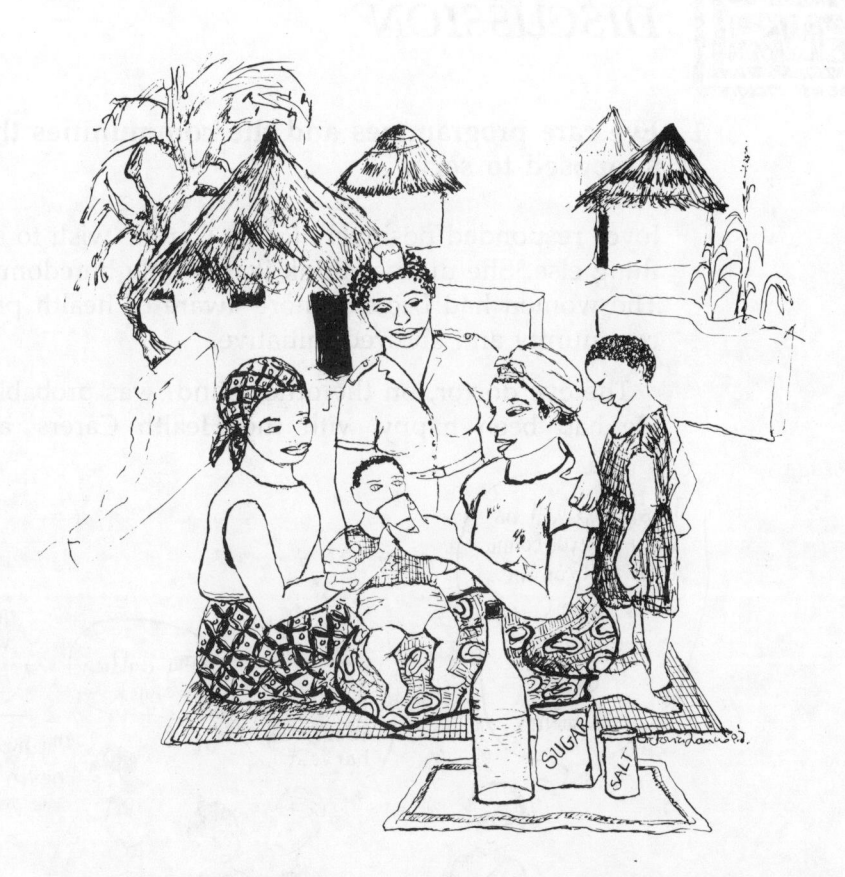

Ma-Anna learnt how to prepare the rehydration drink and saved Musa from dying

Early next morning Ma-Anna knocked at Lerisa's door. Lerisa was scared. Was Musa worse? Had he died? But Ma-Anna stood there, beaming with joy. 'Musa is playing again! He's fine. Thank you, Lerisa. Can I join the Carers now?' Lerisa was overjoyed. She couldn't believe it. She gave her a big hug. 'Of course you can. I've been waiting a long time for this day.'

QUESTIONS

1 What three common environmental factors lead to trachoma and diarrhoea?
2 What is the relationship between xerophthalmia and diarrhoea?
3 How do you prepare the oral rehydration drink?
What mistakes can be made in its preparation?
4 Why did Ma-Anna only join the Health Carers at this stage?

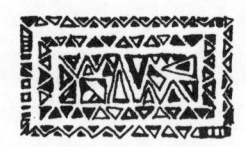

DISCUSSION

1 Eye care programmes and the communities they are supposed to serve

Joyce responded positively to the Carers' wish to start with something else. She did not think it was only boredom with trachoma. The women had become more aware of health problems in their community and showed initiative.

The eye doctor, on the other hand, was probably disappointed. He had been happy with the Health Carers' achievements in

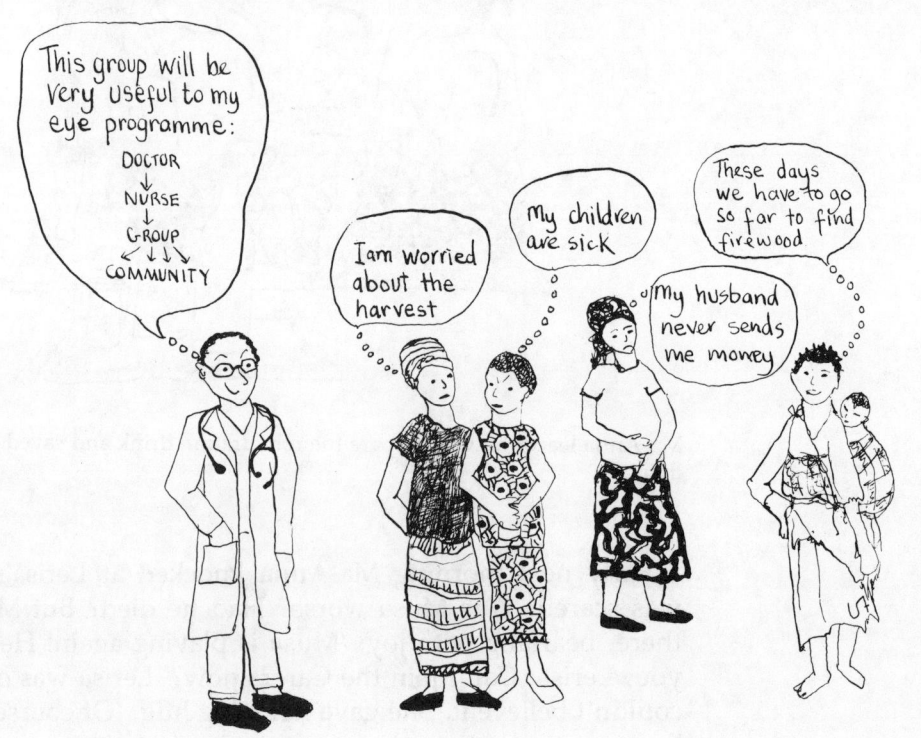

This group will be very useful to my eye programme:
DOCTOR
↓
NURSE
↓
GROUP
↙ ↓ ↘
COMMUNITY

I am worried about the harvest

My children are sick

These days we have to go so far to find firewood

My husband never sends me money

Doctor using community

reducing trachoma. He wanted them to continue with eye care and to address other causes of blindness like xerophthalmia and eye injuries, cataract and glaucoma.

Eye care programmes tend to isolate eyes from other health problems. 'Experts', in their offices, make their own plans to achieve their aims in the control of eye diseases. Health workers and their communities, or voluntary groups like the Health Carers, are then used as vehicles to implement the expert's interests. But such groups are not vehicles. They are the people whose lives are directly affected by health interventions. They have their own views of the world and want to do things in their way.

If voluntary community groups are to be usefully incorporated into an eye care programme, it is important to understand the way they think and work:
a) People see no point in dividing life into different compartments. For them, a healthy life includes good crops, stable families, healthy children, a strong body, etc. The eye is only a tiny part of all this. If one part suffers, all others will suffer too.
b) They have other health problems which are more important to them.
c) When they see an immediate need of any kind, not only health, and if they find their own way to solve the problem, they do so with enthusiasm. But they are loath to carry out someone else's ideas where they do not see the point of them.
d) For the women, the group meetings are also an important social event. They do not talk only about eyes. They discuss village and family matters. They are happy together, singing and dancing. Working for health must be interesting and fun. To repeat the same activity over a long period is boring. To sustain interest, the group's programme must be varied and relevant to their daily lives.

2 'Horizontal' and 'vertical' problems

People see health as something belonging to life as a whole. This, too, is the view of community health experts. Diseases of poverty are linked with each other and result from the environment in which poor people have to live; e.g. trachoma flourishes in dry, dirty conditions. These same conditions are a breeding ground for many more diseases, like diarrhoea, malnutrition, skin diseases or xerophthalmia. Ma-Anna's family is an example of where all these diseases are always present. It does not make sense to try to control only one of these diseases without changing the conditions responsible for its occurrence. Yet, the Carers started with one disease, trachoma. Why didn't they design a programme to prevent all these diseases? Did they waste their time?

There are advantages to starting with one disease, such as trachoma, provided it is a community concern:

a) The disease is well defined and specific interventions are possible.
b) Transmission is easy to understand.
c) The effects of treatment and good hygiene can be seen.
d) The community is more likely to take responsibility for its care and prevention.
e) Its relationship with other diseases of poverty is understandable. It is a good stepping stone for other health interventions and for village development.
f) It demonstrates that primary eye care should go hand in hand with primary health care because the root causes of the most common eye diseases are the same as for most other diseases.

Exercise

The doctor may have been disappointed that the Carers abandoned trachoma control in favour of learning about diarrhoea and its treatment. However, there are some interrelationships between diarrhoea and eye diseases. Find these out by completing Table 22.1 below. Make a cross when the answer is 'yes', as shown with the first examples.

	Diarrhoea	Trachoma	Xerophthalmia
1 Lack of vitamin A in the diet can cause*:	x		x
2 Breast feeding (when the mother is well nourished) prevents:	x		x
3 Flies transmit:			
4 Poor environmental hygiene favours:			
5 Bad water supply favours:			
6 Serving children only *freshly* prepared food prevents:			
7 Washing hands after use of toilet and touching dirty objects prevents:			
8 Measles vaccination prevents:			

* Note also: Xerophthalmia predisposes a person to diarrhoea and diarrhoea may precipitate xerophthalmia.

Table 22.1

SUMMARY

1 Informal groups are part of the communities they serve. They will soon lose interest in health programmes if their own views and understanding of problems are ignored and they are expected only to carry out the plans of 'experts'.
2 A community project must be variable enough to be attractive to the participants.

23

The village fights for clean water – Health Carers activate the community

In the evenings, just before sunset, the women and girls would go down to the river to fetch water. There was always much laughter and talk while the pots were filled and some washing was done. Children would play happily in the water, oblivious to the danger of Bilharzia.

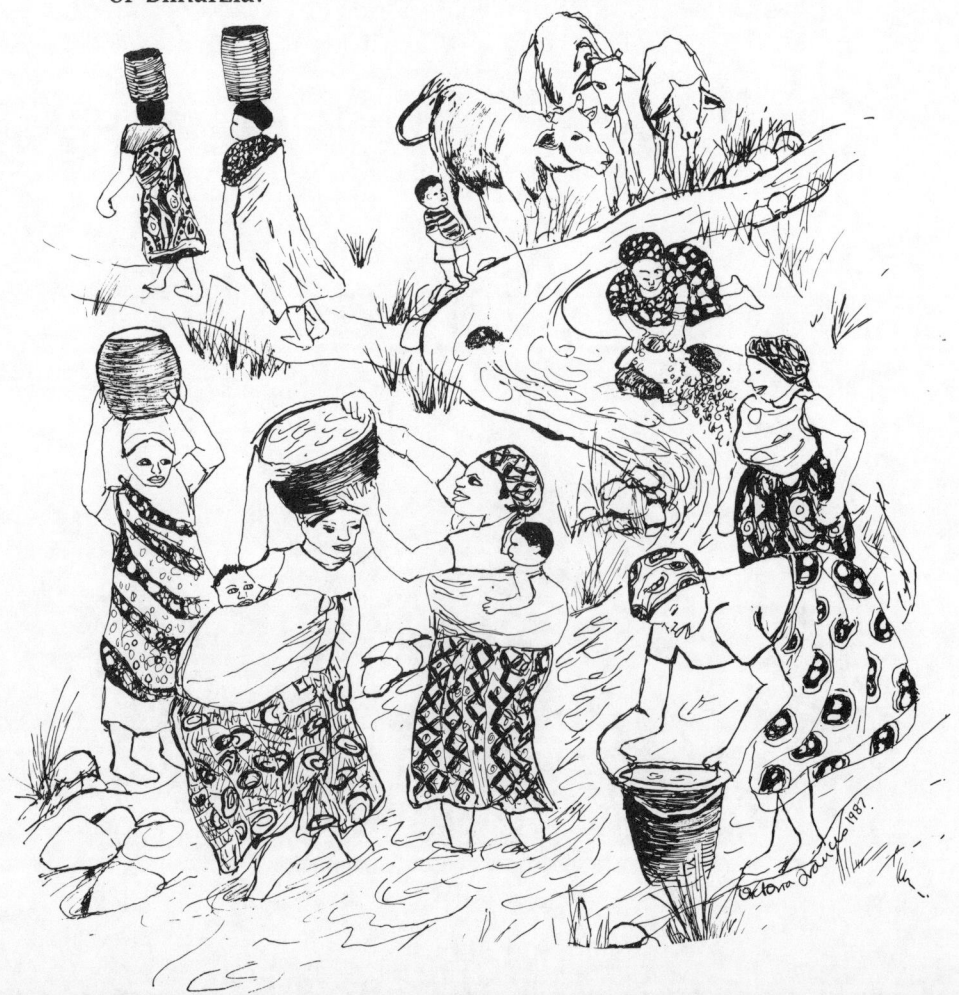

One evening Mavila asked her friends, 'Do you boil this water when you get home?' Nobody did. Even the Health Carers confessed that they seldom boiled their drinking water. It used too much wood and tasted ghastly.

A few paces upstream a little boy urinated into the river. Ruth pointed at him. 'Look at that. Do you realise that we are drinking his pee? How disgusting.'

The Carers shared with the others what they had learned about diarrhoea. Although polluted water is only one of the many causes of diarrhoea, clean water was still important. The only water source for Hanyane was the river. Knowing this, the nurse had advised them to boil it. They realised now that this advice was difficult to follow. It just was not possible to boil large quantities of water.

Lerisa said that she had seen the water pipe in Kulani. 'It's wonderful. You just open the tap and wait for your container to fill up with clean water.'

'Why has Kulani got a tap and we haven't?' one mother asked.

'Probably because nobody here asked for it,' another mother remarked. 'We have always thought the river was good enough.'

One young woman added, 'Of course, our chief is a man. He doesn't know how tiring it is for women to collect water.'

A heated discussion around water, men and government officials followed. They all contributed at the tops of their voices. Someone said, 'You Health Carers must go to the chief. We want a tap like the one in Kulani.' But Lerisa wanted everyone to be involved. After all, it was the concern of all women in Hanyane, not just the Health Carers.

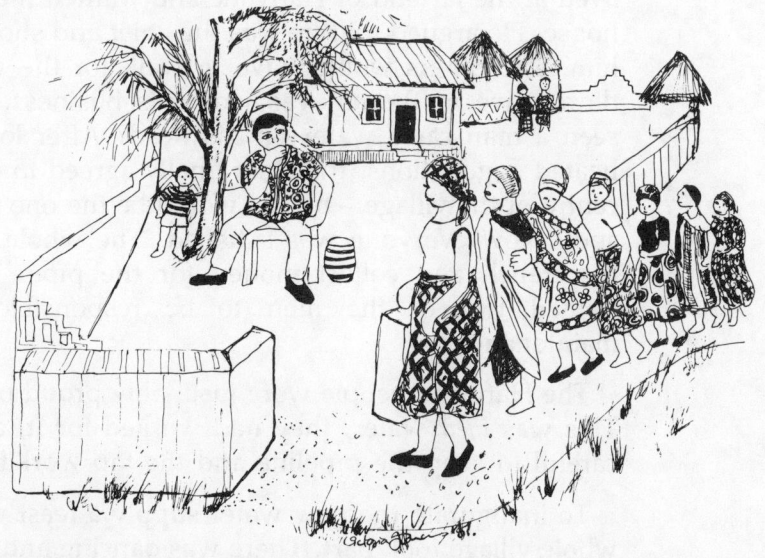

The chief watched the delegation approach his house. What were these women up to now?

The chief watched the village delegation approach his house. What were these women up to now? It must be something serious – other women had joined the Carers this time. He was now accustomed to the fact that women in Hanyane took initiatives. He also had to admit that, in most cases, their requests were very reasonable and for the good of the community.

When he heard their demand for piped water, he made a quick calculation in his mind: the tap would, of course, be placed in front of his house. He sent an application to the water affairs office. After a long time the reply came that a borehole was planned for Hanyane. The machine would not be available for a few years as there was a very long waiting list. The people would have to be patient and wait their turn.

However, the people refused to be patient. For them it meant more children dying of diarrhoea. They wanted clean water now.

The women discussed the matter with Joyce. 'We should find another way to get water. I have heard of people who help villages to build wells. I will find out more about this.'

In the meantime, the community elected a water committee consisting of two men and two women. They would take care of the matter. When the expert arrived he went around the village with the water committee and some community elders to look for springs and suitable places for wells or a borehole. He was impressed by the interest of the people in Hanyane. Together they decided to catch a spring which was some distance away, and lay a pipe from there to Hanyane.

There was still one more obstacle to deal with: the chief. He lived at the far end of Hanyane and wanted the tap in front of his house. He argued that he was the chief and should have it close to him. The others would have to walk for the water. The women didn't give in. Water was women's business. Had anyone ever seen a man carry water on his head? After long and sometimes heated negotiations, the chief finally agreed to have the tap in the centre of the village – but he would be the one to choose the exact spot. Now everyone was satisfied. The whole village helped dig the trench and collect money for the pipe. The water experts trained two of the men to be responsible for repairs and maintenance.

The Hanyane people were justifiably proud of their clean water. This was *their* water, they had worked for it, and they would be careful to keep the pipeline and the tap working well.

To inaugurate the new water supply a feast was organised. The whole village took part. There was dancing and singing and lots to eat and drink. The best drink they all tasted was the fresh clean water from the tap. At the end of the feast the chief stood up and paid tribute to the Carers. It was they who had managed to shake Hanyane out of its apathy and indifference and it was thanks to them that Hanyane now had its own clean water.

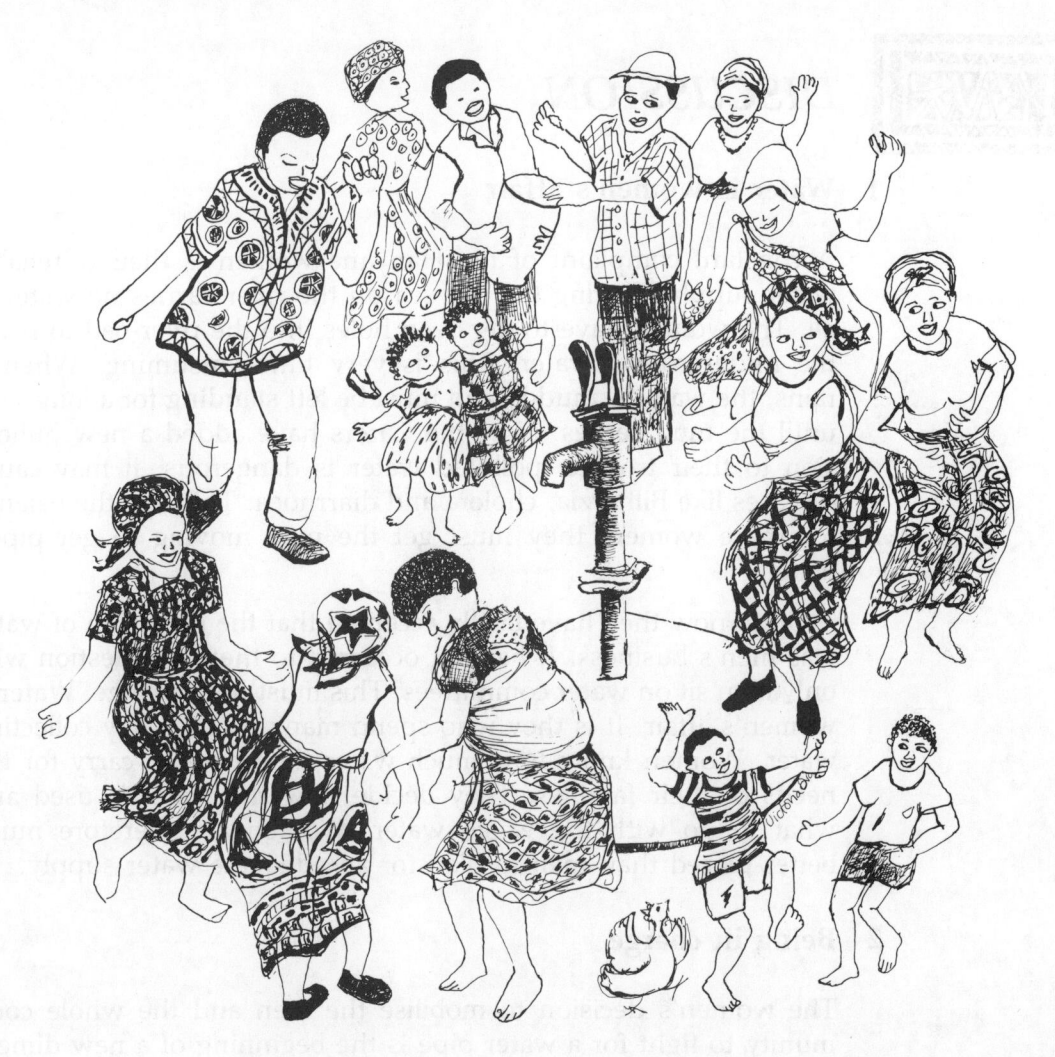

QUESTIONS

1. Do you think it is practicable in your area to boil all drinking water? What are the constraints?
   Do you know other methods to purify polluted water? Describe them.
2. What diseases can be caused by polluted water?
3. Why are women more motivated to improve the supply of clean water than men?
4. What action do people take in your area to gain access to enough clean water?

DISCUSSION

1 Water is women's affair

A constant complaint of the Hanyane women is their unreliable water supply. During the dry season the river carries no water at all. The women have to dig deep holes into the river-bed to reach the underground water. This is very time-consuming. When it rains, the water is muddy and must be left standing for a long time until the mud settles. Now the Carers have added a new dimension to their trouble: polluted water is dangerous, it may cause diseases like Bilharzia, cholera and diarrhoea. This tips the balance for these women: they must get the men moving to get piped water.

Up to now they have tacitly accepted that the provision of water was men's business. It has not occurred to them to question why only men sit on water committees. This must now change. Water is women's affair. It is they who spend many hours a day collecting water. Women know how much water they have to carry for the needs of their families. They decide how the water is used and what to do with the waste water. Women are therefore much better placed than men to plan for an adequate water supply.

2 Being in charge

The women's decision to mobilise the men and the whole community to fight for a water pipe is the beginning of a new dimension in the Carers' work.

They started as a project directed by the doctor and the nurse. Now they have become self-directed community developers. In the beginning the group was exclusive – you remember the 'Tidy Ladies'. Later on it opened up to include women of all sections of the village, from the teacher's wife to Ma-Anna. The group has become well established and accepted. Now, at the river, the Carers have taken the next important step: they are no longer jealously guarding their group identity. They are now willing to include all members of the community. This standing together and joining hands has made them strong. They do not need the nurse anymore to tell them what to do.

The Hanyane people, men and women, have captured the spring and laid the pipe. They have fought for the proper site of the tap. The water is theirs. They are proud of it and will look after their water supply. The Kulani people were not involved in getting their water pipe. It was given to them. They did not look after it

The chief wanted the water tap here

Water experts located the spring here

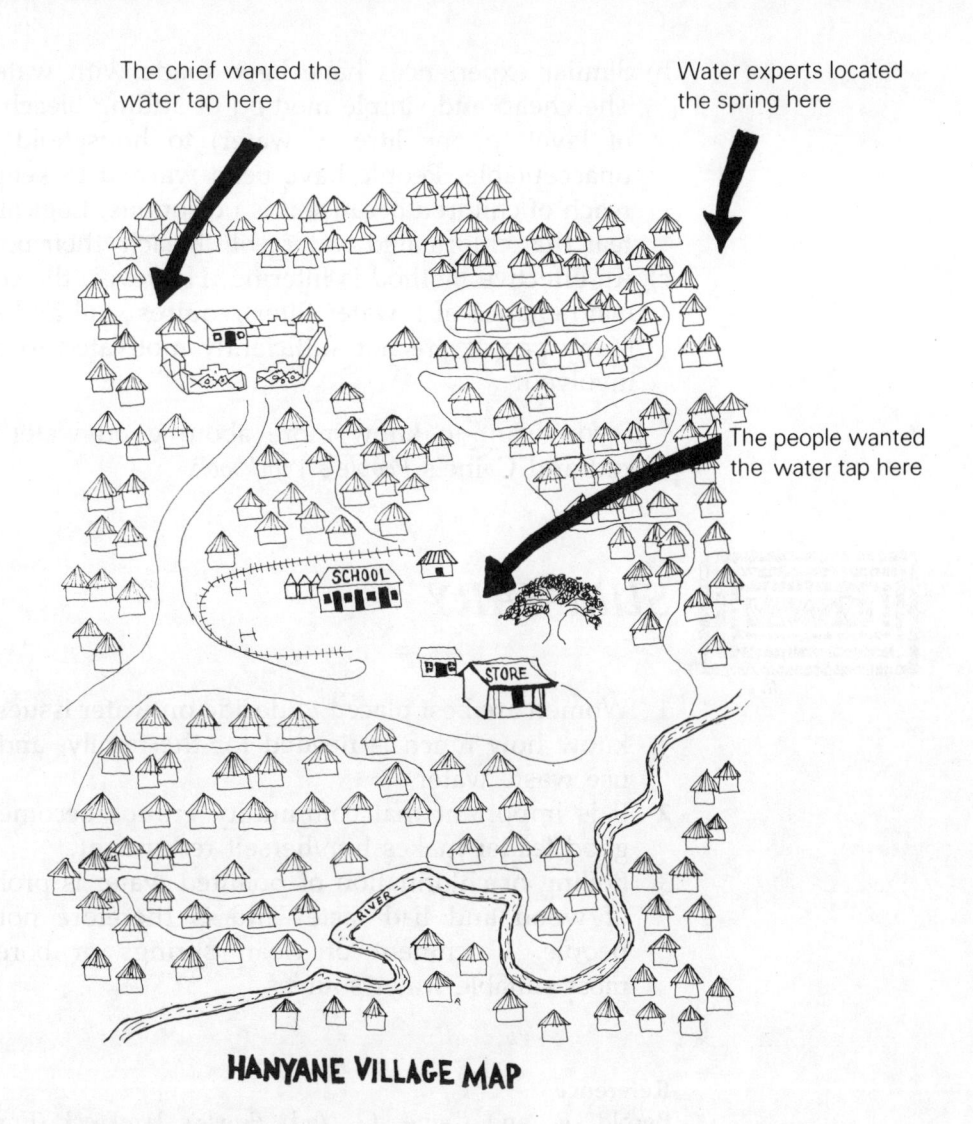

The people wanted the water tap here

HANYANE VILLAGE MAP

Where should the water tap be?

and depended on the government to repair the broken pipe. It is tempting (and often easier) to act as 'provider' for a community. But if you really want to help people gain independence, your most important task is to help them to achieve things in their own way.

3 Methods of water purification

It is difficult to obtain good water from a polluted source such as a river, and it is even more difficult to find a method which is both acceptable and feasible for rural communities.

a) The women at the river have given their reasons why boiling water is not realistic: it uses too much wood and it spoils the taste.

b) Similar experiences have been made with water chlorination. The cheap and simple method of adding bleach (e.g. one drop of Javel to one litre of water) to household water is often unacceptable. People have been warned to keep bleach out of reach of children because it is poisonous. Logically, people then fear that chlorinated water will 'bleach' their bowels.
c) An effective method is filtering. However, the construction and maintenance of a water filter requires skill and understanding. Many people are not sufficiently motivated to make the effort involved.

If you want to know more about good water supplies, read Berold and Caine's *People's Workbook*.

SUMMARY

1 Women are best placed to decide on water issues. They carry it, know how much is needed for the family, and know how to use waste water.
2 It is important that community groups become self-reliant. A good leader makes him/herself redundant.
3 Boiling or chlorination of polluted water is problematic (waste of wood and bad taste) and is therefore not acceptable to people. Catchment of clean springs or boreholes are the most suitable water sources.

Reference
Berold, R. and Caine, C., (ed) *People's Workbook* (Environmental and Development Agency, Johannesburg, 1981)

24

Joyce is sick
– Coping by ourselves

Joyce felt very tired. She had worked hard. The Health Carers had done a good job. There was now less trachoma and diarrhoea to treat. Health in the village had certainly improved. The water pipe had made life easier for the women and boosted their morale. But all of this had not diminished Joyce's work. More people came to the clinic because they were more aware of the services and they trusted Joyce. Word had gone around that blind people could recover their sight with an operation. There were also regular meetings with the Hanyane Health Carers. She loved the group and considered it to be the most worthwhile thing she had ever done in her life.

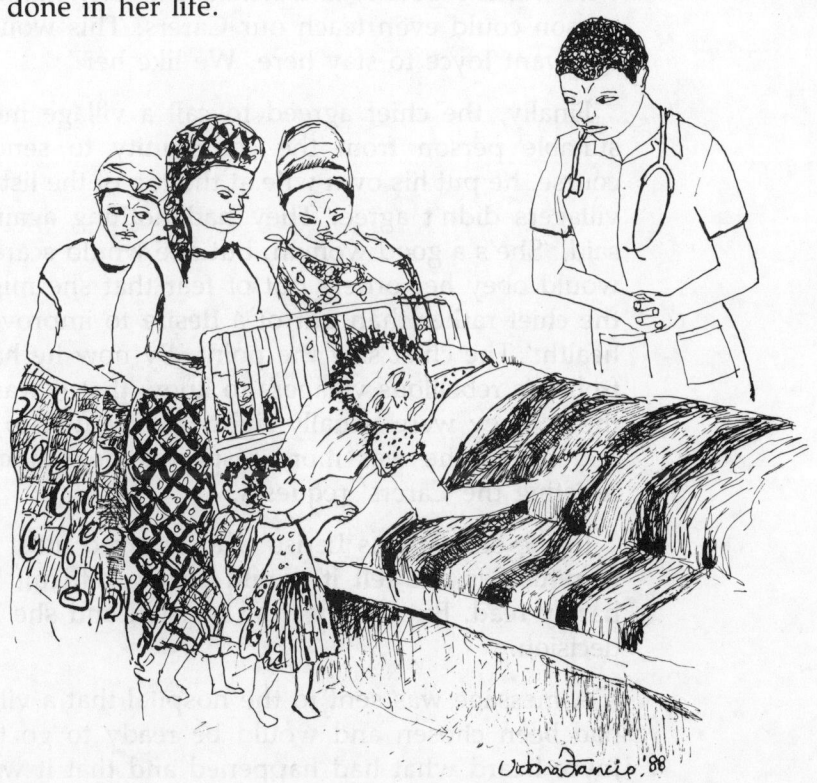

141

But now she was tired and every movement made her sweat. She was shivering and thought something must be wrong. She took her temperature and found she had a fever. Joyce was taken to hospital. She was away from work for three months. She had been overworking. This was clear to both the doctor and the people of Hanyane. They wondered how they might help her. The doctor suggested that an assistant nurse could help her at the clinic. Also, the idea of village health workers should be taken up again with the various communities. Little did the doctor know that the people of Hanyane had already acted.

People were worried that there was no nurse to replace Joyce while she was sick. They couldn't be without a clinic for so long. In Hanyane the elders called on the chief. They wanted him to put pressure on the matron to send a relief nurse. The chief had done so already, but to no avail, he said.

The teacher thought that the time was right to choose a village health worker. The Carers were proof that not much formal education was required to do a good job. The chief was still reluctant. A village health worker had to be paid, while the Health Carers worked free of charge. Couldn't they do the job of a village health worker?

The elders objected. 'We respect our ladies but they work when they have the time and when they feel like it. We need a person who works regularly and who is properly trained for the job. This person could even teach our Carers. This would help our nurse. We want Joyce to stay here. We like her.'

Finally, the chief agreed to call a village meeting to choose a suitable person from the community to send for training. Of course, he put his own wife at the top of the list of candidates. The villagers didn't agree. They had nothing against his wife. They said, 'She's a good woman, but she would scare the people – they would obey her orders out of fear that she might report them to the chief rather than out of a desire to improve the community's health.' The chief saw the point. By now he had learned enough from his rebellious villagers to know that it was better to listen to them. They were usually right. He wanted to remain their chief and he felt he was more respected now since he had stopped resisting the Carers' requests.

In the end, it was Lerisa who received most votes. She wanted to refuse as she felt it would be too difficult for her. She could hardly read. But the meeting insisted and she had to accept their decision.

A message was sent to the hospital that a village health worker had been chosen and would be ready to go for training. When Joyce heard what had happened and that it was Lerisa who had

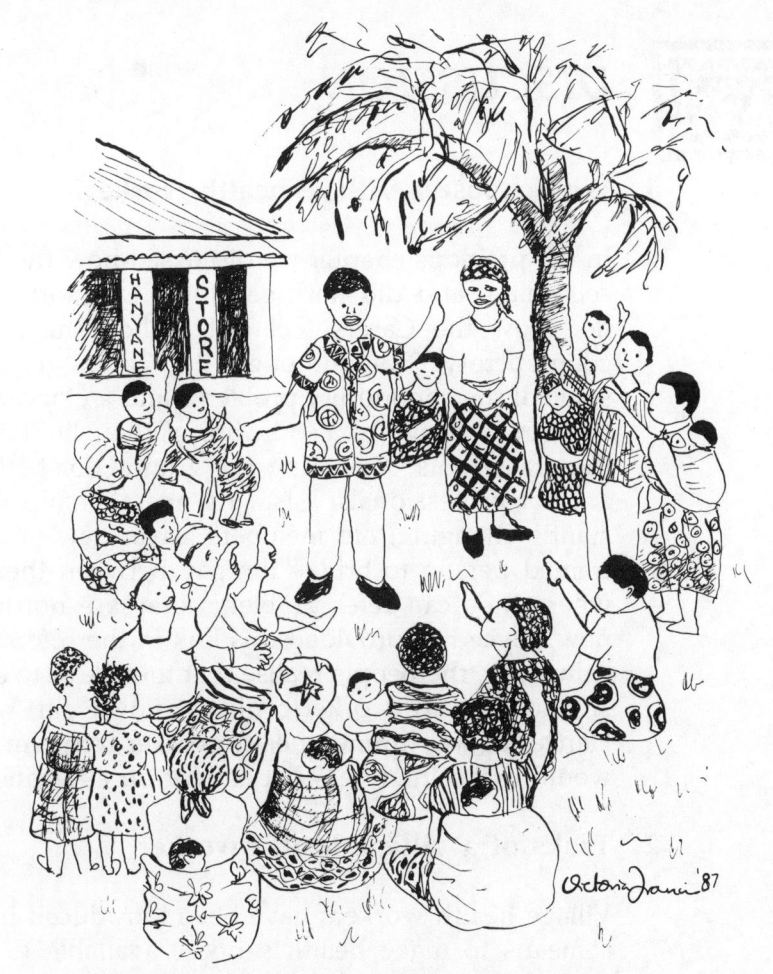

Lerisa was chosen to become their village health worker

been chosen, she cried with joy. From then on she made a speedy recovery.

QUESTIONS

1. What qualities should the ideal village health worker have? Has Lerisa been a good choice?
   How would you advise a community about choosing their village health worker?
2. Should the village health worker be a member of the community or an outsider? Why?
3. Do you think the choice of Lerisa will cause conflict between her and the other Carers? In what way?
4. How could the Carers take over the role of a trained village health worker?

DISCUSSION

1 Why choose a village health worker?

In the previous chapter we discussed how the Carers have become self-reliant and did not need Joyce anymore to tell them what to do. Now the Carers feel lost without her. This appears to be contradictory. But, although the Carers have become aware of some of the community problems and feel more confident to act on their own, they are also aware of their limitations. They work at the grass roots, preparing the ground for better health. But they are not professionals. Also, the membership in the group is constantly changing, old members leave, new ones join. They need a trained person to bridge the gap between them and the hospital, where they can refer problems they are not able to solve. Up to now, Joyce has provided this link in the referral chain. With Joyce being sick, the people realise that they have to strengthen that link. A village health worker could take over part of the nurse's job. If Hanyane has a trained health worker from amongst themselves, it would make them less dependent on assistance from outside.

2 Tasks of a village health worker

Village health workers have been introduced in many countries as a means to make health services available to all. Many things a nurse has to do can be done just as well or even better by a lesser trained person, e.g. a village health worker. He or she can treat some common minor ailments and refer those requiring more care to the health post. They can also be trained to recognise and manage or refer common eye problems and advise on their prevention (see also Part 2).

The village health worker should fill the gap between the community and the health services. She or he is the mouthpiece of her/his community. His/her voice carries weight because the village health worker, as a member of the community, has personal experience of the village's problems. A good village health worker can thus contribute towards a fruitful partnership between the people and the health services. Instead of health officials giving one-way directives or orders, both sides might become engaged in dialogue and work together.

You may argue that such a situation is too idealistic. You are probably right in most instances. Village health workers are often employees of the government or of a non-government organisation, just as professional health workers are. Naturally, the employee's loyalty is strongest towards the one who pays his/her salary. For fear of losing his/her job a village health worker will avoid offending the employer with sensitive issues, e.g. when people have complaints about the health care provided.

In many countries, the health care organisers are aware of this danger. They therefore encourage the communities themselves to employ their own village health worker. The community is then responsible for their chosen person, and he or she will feel responsible for the community. Unfortunately, many such schemes are not as successful as anticipated. Rural communities, such as Hanyane, are usually poor and fail to compensate their village health worker for the work done. Few people who are dependent on an income will work for nothing. The village health worker will simply stop working.

3 Choosing a village health worker

Mistakes may be made when people are not clear about the tasks of a village health worker. In Hanyane, people were well prepared and managed to avoid some of the common pitfalls, like the two below:

a) A relative of a powerful person (chief, landowner, teacher, etc.) is chosen. Such a person will be more interested in pleasing the powerful than assisting and representing the poor.

b) A very young person with higher schooling is chosen. Most older people will not trust him or her because she lacks experience. Young people are also likely to leave the community for a better job at a later time.

We will talk more about village health workers in Chapter 26. In the meantime, read the short informative chapter on the subject in Werner, *Helping Health Workers Learn* (Hesperian Foundation, 1982), Ch 2.

Exercise

What is the difference between a village health worker and an informal group like the Health Carers?

Imagine that you have to explain to the chief of Hanyane why, at this stage, a village health worker is needed in addition to the Carers.

To clarify your points complete Table 24.1. For each item, mark with a cross what type of health worker (group or individual village health worker) you think would be most effective in the control of trachoma.

	Health Carers	Village health workers

1 Addressing the root causes of trachoma
a) Improve water supply
b) Fly control through
  i) building toilets
  ii) waste disposal
  iii) keeping animals away from homestead
c) Personal hygiene (hand and face washing)
d) Fight poverty (job creation)		

2 Control of trachoma a) Case finding b) Treatment of active cases, and c) young children d) Treatment or referral of entropion cases		
3 Long-term maintenance of low incidence of trachoma a) Maintenance of good hygiene b) Treatment of new cases		
4 Community involvement in scheme a) Acceptance by community b) Inclusion of the poorest c) Decision-making by community		

Table 24.1

SUMMARY

1 Choosing a village health worker from the community can make people more self-reliant and ensures the maintenance of a referral chain.
2 A good village health worker is the mouthpiece of the community and can encourage dialogue between the health services and the community.
3 In practice, village health workers often feel more loyal towards their employer than to the community.
4 Badly chosen village health workers are often a failure.

Reference
Werner, D., *Helping Health Workers Learn* (Hesperian Foundation, 1982)

25

Green vegetables prevent xerophthalmia –
Gardening without water

After being chosen as village health worker, Lerisa went for training. Joyce recovered and returned to work, but was advised by the doctor to take things easy. In spite of the two key people being away, the group continued to meet.

This time the Carers met at Mavilá's home. It was a hot afternoon. Conversation in those days revolved around the drought. It was the second year running that there had been no rains. The maize plants dried out before they could flower. The Carers wondered what they would eat the following year. It was not even possible to plant a few vegetables around their houses. The soil was too hard. Ma-Anna was especially worried. She remembered only too well what the nurses at the hospital had told her: young children need green vegetables for their eyes. She had seen other children at the hospital who were blind like Musa. They had all had measles and none of them had been given green vegetables to eat.

The other mothers were frightened too. If the drought continued more children could go blind.

'I was in Kulani recently,' said Leah, the teacher's wife. 'I passed Mr Sibila's office. He's our new agricultural extension officer. He had fresh green vegetables in his garden.'

The group didn't believe her. 'That's not possible. He must surely be using witchcraft.'

At that very moment, Mr Sibila passed by. Ma-Anna jumped up and called him. He must tell them his secret. What sort of magic did he use?

Mr Sibila assured them that he had no secret source of water and that there was no magic involved. He called his method of vegetable growing 'deep trenching'. He had learned it not long ago. He wanted to try it out first to see whether it was suitable for the local area before instructing others. The method involved hard work so he wanted to be certain it would work.

'We are not afraid of hard work,' Mavila said. 'Couldn't you show us this method right now, in my garden?'

Mr Sibila took a lump of hard, dry soil. He crumbled it tenderly in his hand. 'The soil is our mother. She feeds us and gives us life. So, we must love her and take care of her. When nature fails, we must help. One way of helping the soil is through the method of deep trenching.'

Mr Sibila asked for a pick and a few spades. He then marked out the area of the vegetable plot, one metre wide and two metres long. They had to dig this whole plot two spades' deep. The top soil was put on one side of the trench and the deeper soil on the other side. It was hard work. To make it easier, the women chanted songs about Mr Sibila and his green vegetables.

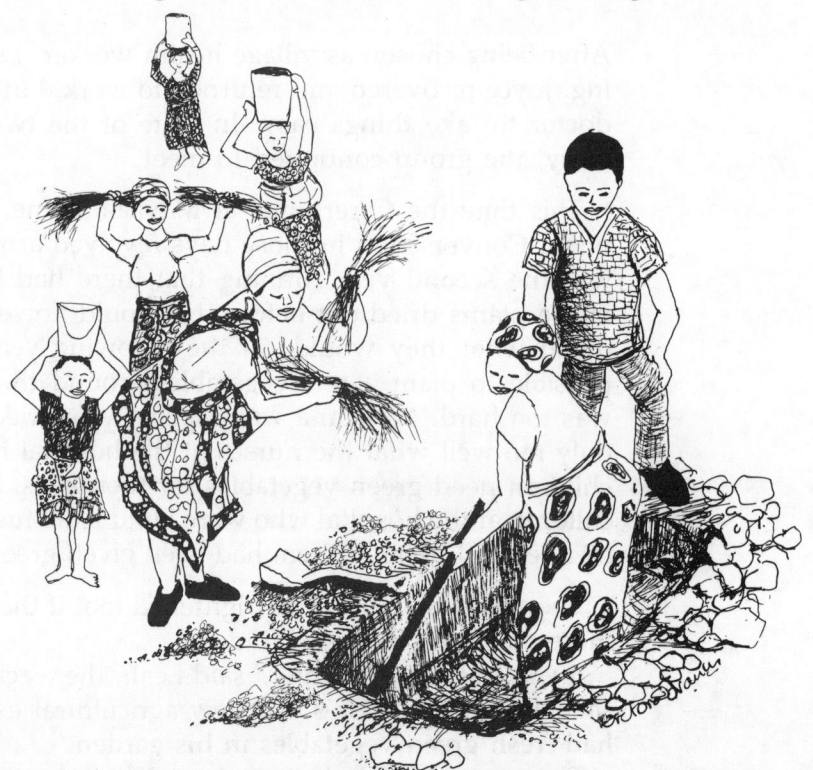

While some of the Carers were busy with the spades, the others had to fetch grass and leaves – whatever they could find. Then, when the trench was dug, it was filled in again: one thick layer of grass, one layer of soil, repeated until the trench was full. At this stage a few buckets of water had to be poured on the grass to get it thoroughly moist. The top soil was put back at the very end.

Now Mr Sibila pulled a handful of bean seeds out of his pocket. He planted the seeds in the top soil. Ma-Anna watered them carefully.

'You must now wait for the beans to grow. When they are about one foot high, dig them under.'

'What a waste!' the women shouted.

'Why not harvest the beans first and then dig the stalks under?' one of them asked.

Mr Sibila explained that the young bean plants are excellent food for the soil.

'Why don't you use fertiliser?', the women asked.

Mr Sibila had several good reasons for not using fertiliser. First, fertiliser costs money. Second, one has to know exactly how to use it otherwise it does more harm than good. Third, with this particular method, the fertiliser would be too concentrated and would poison the plants.

'When you use this method,' he added, 'all you have to do is to add compost from time to time. You will only need to water the vegetables occasionally.'

Mavila's garden made news in Hanyane. Everyone came to see the beautiful green patch in the midst of dry and dusty land. It was difficult to believe that this could happen without witchcraft, but there it was. From then on the sound of spades was heard all over Hanyane, and small green patches started to appear here and there.

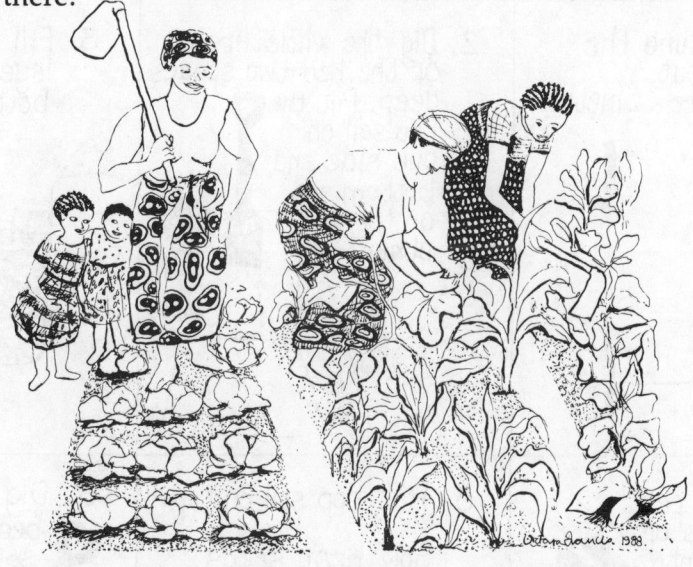

Small green patches started to appear all over Hanyane

The question they had to answer next was how to persuade the young children to eat the spinach. They were not used to the taste and spat it out. Most mothers were discouraged and they wouldn't force the children to eat what they didn't like. So, in spite of having green vegetables, the children's eyes were still in danger.

How would you solve this problem?

QUESTIONS

1. Which vegetables, growing in your area, are good for the prevention of xerophthalmia? Which ones are of little value?
2. How would you advise mothers to feed green vegetables to small children? At what age should they start to add vegetables to a child's diet?
3. Does the addition of skimmed milk to the child's porridge prevent xerophthalmia?
4. Do you think the method of trenching described here could be suitable where you work? In what type of climate would it not be suitable?

What other improved methods of vegetable gardening do you know?

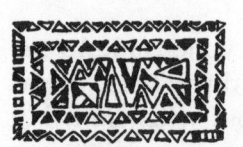

DISCUSSION

HOW TO MAKE A TRENCH FOR VEGETABLE GROWING

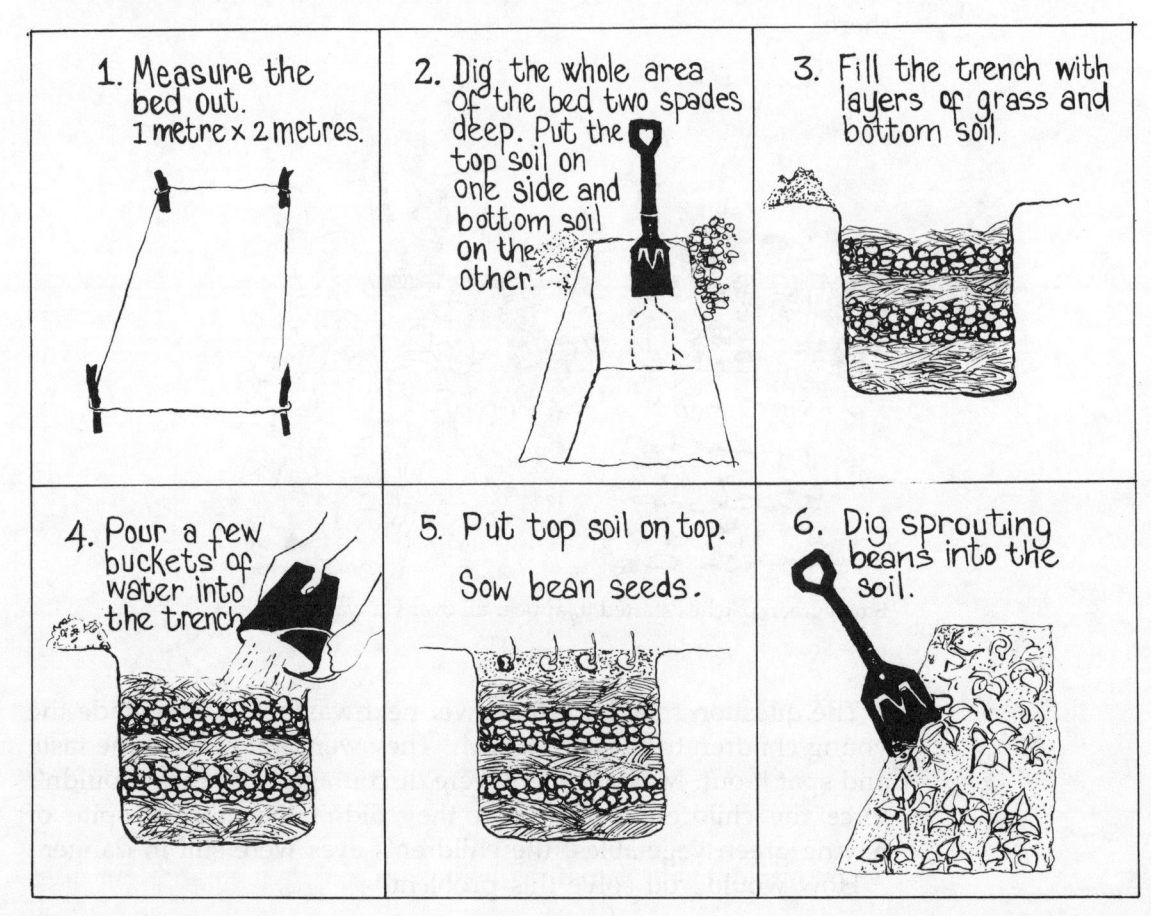

1. Measure the bed out. 1 metre × 2 metres.
2. Dig the whole area of the bed two spades deep. Put the top soil on one side and bottom soil on the other.
3. Fill the trench with layers of grass and bottom soil.
4. Pour a few buckets of water into the trench.
5. Put top soil on top. Sow bean seeds.
6. Dig sprouting beans into the soil.

1 Deep trench gardening

The method of 'deep trenching' described in the story has been well tried and proved to be successful in a dry climate.

Care should be taken to make sure the planting bed is slightly deeper than the surrounding terrain. This will hold the water whenever it rains so that it will not run off and carry the good soil and seedlings with it.

With the method described it is possible to grow vegetables even during prolonged periods of drought. In areas not too far from the sea, the night-time dew suffices to provide enough moisture for plants, but if there is no dew, the vegetables require weekly watering.

In the area where you work, some other method may be more appropriate. Discuss this with someone who has experience, e.g. an agricultural extension officer.

2 Eye health and growing vegetables

Refresh your memory about xerophthalmia by reading Part 3, Section C. While reading this book, you may have realised that mere knowledge about eyes is not enough if you want to be a good primary eye care worker. You must know about refuse disposal and how to build a toilet. Now you are learning about agriculture. If you want to prevent xerophthalmia you should know how to grow green vegetables in your area.

Nobody expects you to be an expert in everything. But you should know who you can turn to for advice. Good food is essential for eyes and general health. Therefore you must use the best possible method of food production in your area. It must be feasible for the poorest villager. This means artificial fertiliser should be avoided and natural compost from refuse (the Carer's refuse pits!) used instead. There is also another reason for not using fertiliser: most people use too much for too long. This spoils the soil and can even poison the water you drink.

> HEALTH CARERS MUST WORK TOGETHER WITH FOOD PRODUCERS

3 Ma-Anna takes initiatives

Ma-Anna took a long time to join the Carers. Did you notice that even after she joined she kept very quiet? What makes her now take the lead with the vegetable gardens?

Once Ma-Anna felt accepted in the group she became more self-confident. She began to believe in her own abilities. In questions of child nutrition she has become more confident because of all the information she received at the hospital. It is her own concern and she is determined to take the Carer group along with her to solve the problem of growing vegetables in their poor soil and dry climate.

But the Health Carers have still to learn more about working as a group. Why has each member got her own little garden? Few of them have enough money to make a solid fence to keep goats and chickens out. If they had got together to make a communal garden, good fencing would have been affordable. They have not done so because they were afraid one or the other might steal the vegetables. They did not yet fully trust each other. It takes a long time for a relationship of trust to grow within such a group.

If you want to know more about working in groups, the three volumes of *Training for Transformation* by Anne Hope will give you excellent guidance.

SUMMARY

1 The deep trenching method for vegetable growing is suitable for dry climates.
2 As an eye health worker, you have to know about more than eyes: toilets, refuse pits, clean water supply and vegetable growing are all essential to prevent unnecessary blindness.
3 Working in groups helps the weaker members to become strong and confident.

Reference
Hope, A. and Timmel, S., *Training for Transformation* (Mambo Press, 1984)

26

Lerisa's new found knowledge – Acceptance or jealousy?

Three months later Lerisa returned from her training. She was worried about how she would be received in her new role. Would her fellow Carers want to learn from her? Would the chief and the elders welcome her back? Would the people trust her to do the things that Joyce had done before?

Joyce helped Lerisa to overcome some of these fears at a big party held on her return. She explained what the villagers could expect from their village health worker and what kind of illnesses she would have to refer to the clinic. She wanted to have this very clear from the start to avoid misunderstandings and unhappiness on both sides. Then it was Lerisa's turn to speak about the things she had learned. Proudly she opened her little suitcase which contained a first aid kit, a baby scale, Road To Health Charts, some aspirin, malaria tablets and tetracycline eye ointment. The babies could now be weighed and checked in Hanyane. The long journey to the clinic would only be necessary if there were problems she could not solve. The people of Hanyane were delighted to hear this and were surprised at what Lerisa could now do. But Lerisa was still nervous about how the Carers would react to her in her new, paid position.

Not long ago she had been just an ordinary member of the group. Now she had to take over part of Joyce's role in the group. Would they be jealous?

Lerisa went to visit her oldest friend, Ma-Anna, for advice. Ma-Anna said, 'My friend, we will not be jealous of you. It was we who chose you. But you must be careful not to become too proud of yourself and start acting like those nurses at the hospital.'

Then the Carers wanted to know all about her training at the Health Centre. Could she deliver babies or set broken limbs? They were suprised to hear that the training included a lot of useful home crafts – how to cook vegetables and prepare a healthy baby porridge which could almost replace milk. She even knew how to build a good toilet and make a stove out of mud bricks. This stove, if properly built, would save a lot of wood. Mothers would then use less time collecting wood and save money. Everybody wanted to have such a wonder stove and to cook on it for their children.

The group would be busy for a long time with the new things Lerisa could teach them.

During the following weeks and months, Lerisa settled well into her new job. Joyce and Lerisa met often to discuss problems. The chief and village elders were helpful whenever Lerisa had difficulties.

Every month she spent two days at the Health Centre for a refresher course. Village health workers from various areas met and exchanged their experiences. It was comforting to see how all of them faced similar problems. Sharing their difficulties made it easier to find solutions.

Two problems were frequently mentioned: sore eyes and eye injuries from thorns. Lerisa suggested that Joyce, who had special training in eyes, could teach them. This was arranged with the doctor and Joyce was given some time to prepare a course for village health workers on eye care (see Part 2).

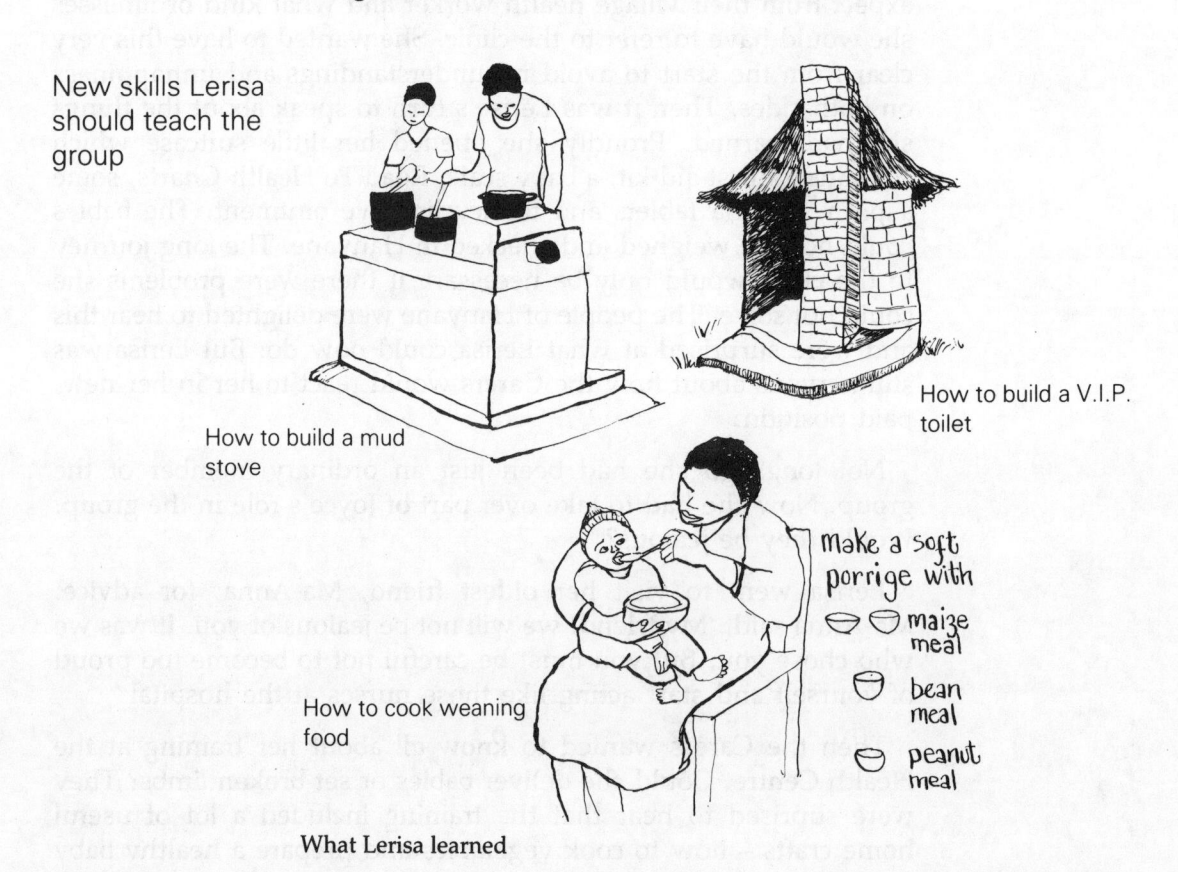

New skills Lerisa should teach the group

How to build a mud stove

How to build a V.I.P. toilet

How to cook weaning food

make a soft porrige with
maize meal
bean meal
peanut meal

What Lerisa learned

QUESTIONS

1. What fears do you have when you return to your place after a long absence for study? How does this relate to Lerisa's experience?
2. How do you support and supervise your village health workers in their work in your area?
3. What should a village health worker know about eye care? Draw up a syllabus for the village health workers in your own area.
4. What weaning foods are traditionally used where you work? What foods do you suggest?

DISCUSSION

1 Lerisa's problems

When Lerisa returns from training she has to face two potentially difficult situations:
a) With the people, and
b) With the Health Carers.

The people of Hanyane have known Lerisa since childhood

They knew that she attended school for only two years. She could not have learned much in a short three month training period. She is not a nurse. They will have to wait and see before beginning to trust her.

For these reasons, village health workers working in their *own* community have more difficulty starting work than do outsiders. However, once established they are usually more committed and more stable than a person from somewhere else who may change jobs as he/she pleases. Lerisa has her family in Hanyane and is unlikely to leave her home village in the foreseeable future. This makes Hanyane independent from outside assistance and promotes its self-reliance.

Lerisa had been an ordinary member of the Carers

The positions of chairlady, treasurer and secretary had been given to the teacher's wife, the chief's wife and to Mavila, who had completed primary school. Being a village health worker, Lerisa should now replace Joyce for almost everything concerning the group. Would the group accept her in her new role? Wouldn't the others, especially the three office bearers, be jealous of her? How would the group accept that she, Lerisa, was now paid for her work while the group members remained unpaid volunteers?

2 How can Lerisa's and other village health workers' problems be met?

a) People are sometimes unhappy about their village health workers because they have wrong expectations about them. It is therefore important that the community is well informed from the beginning. Joyce has ensured this. Hopefully this will avert future misunderstandings.

b) People expect *curative* care. In many primary health care programmes the role of the village health worker is restricted to *preventive* and *promotive* work. We have already discussed the pros and cons of these limitations in Chapter 19.

c) It is important that there is a well functioning *support structure* for each village health worker. Many primary health care projects go wrong because the field workers are left without support. The post of a village health worker is a lonely and isolated one, usually miles away from a clinic. Regular visits by an experienced health worker are therefore important to sustain the village health worker's morale as well as the quality of performance. If you will be in charge of village health workers, make a point of taking enough time when you visit them. Do not just hurry past with a quick glance at the records or an unfriendly remark when you find mistakes. Sit down with your village health worker and listen first to what he/she has to say. Then, together, try to find a solution to the problems. Joyce has given you an example of how it can be done. You will have to find your own method for your particular situation.

d) Lerisa and the Carers will have to design a plan for their new relationship with each other. The Carers should clearly define their own and Lerisa's roles and record them for future reference.

Also, Lerisa's paid employment must be thoroughly discussed, so that everyone is clear about the difference between a permanent job with well defined tasks and the Carers' informal activities. This will be discussed further in Chapter 28.

3 Lerisa's new found knowledge

In the illustration on page 154 you can see some of the things Lerisa has learned. One of them is the preparation of **weaning food**.

Usually mothers are advised to add milk powder to children's diet or even to use milk as a main food. This benefits manufacturers of powdered milk who, by promoting their products with glossy advertisements reap financial reward. Most mothers who need food supplements for their babies would have to spend the greater part of their household budget on milk powder. The usual outcome is that insufficient milk is used for the baby. Even then the extra money spent on milk means poor diets for older children.

Lerisa learned to prepare **weaning food** as follows: take 2 parts of maize flour, 1 part bean flour and 1 part ground peanuts. Prepare a soft porridge with these ingredients.

The advantage of this food is that it is about 20 times cheaper than milk, the ingredients can be grown at home, and it tastes delicious. Its disadvantage is that it does not contain sufficient vitamin A. Therefore, *green vegetables* (or another vitamin A source) must always be added.

But be careful. All weaning food should be freshly prepared for each meal. Microbes which cause diarrhoea grow fast if the porridge is allowed to stand for more than an hour, even if you protect it from flies.

If you want to know how to build a **mud stove** you will find instructions in: 1) GATE, *Helping People in Poor Countries Develop: fuel-saving cookstoves*, (available free of charge); and 2) Volunteers for Technical Assistance, *Wood Conserving Cook Stoves: a design guide*. On **VIP toilets**: 1) D.M. Duncan, 'The Design of Ventilated Improved Pit Latrines' in *TAG Technical Notes no. 13* and 2) Collins et. al. *Where there is no toilet*.

SUMMARY

1 Village health workers from their own community have more difficulty starting work than outsiders. But later on they are more stable and committed.
2 The tasks of village health workers should be well defined and explained to the community to avoid wrong expectations.
3 Village health workers must be well supported by the health services.

References
Collins, R. et. al., *Where there is no toilet* (in press, David Philip Publishers, expected 1989)
Duncan, D.M., 'The Design of Ventilated Improved Pit Latrines' in *TAG Technical Notes no 13* (World Bank, Washington, D.C., 1984)
GATE, *Helping People in Poor Countries Develop: fuel-saving cookstoves* (German Appropriate Technology Exchange, 1980)
Volunteers for Technical Assistance, *Wood Conserving Cook Stoves: a design guide* (Maryland, USA, 1980)

27

Starting a cooperative – Development and health

Lerisa's baby clinic was running well. Most of the mothers brought their children regularly for weighing and a check-up. Lerisa didn't forget to examine the children's eyes for conjunctivitis and trachoma. She was satisfied that trachoma cases were now rare and hadn't increased since the Health Carers had turned to other health problems.

However, the children's state of nutrition had not improved. Lerisa was worried. According to the Road to Health Charts nearly every third child was underweight. Why? People knew how to make good weaning food and had vegetables. Yet malnutrition remained. She decided to bring the problem to the Carers' meeting.

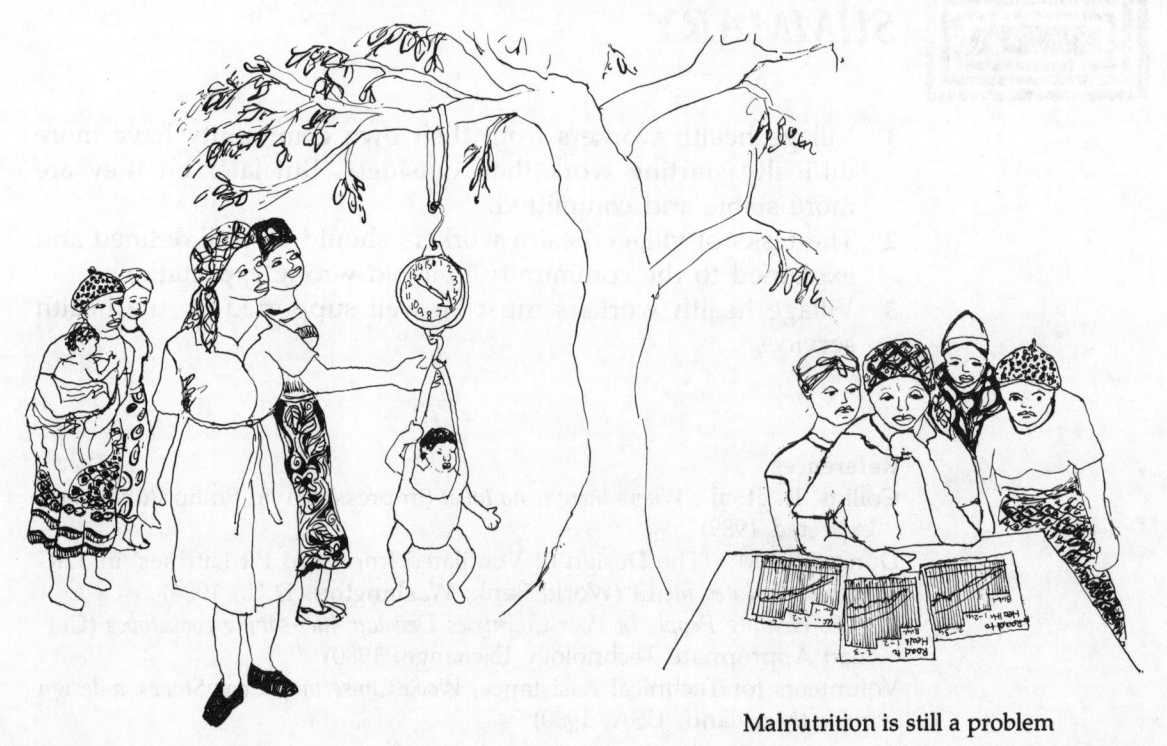

Malnutrition is still a problem

158

The group members voiced many suggestions:

'Most mothers are careless and don't want to change their ways.'

'It's easier to give a child maize porridge from the family pot than to cook a special mixture just for the baby.'

'Maybe our teaching isn't good, and the people have not understood our message.'

'Some of the mothers work on the farm and are away all day. The grannies don't look after the little ones well enough.'

Ma-Anna listened quietly to what the others had to say. Her own experience had been different. 'I think a lot of what you say is true. But look at my children. I know how I should feed them and I try hard. But Rose and Musa are still below the line on the chart. My problem is money. We couldn't grow beans and peanuts in the drought, and I can't afford to buy them at the shop.'

There was an uneasy silence after Ma-Anna spoke. Ma-Anna was right. The problem was not ignorance. People simply did not have the money to practice what they knew.

They felt helpless. They could not wipe out poverty. The chief's wife confirmed that there were no jobs.

'How can we get money?'

'We used to sell handicrafts.'

'But nobody buys them anymore.'

'What about our vegetables? I'm sure people would buy them.'

'But what will our children eat?'

Ma-Anna had a good idea. She introduced it carefully. 'We should work together and try to grow more vegetables to sell.' She saw the worried faces and knew what they were thinking. 'Not on our own plots. We must find another big plot to share.'

They decided to ask the chief for a plot for a communal garden and work together to grow vegetables and peanuts for everyone to buy at a price they could afford.

'We'll make money and the people can make good baby food.'

The plan became reality. The chief allocated a plot of land big enough for vegetables, peanuts and beans. Mr Sibila managed to provide fencing at the wholesale price. Hanyane people, and many from neighbouring villages, were eager to buy fresh vegetables directly from the fields. The growers worked collectively and shared the profits equally. Naturally, quarrels occurred, especially about who was allowed to take part in the cooperative and who was not. However, the group had grown in the spirit of cooperation and learned how to settle their own differences.

Neighbouring communities had heard of the Hanyane Carers for some time but never bothered to go there and find out more. Now that they knew they could buy fresh vegetables at a fair price, they came to Hanyane and met the Carers. They learned about their diverse activities and could see the results. This stimulated them to start their own 'Carer Groups'. The Hanyane group helped them, sharing their experiences.

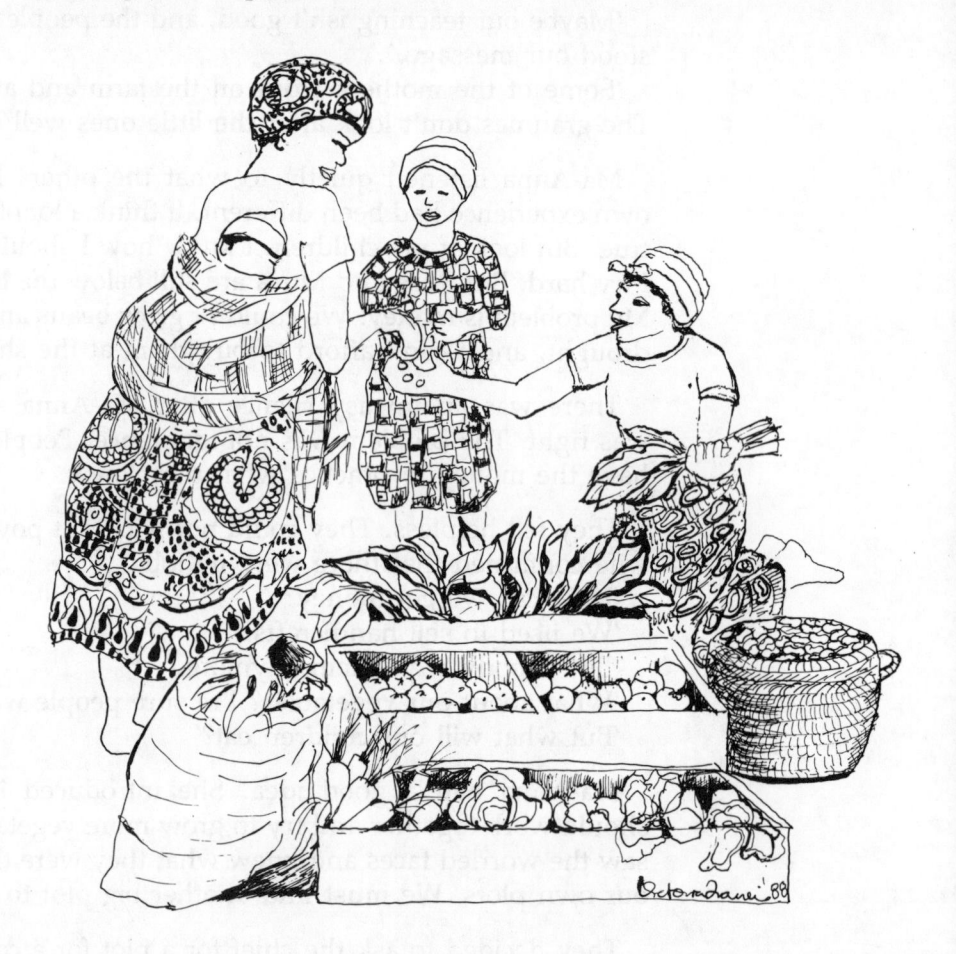

A whole network of Health Carer groups developed, linking together and learning many things from one another.

QUESTIONS

1. What could be the reasons in your area for malnutrition remaining a serious problem?
2. What is a cooperative? What are its advantages and what are its pitfalls?
3. What could you do in your area to help people to get some income?
4. Is the gardening cooperative in Hanyane all that is needed to solve the people's problems?

DISCUSSION

There is disagreement in primary health care thinking about the best way to start a project. Some think you should begin through village development activities – this is the development, or 'bottom up', approach. Others think programmes should be directed by a medical person from above – these are 'top down' projects.

The two approaches look like this:

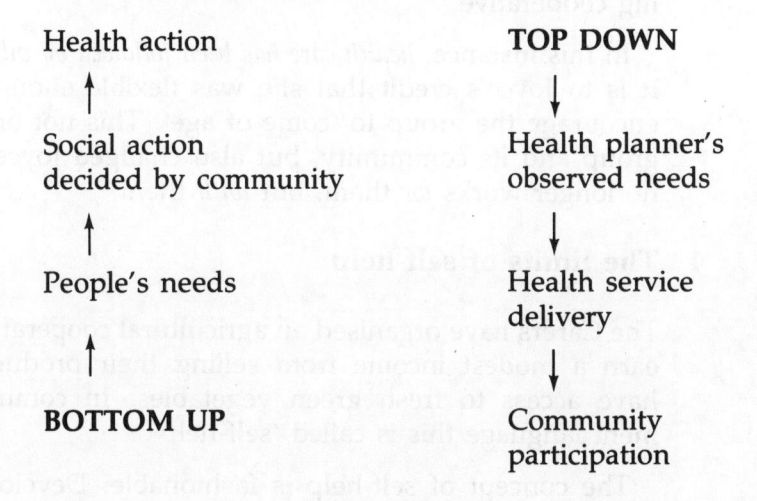

Health action	**TOP DOWN**
↑	↓
Social action decided by community	Health planner's observed needs
↑	↓
People's needs	Health service delivery
	↓
BOTTOM UP	Community participation

1 The 'bottom up' approach

Projects starting with development from the 'bottom up' approach have the advantage that people learn faster to plan and work together. They learn to see which essentials of life they are lacking and what they can do about them for themselves. This also makes them more aware of health needs. Their experience in development activities enables them to be more self-assured about making their demands on health matters to those in control.

2 The 'top down' approach

The opposite, the 'top down' approach, starts with health workers telling people what to do. People are made dependent and adopt an attitude of 'sit-and-wait' for health to be delivered to them.

The traditional and commonly adopted method in health care is the 'top down' approach. It is easier for everybody. Health workers can pass on what they have learned without much imagination. The people do, or more often don't do, what they have been told. Health officials may believe that this is effective primary health care with 'community participation'.

3 The integrated approach

The Hanyane project does not fit into either of the two categories described above. When Joyce started work at her clinic she used the traditional 'top down' method. Her own training experience had been to be ordered from above, so she did the same to those in her care. She told the people how they had to change their ways. But gradually the Hanyane people began to take things into their own hands. Over the years the group has attained sufficient self-assurance and strength to be able to organise its own well functioning cooperative.

In this instance, *health care has been followed by village development*. It is to Joyce's credit that she was flexible enough to allow and encourage the group to 'come of age'. This not only changed the group and its community, but also changed Joyce's attitude. She no longer works *for* them, but *with* them.

4 The limits of self-help

The Carers have organised an agricultural cooperative. The women earn a modest income from selling their products, and people have access to fresh green vegetables. In community development language this is called 'self-help'.

The concept of self-help is fashionable. Development agencies prefer to support self-help programmes rather than any others. Poor people should not passively wait for charity. They should make their own efforts to improve the quality of their lives through improving their own socio-economic situation.

How realistic is this expectation? Do you believe the cooperative has really changed the 'socio-economic position' in Hanyane? You will agree that at best the improvements in terms of income are minimal. Vegetables are sold at a low price so that the people can afford to buy them. As a result of this the earnings are little more than the cost of seeds and fencing.

It is unrealistic to expect those who struggle to survive to help themselves out of proverty. The benefits of self-help programmes will be severely limited as long as economic and political powers continue to control and exploit the poor. Having said that, we must stress that in terms of human values and the morale of a people, self-help programmes can have a tremendous impact. In Hanyane, people have found their dignity. They now have hope and trust that things are changing when they join hands. This has not only changed life in Hanyane, it has also had a ripple effect on neighbouring villages. In addition the newly acquired organisational skills may equip the people to work for more fundamental changes if and when they see a need for it.

SUMMARY

1. The 'bottom up' approach in health care starts with community development, leading to self-directed health action. The 'top down' approach starts with health care directed from above. In many projects, health care and community development overlap.
2. Self-help projects by poor communities are limited by social, economic and political structures. But self-help programmes can develop skills in people to work for more fundamental change.

28

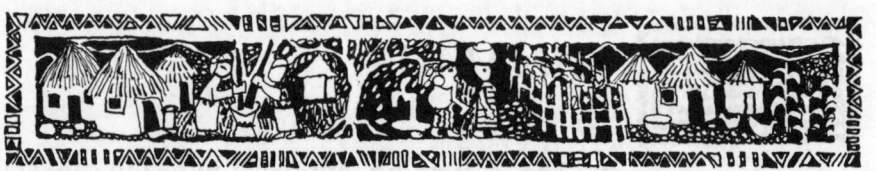

Who are we working for?
– The question of payment

Not all the new Health Carer groups were in Joyce's clinic area. Some were in villages belonging to a different clinic where the nurse in charge was not aware of the way the health carers functioned.

One of these groups was keen on teaching the people how to prepare the 'diarrhoea drink'. Diarrhoea was their main worry. They did a good job. Many mothers saved their babies' lives with the drink. They told the nurse about their successes. The nurse, too, had noticed that less children were taken to the clinic with diarrhoea. So she told the group that it was not fair for them to work for the health of the people without being paid. She and the community health worker, who did the same job, had their regular salary.

From then on the group was unhappy. They stopped working and continued to ask the nurse for money. The nurse didn't know what to do because she had no idea where she could find it. The group decided to ask Lerisa and the Hanyane group to help them solve their problem. They joined the meeting in Hanyane on a day when Joyce was with the Carers.

The Hanyane group was surprised about the idea of payment. They had never thought of such a thing. Their group had grown out of the need to know more about trachoma. It was natural for them to try to do something to protect their children and themselves from the disease. It was for their own benefit that they helped each other.

Ma-Anna added, 'Every mother wants to have healthy children. Have you ever heard of a mother being paid for caring for her own house and children?'

'We felt the same when we started,' the leader of the new group said. 'It was only after the nurse told us that we should be paid that we noticed that the others working in the community are paid.

They are just like us – why shouldn't we get paid?'

Joyce did not want to interfere. It was a delicate and important issue each group had to work out amongst themselves. Her worry was that suddenly all groups would want to be paid. This might be the end of the Carers. A story came to her mind which she thought could help. Look at the illustrations below and on page 166 to see her story.

The Question of Payment. Joyce's Story.

1. Once upon a time there was a very poor family. The father had died many years before. The mother, her sister-in-law and her five children had nothing to eat. They could do nothing because they had nothing.

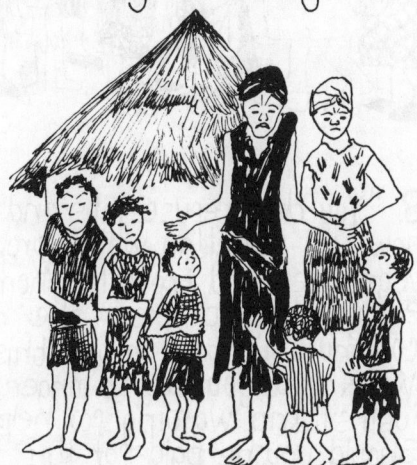

2. For a while the neighbours helped them but they were too poor themselves to go on helping forever. One day they stopped helping them altogether.

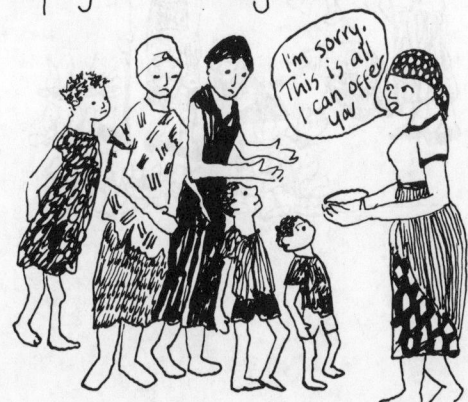

"I'm sorry. This is all I can offer you."

3. The family got more and more miserable, the children cried for food. One day the shopkeeper happened to pass near their house. He heard the children crying and went to see what was wrong.

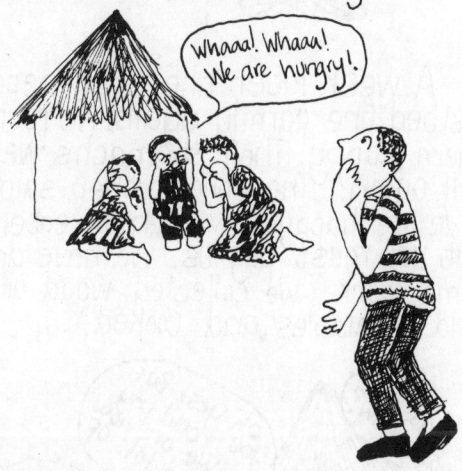

"Whaaa! Whaaa! We are hungry!"

4. He felt great pity for them and brought them a big bag of maize from his shop. The family was very happy.

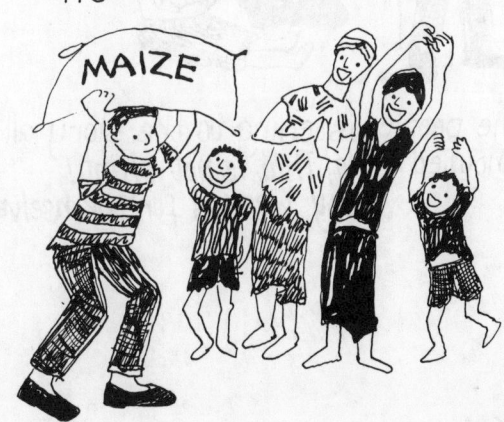

5. They cooked the maize and fetched some wild vegetables to add as a relish.

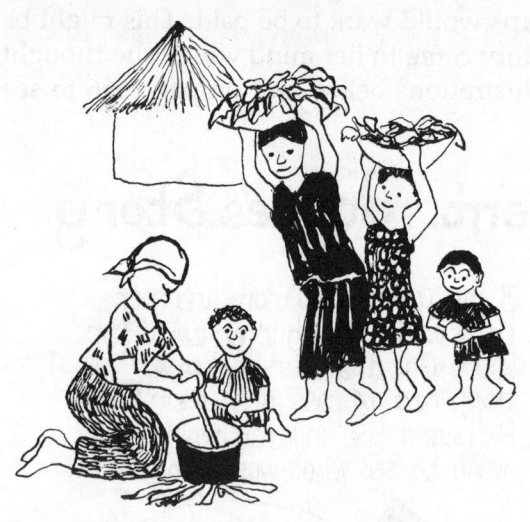

6. A week later the shopkeeper visited the family again. He found them happy! Their stomachs were full again. Then the mother said: "We are happy now we have eaten. But you must pay us. We have done some work. We collected wood and wild vegetables and cooked."

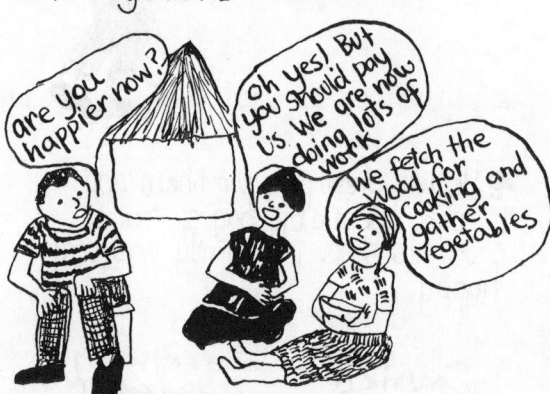

are you happier now?

Oh yes! But you should pay us. We are now doing lots of work

We fetch the wood for cooking and gather vegetables

The people listening to the story all shouted: "No! That is not right! They worked for themselves!"

7. Nurse Joyce said: "When you were burdened with the problem of eye disease, you were like the poor family— you could do nothing because you had nothing; you had no knowledge. You could only wait for help. Then we brought you knowledge about Trachoma. With this knowledge you could do many things."

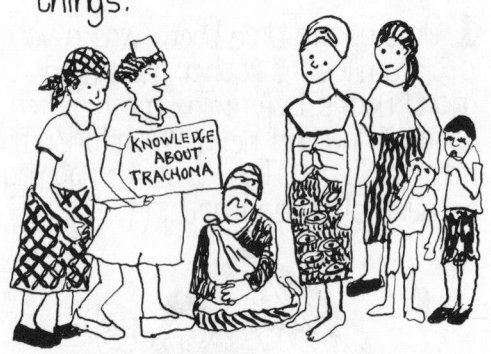

KNOWLEDGE ABOUT TRACHOMA

8. "You dug refuse pits and now you use clean water, grow vegetables and treat trachoma early. Many people in the community take part in this work and you are no longer just sitting waiting for help. Should you be paid for it?"

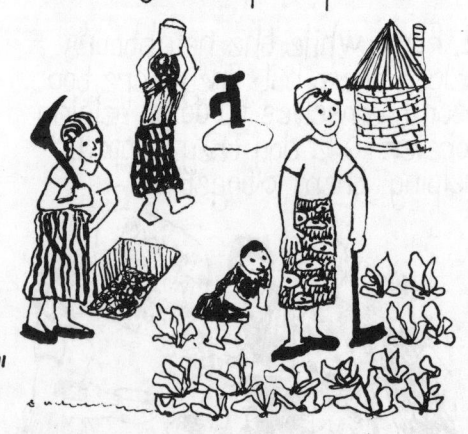

QUESTIONS

1. Do you think groups like the Carers should be paid? If yes, who should pay them?
2. Can you think of other ways of showing appreciation of the Carers' work?
3. If you want to start a Health Carer group in your area, how would you go about it? What would be suitable for your area?

DISCUSSION

The issue of payment is a serious source of conflict in most community health projects. It is bound to come up as soon as movements such as the Carers expand and become established. Welfare and religious organisations would like to see more voluntary work done in under-served communities. Financial resources are scarce in most developing countries. In addition, social services are often the first and hardest hit when government expenditure is cut. Therefore social development depends, to a large extent, on voluntary input.

In our story we have introduced two different types of grassroots health workers:
1) the group of Health Carers, and
2) Lerisa, the village health worker.

When Lerisa returned to Hanyane we mentioned that tensions between her and the Carers might arise over the question of payment. Lerisa is paid while the Carers are not. In Hanyane this has not caused any problems. Lerisa and the Health Carers discussed the matter and accepted the difference. What do you think has been the outcome of their discussions? Before reading on give your answer to the questions in Table 28.1 on page 168.

Voluntary care or paid occupation?

According to Lund, there are some valid arguments for and against unpaid voluntary work:

a) It is, in itself, a good thing to work for the welfare of the community. Many voluntary workers find a personal joy and feeling of pride in contributing to their community's future.

b) Many societies have had a culturally inherent sense of caring for needy members in their community like the old, the sick, the

Topics discussed	Outcome of discussion for	
	Lerisa	Health Carers
1 How much time should be spent on health care?		
2 Should there be fixed working hours?		
3 Who decides on tasks to be carried out?		
4 Who are they responsible to?		
5 Can she/they be dismissed? By whom?		

Table 28.1

orphans. Reviving and nurturing these old traditions could counteract destructive effects of modernisation. In contrast to the rich, poor people have a wonderful capacity to help each other and share resources.

c) Payment – usually from outside sources – fosters dependency on the sponsoring organisations or institutions. This would hamper the development towards self-reliance of a people.

The Carers have learned to recognise the roots of their problems and to take decisions about what they can and cannot do to improve things. When they see that a task needs to be done, like digging refuse pits, they do it with an enthusiasm which does not count the hours spent.

However, the Carers are mothers and wives whose first task is to look after their family and work in the fields. Some also have income generating activities like chicken rearing. Other things like sharing knowledge with their neighbours and working for community projects must be done in their spare time. During ploughing and harvesting seasons there is no spare time. So these activities come to a halt.

Village health workers must be able to devote time, during all seasons, to attend to the various needs of the people. Like Lerisa, they have their well defined programme of home visiting, child health clinic, and attending to minor ailments. Lerisa is expected to work at least half-time. This means that she has less time to pursue the productive activities she used to do to get the extra cash she desperately needs. If compensated, she will give of her time without losing vital income. It is unrealistic to expect regular routine work on a voluntary basis.

What about the Carers who remain unpaid volunteers? They certainly would deserve some kind of encouragement and signs of appreciation. You may have some ideas, like competition parties between various groups, or scarves or badges to identify group members. A pat on the back encourages us to continue.

SUMMARY

1 In poor countries financial resources for social and health services are scarce. Social development therefore relies to a great extent on voluntary work. However, those most in need of development are the poorest who struggle to survive. It is unrealistic to expect them to spend time on unpaid work.
2 Health Carer groups and village health workers differ. Groups do their work if they feel a need and when they have time and feel like doing it. A village health worker has his/her definite programme and regular work and is in a position of employment. This ensures continuity.

Reference
Lund, F.J., *The Community-Based Approach to Development* (Dissertation, 1987) – available through Centre for Social Development Studies, University of Natal, Durban, South Africa)

29

Learning from the past
– The Health Carers look back

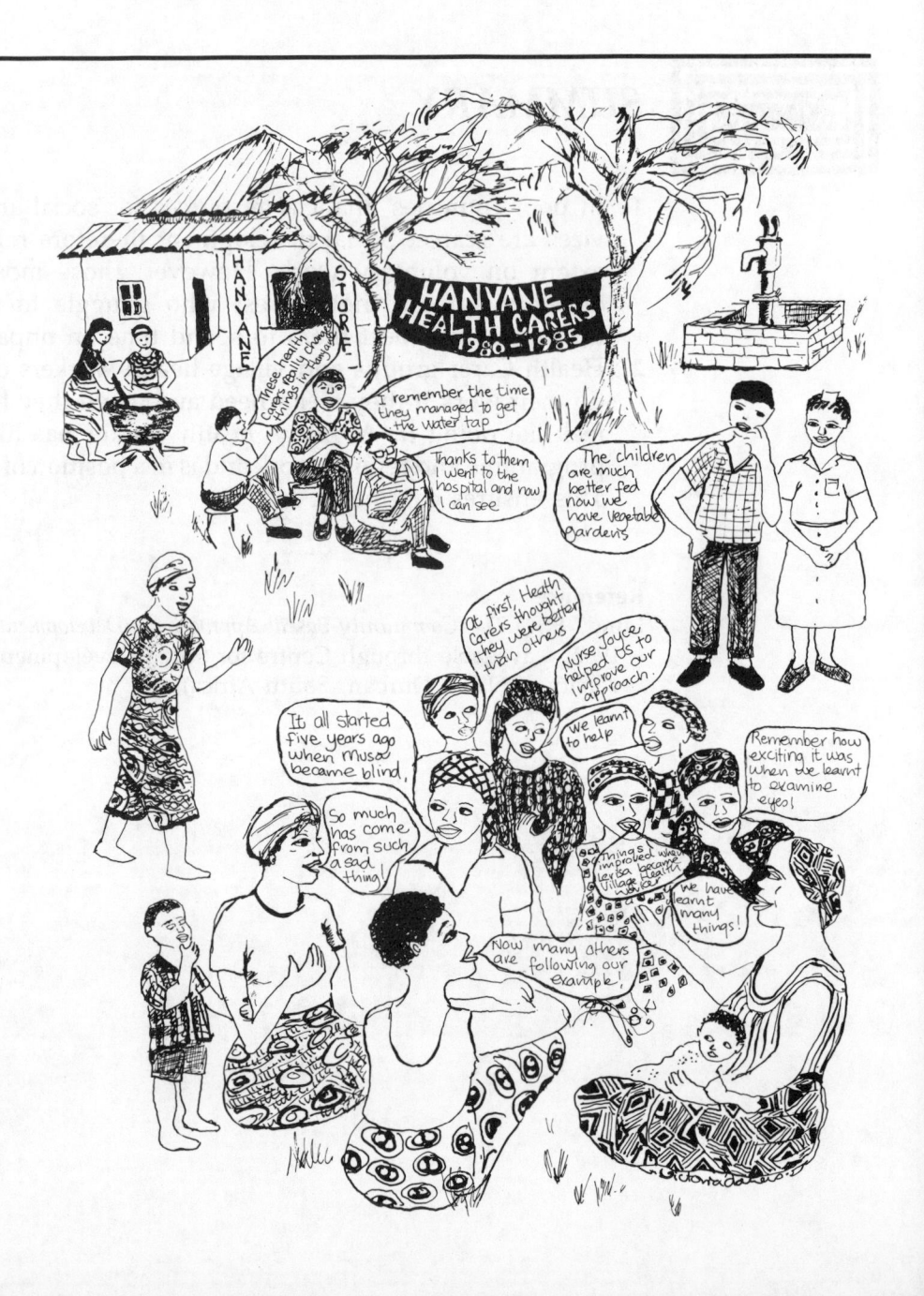

The Carers celebrated the group's fifth birthday. Their thoughts went back to the past, how it all began, how they progressed, the ups and downs. Memories came back, pictures appeared and disappeared in their minds like a slide show. They shared their stories which were interrupted with bursts of laughter when they recalled funny events or realised what silly things they had sometimes done.

Joyce and Lerisa wanted to make the most of this large gathering. The people there had a wealth of experience to look back on. They could use these experiences – both good and bad – to learn from and to plan for the future. Joyce and Lerisa prepared an exercise for the Health Carers to look critically at their successes and failures while still having fun.

Lerisa gathered the group around a board on which was written 'Hanyane Health Carers – five years on. Self-evaluation.'
'What is this?' asked one of the women.
'Are you going to teach us something here at this party?'
'What is written on that paper?'

Lerisa reminded them of the time they used the beans to evaluate their success in the fight against trachoma. Now they would look back at what had happened with the progress of their group. She turned over the paper and showed the picture she had drawn. 'This is Hanyane five years ago. My drawing is not very good but what do you see?'
'The people are crying.'
'Some are rubbing their eyes.'
'They are crying alone.'
'There is a blind person.'
'There are flies.'

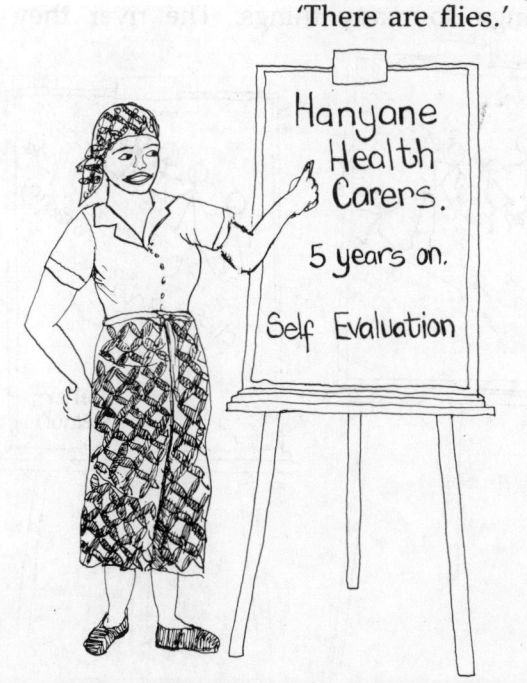

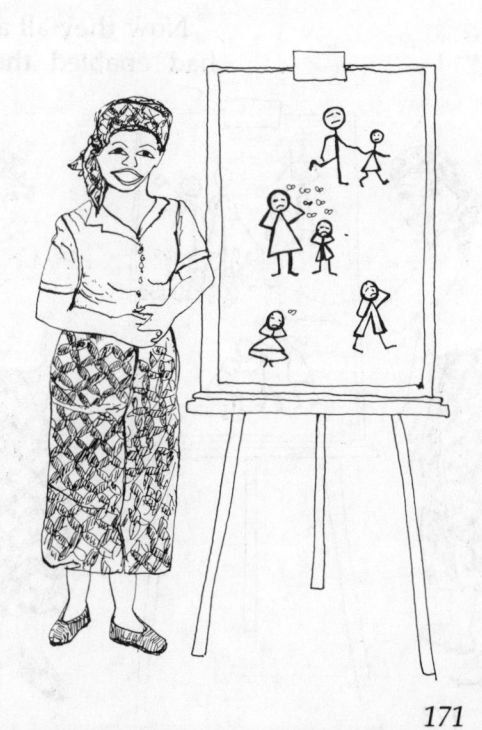

171

The picture reminded them of the time when there were no toilets, no refuse pits, no vegetable gardens; when they were afraid to go to the clinic and when they were even more afraid of the chief. At that time people felt hopeless and powerless and alone in their troubles.

Lerisa turned over the page again to show her picture of Hanyane today. They were delighted with her attempts and pointed out all the things which had changed:
'The people are happy.'
'There is clean water.'
'We have vegetable gardens.'
'We are helping each other.'
'We are proud.'

The next question was: 'How do you think we have managed to change things so much?' This led to much discussion in which people praised the efforts of Joyce, the chief, Lerisa, Mr Sibila, and the doctor.

Joyce stood up and said, 'Thank you for your compliments but you are forgetting the most important people. Look around you.'

The Carers began congratulating each other and said, 'We could do nothing when we were alone. When we began working together we could change things.'

Lerisa turned to the next picture. It showed people crossing a river. The crowd was delighted with this and spontaneously began singing the well known song about how it is impossible to cross a river alone.

Now they all agreed that it was their strength as a group which had enabled them to change so many things. The river they

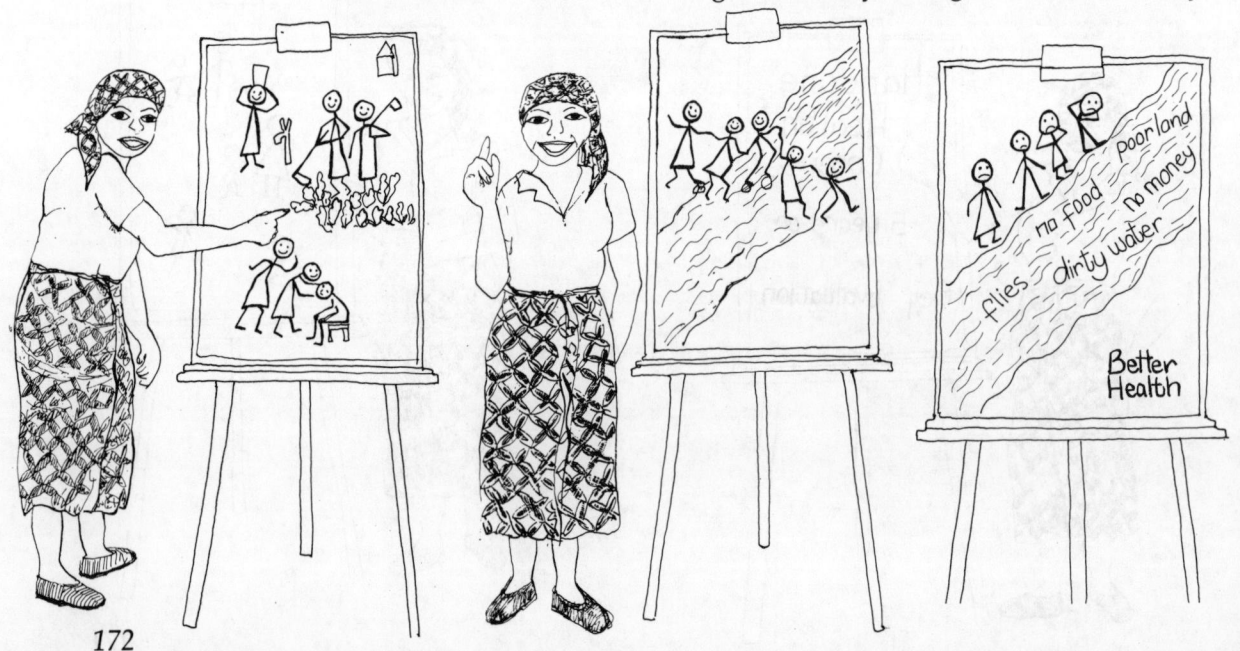

172

crossed represented the many problems separating them from better health. The first part of the evaluation exercise was to name some of these problems.

In order to cross this river, they had joined hands. But there had been problems with that too. The second part of the exercise was to name some of the things which had prevented them from joining hands and working together, like:
- Isolation of the poor – people like Ma-Anna did not join in at first.
- Despondency – people believed that there was nothing they could do.
- Elitism – the Tidy Ladies did not want others to join them.
- Superiority – some felt better than others and behaved like policemen.
- Lack of trust – people were reluctant to share in a communal garden.

The last part of the exercise was to share ideas about what they had to do in the future. These were listed under two headings – 'Health and Village Development' and 'Health Carer Movement' – as shown in Table 29.1:

Health and village development	Health Carer movement
Maintenance of water tap	Ongoing self-evaluation – group should meet four times a year to look at health problems and inter-group difficulties
Cooperatives should develop more income generating projects, e.g. brick making, grain milling	Networking with other groups
Training of traditional birth attendants	Leadership training
Water reservoir for the gardens	Workshops to introduce new skills e.g. weaning food preparation, teaching methods, chicken rearing
Pre-school activities for children	
Literacy classes for adults	

Table 29.1

QUESTIONS

1. In what ways does the self-evaluation differ from the evaluation discussed in Chapter 20?
2. As an outsider, how would you go about evaluating the Hanyane Health Carers' project?
3. Do you know a traditional song about working together from your own area?

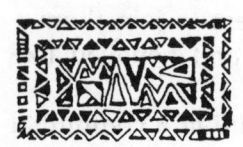

DISCUSSION

1 Primary eye care and primary health care

In tracing the pathway of the group we recognise these stages:
a) Control of trachoma.
b) Improving general health.
c) Improving the quality of life in the village (development).

Are we then right to say the book is about community eye health? Except for a few chapters, there was not much talk about eyes.

What we have been discussing so far in this book is how eye health is *included* in the general health of both the individual and the community. Eye health in a community and the prevention of blindness are dependent on:

- Good environmental hygiene
  (to prevent trachoma, seasonal conjunctivitis).
- Good nutrition, availability of fruit and vegetables
  (to prevent xerophthalmia).
- Accessible health services
  (measles vaccination to prevent post-measles blindness; entropion repair; cataract and glaucoma operations; treatment of conjunctivitis of the newborn and of ocular trauma).
- Good education
  (early diagnosis of glaucoma at the time when people first notice a change in vision or ask for reading glasses).
- Development to relieve poverty
  (to eliminate the root cause for the lack of the items above).

> GENERAL HEALTH AND DEVELOPMENT
> ARE ESSENTIAL FOR EYE HEALTH

2 Evaluation

Joyce and Lerisa worked out a simple evaluation exercise to help the Carers look at their strengths and weaknesses. The exercise in which they all participated gave them a framework to organise their experiences and use them in a positive way. The exercise could be adapted to help people look critically at their own projects.

It is sometimes useful to look separately at **task functions** and **group functions**.

Task functions

In looking at task functions, we examine how well the task, in this case health and village development, is being accomplished.

Group functions

In looking at group functions we are more concerned with how the group is functioning. Are people working together? Are decisions taken democratically? Who are the leaders? What tensions exist in the group? Does the group include members from all sections of the society?

It is not always easy to get people talking openly about these things. Games and exercises, such as the one Lerisa devised, can help. You will find more ideas in M.T. Feuerstein's, *Partners in Evaluation*.

3 Visual aids for self-evaluation

Lerisa's drawings, simple as they were, helped to focus the group's attention on the self-evaluation and acted as a trigger for discussion. Make a series of simple pictures that might encourage this sort of discussion amongst your own working team.

SUMMARY

1. It is important for groups to look critically at their progress.
2. In conducting a self-evaluation programme, it is useful to examine both task accomplishments and group processes.
3. Factors on which eye health depend are listed on page 174.
4. Factors which hamper group cooperation are listed on page 173.

Reference
Feuerstein, M.T., *Partners in Evaluation* (Macmillan, London, 1986)

30

Planning for the future – The struggle continues

Health Carer groups continued to be formed in most villages in the district. These groups helped to bring about subtle changes in the villagers' attitudes. Ma-Anna was a good example of how even the poorest gained confidence and strength from joining with others. Five years earlier, she was the silent victim of poverty and disease. She felt too ashamed of her status to join in any community activities. She had lost one son and Musa had become blind. She must have felt that life treated her harshly and there was nothing she could do about it. When she saved Musa with the rehydration drink, she discovered for the first time that she *could* do something and this gave her faith in herself and in the Health Carers. She joined them and gained in confidence and vision: it was she who saw the potential for a vegetable growing co-operative and took a leading role. Her circumstances had not changed through a miracle or the much longed-for return of her husband, rich from the city. She had changed in her ability to cope with, and improve, her life. The Health Carer groups were made up of people just like Ma-Anna.

As the movement of Health Carers was growing rapidly, some sort of overall organisation became essential. The groups wanted to keep in contact with each other to co-ordinate their activities and to learn from each other. They decided to form a Health Carers' Association with their own office holders. This meant they were no longer dependent on Joyce as a leader and teacher. They were strong enough to continue on their own.

Through all these years, the doctor had watched the events with keen interest. He often discussed it with Joyce and helped her to meet people with special knowledge about village improvement. Together they learned a lot from their successes and even more from their mistakes. They found they were most successful when they had the patience to go at the pace of the people, with a gentle push here and there. Most of the disasters happened when they pushed too hard or ignored the opinions of the Carers and imposed their own ideas.

The successes in Hanyane encouraged the doctor to train more nurses in eye care. Joyce had been promoted to the main health centre. She was now responsible for the community eye care of the whole district, including Hanyane village. She trained the new ophthalmic nurses in community and preventive work and taught basic eye care to the village health workers.

Now not only Hanyane but many other villages could join in the struggle for eye health. The doctor was no longer alone in his fight aganist blindness. The communities were all part of it. He discovered that he learned more from the people of Hanyane and other places than he could teach them. The eye nurses and community health workers formed the essential link between the people and the hospital. The doctor supported and supervised the whole blindness prevention scheme. He had more time now for patients with serious problems who needed special care.

Look at the illustration below to see what eye care in the area looked like.

Joyce was glad that her new job allowed her to keep in touch with her old clinic and with Hanyane. The bond of friendship remained. Although the Carers were obviously able to function without her, she often went there to visit them. There was another good reason for maintaining ties with Hanyane: she was soon to be married to Mr Sibila, the local agricultural extension officer.

REFERRAL AND KNOWLEDGE CHAIN

Rural Blindness Prevention Scheme

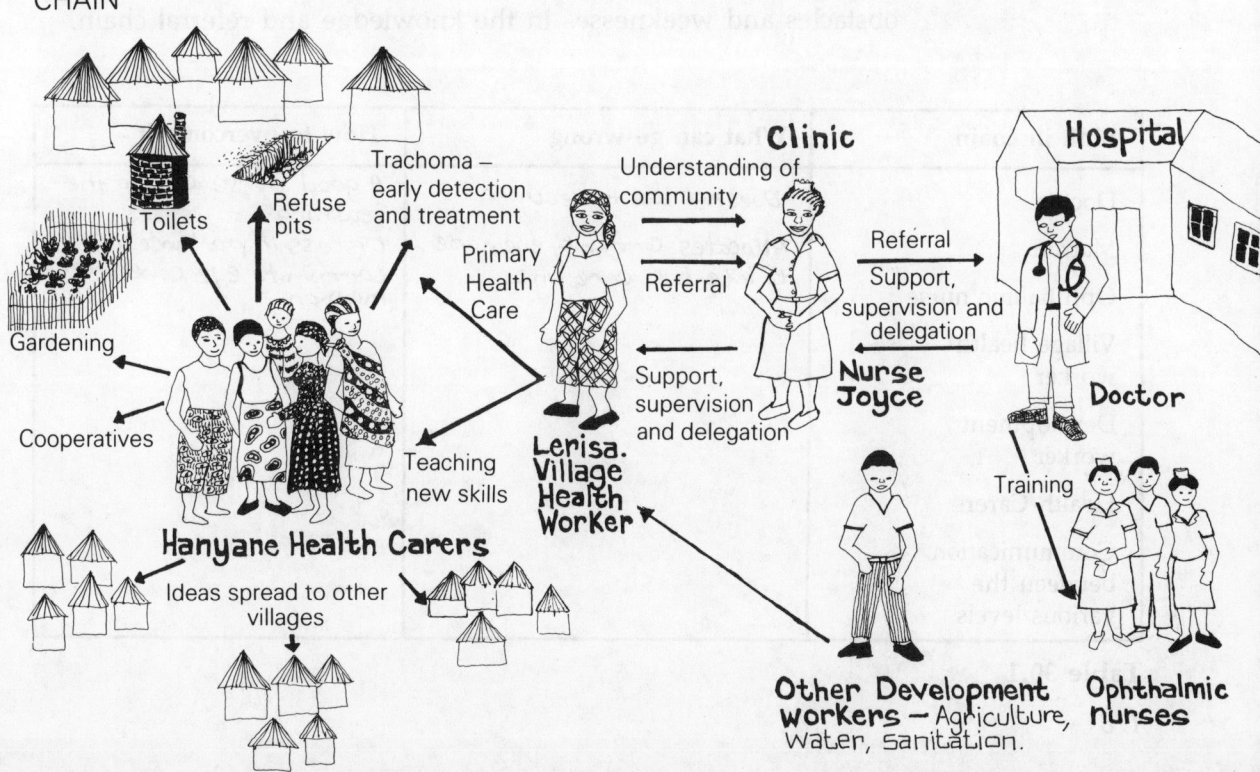

And what about Musa, who started it all? He was admitted to a school for blind children and is learning to walk by himself using a stick, to look after himself and even to cultivate and farm a plot of land. He is also learning to read with his fingers.

QUESTIONS

1. What are the constraints concerning health promotion and community organisations in your area?
2. Are you working within a blindness prevention scheme? How could it be improved further?
3. How do you understand your own role as a primary eye care worker?

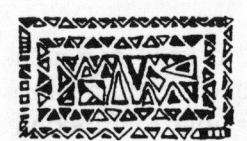

DISCUSSION

1 The limitations of blindness prevention programmes

We have reached the end of the story. It started with a blind child, Musa, and ends with a promise of good eye care for a whole district. The rural blindness prevention scheme in the illustration on page 177 shows an ideal situation. In practice, there are many obstacles and weaknesses in the knowledge and referral chain.

Link in chain	What can go wrong	How to overcome it
Doctor	Does not like to teach.	A good nurse can do the teaching.
Matron	Allocates community eye nurse to intensive care unit.	Discuss importance of community eye care with matron.
Ophthalmic nurse		
Village health worker		
Development worker		
Health Carers		
Communication between the various levels		

Table 30.1

Exercise

With the help of the illustration on page 177, list what could go wrong at each link in the referral chain, and how to overcome it. The examples in Table 30.1 show you what we mean.

Having done that, answer the following questions for yourself:
a) In your own situation where do you fit in to such a scheme?
b) What are your personal problems with referrals and communication?
c) What can you do to improve the function of your scheme?
d) Are you free to exercise all your abilities, or are you restricted by regulations or superiors who do not trust your skills?

2 Delegation

This last question leads us to the art of *delegation*. Few people are good at it. David Morley makes some useful comments about delegation in the book *Paediatric Priorities in the Developing World*, p. 386 ff. Read through the following points. For each one try to find an example from the story.

- Delegation is *not* ordering somebody to do a certain job in a certain way.
- Good delegation means trusting the lesser skilled to do a job well.
- Trained people fear delegation because:
  i) The job may not be done well enough.
  ii) It is easier and quicker to do the job themselves than to train someone else.
- The lesser skilled may fear taking responsibility. Good training helps to overcome fear and leads to greater job satisfaction and confidence at all levels of health care.
- The person who delegates must continue to support the lesser skilled.
- Good delegation increases the efficiency and scope of a programme.
- The more people are trained and allowed to exercise their skills, the greater is the chance that a community-based eye care project will continue into the future.

3 Continuity

You have followed the growth of the Hanyane Health Carers. You may have some doubts about whether the groups will continue to function in the future. Many projects collapse as soon as the initiator leaves.

A village organisation is composed of people and is therefore a living body with its own unpredictable dynamics. It is to be expected that there will always be ups and downs, happy surprises and sad disappointments. Experience has shown that the effectiveness and stability of such groups depends, to a great deal, on their structure and the quality of leadership.

Structure

After Health Carer groups spread to other villages, they decided to form their own association. This was an important act of self-reliance. Without it the groups would be dependent on Joyce and the health services. Should they withdraw their support, the groups might easily disband.

Leadership

There are different types of leaders. Some make all decisions themselves and tell their group what to do. This type of leader is usually an authoritative person. He or she might hold an important position in the community and like to be in control of all activities taking place. Usually such a person is chosen as leader because people believe that no one else can do the job, and because they fear offending that person. Once in office, you will never get rid of him/her.

Other leaders encourage the group members to explore the situation themselves, to discuss the various possibilities of action and to take their own decisions. Such leadership fosters self-reliance.

You have learned enough in the course of the discussions to choose the type of leader you would like to have for your community groups. It may take years for groups to learn from experience how to choose their leaders. Unsuitable leaders may destroy the spirit of a group. You should therefore discuss the qualities of leadership with the group and make them conscious of its value.

It is a common problem for groups to be stuck with an unsuitable authoritative leader of whom they cannot be rid without getting into trouble. Here are two helpful strategies to overcome this problem:
a) Introduce rotating leadership, e.g. rule that no leader is allowed to stay longer than two years.
b) Create a number of sub-committees, e.g. a garden committee, a water committee, etc. Good leadership talents may be discovered when more people have a chance to take responsibility.

If you want to know more about leadership, read Anne Hope's *Training for Transformation* books 2 and 3.

SUMMARY

1 The functioning of a blindness prevention scheme integrated into general health care depends on the reliability of every member of the scheme and good communication between all levels of care.
2 Good delegation increases the efficiency and scope of a programme. Delegation means trusting the lesser skilled to do a job well.
3 The continuation of a community programme depends on a self-reliant structure and good leadership from within.

References
Hope, A. and Timmel, S., *Training for Transformation: A handbook for community workers* (Books 1–3, Mambo Press, Gweru, Zimbabwe, 1984)
Morley, D. *Paediatric Priorities in the Developing World* (Butterworth, Guildford, 1983)

CONCLUSION

While we wrote about the Hanyane Health Carers we had an actual project, the Elim Care Groups, in mind. The story is a summary of some of the successes and failures of these groups. There, a few women in three villages began with their activities to prevent trachoma. Thanks to people like Joyce and Lerisa, the project has grown from its modest beginnings into a large movement, engaging in health promotion and, in a number of places, in community development.

The Joyces, Lerisas and doctors of the Elim Care Group Project had to learn many things the hard way. They want to share with you the lessons painfully learned from mistakes they made so that you will not repeat them. The many happy experiences they had should encourage you not to give up when things go wrong.

> So, when you close this book:
>   Stand up and go to your people, work with them,
>   Believe in their abilities even when they disappoint you,
>   And you will discover
>   Hidden qualities in people who have learned
>   To move rocks
>   By joining hands.

PART 2
Common eye problems for village health workers

Contents

Introduction to Part Two — 185

SECTION A: How to examine an eye patient — 186
1. Taking a history — 187
2. Taking the visual acuity — 187
3. The normal eye — 188
4. Examination of the eye for abnormalities — 189

SECTION B: Making a diagnosis — 190
1. Acute red eye — 190
   - in babies — 190
   - in young children — 190
   - at any age — 192
   - due to injury — 194
2. Blindness — 195
3. Presbyopia – difficulty in reading — 197
4. Other eye diseases — 198

SECTION C: How to work in your eye clinic — 201
1. Equipment — 201
2. Medicines — 202
3. How to put eye medicine in the eye — 202
4. Keeping records — 202

SECTION D: Health teaching to prevent blindness — 204

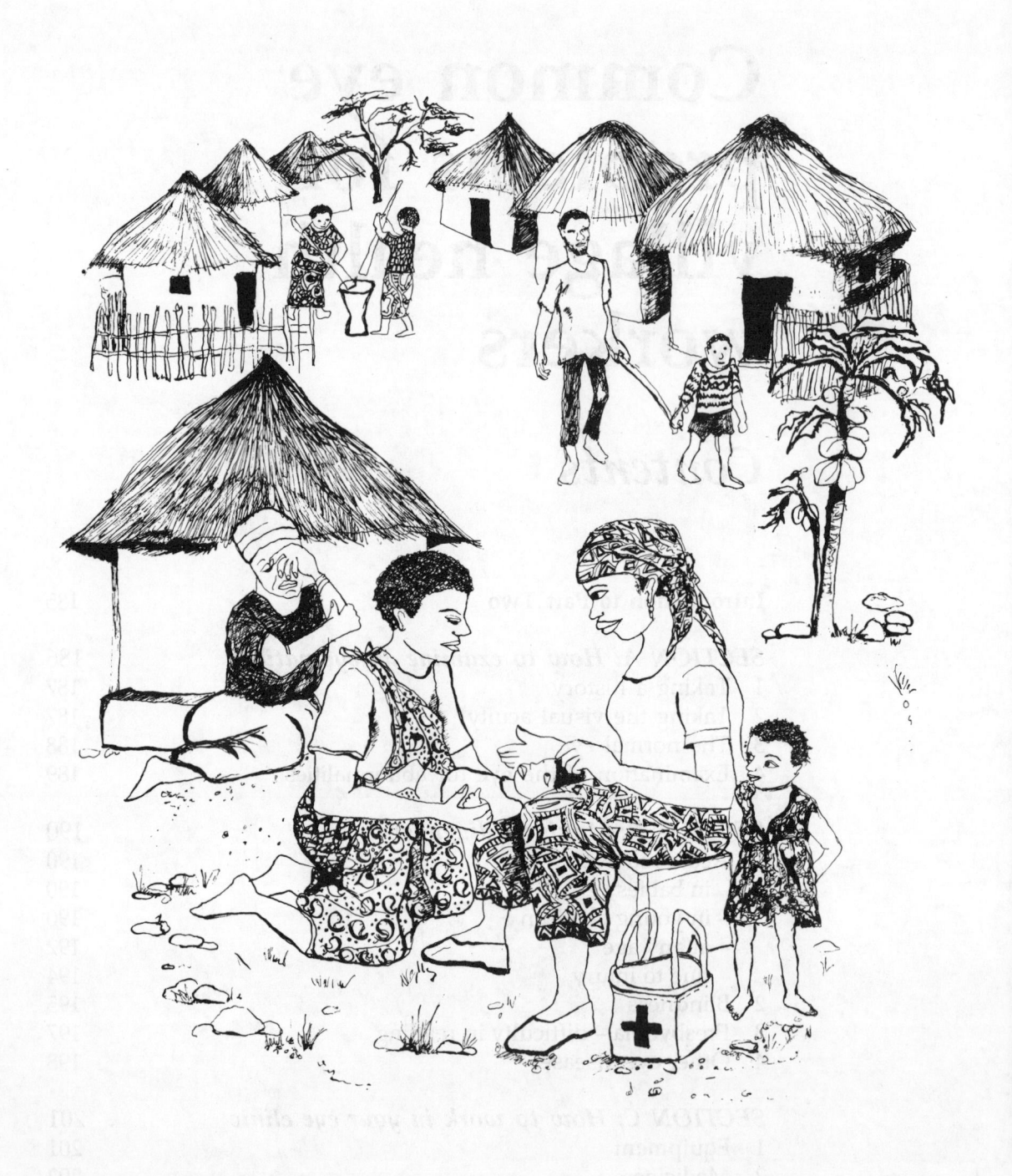

Introduction to Part Two

This part of the book is intended for health workers, like Lerisa, who work at the village level, have little or no formal teaching in eye care, and who have only basic equipment and medicines.

It is set out in four sections:

A – The first section shows the basic examination of an eye patient.
B – The second section is how to make a diagnosis and manage a patient with an eye problem.
C – The third section gives some advice on how to work in your clinic.
D – The fourth and last section gives some important information which can be taught to your individual patient and to the community at large in order to prevent eye disease and blindness.

Some eye conditions can be treated in the village with antibiotics. Some eye patients can be examined, diagnosed and reassured that there is nothing too serious. However, if a patient has a red *very* painful eye from whatever cause, or if the patient is blind in both eyes, he should be referred for more expert help.

SECTION A:
How to examine an eye patient

There are **four** steps to know and follow when you examine eye patients (Figure 1):
1. Take a history of the patient's eye problem.
2. Measure the visual acuity in each eye.
3. Know the findings in a normal eye.
4. Examine your patient for abnormalities of the eye.

1. TAKING A HISTORY

2. TAKING THE VISUAL ACUITY

3. THE NORMAL EYE

4. EXAMINING THE EYE FOR ABNORMALITIES

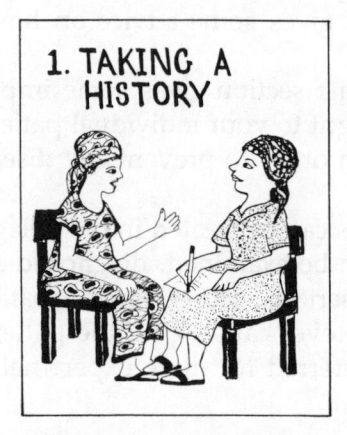

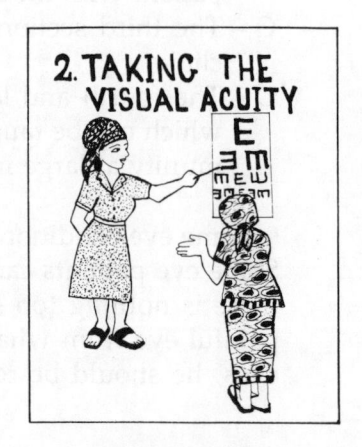

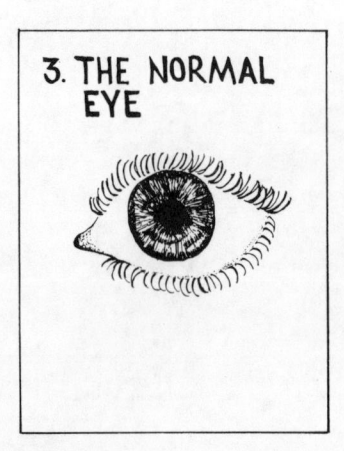

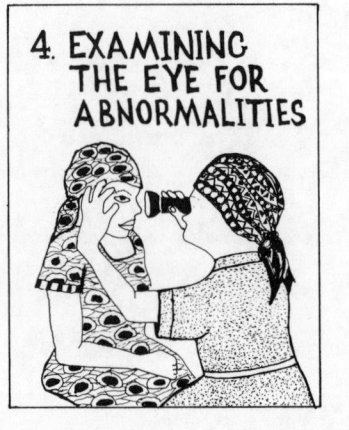

Figure 1
Four steps in examining an eye patient

1 Taking a history (Figure 2)

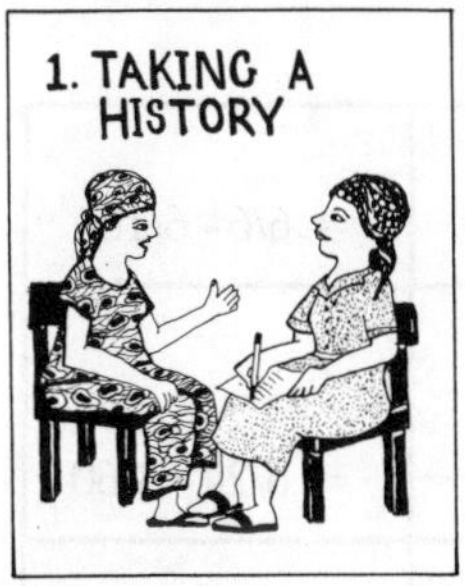

Figure 2
Taking a history

Start by asking your patient what his eye problem is. Eye complaints can be divided into **four** major groups:
1. The eye is red and painful   ACUTE RED EYE
2. The patient cannot see   BLIND
3. The patient cannot read clearly   PRESBYOPIA
4. Any other specific complaint   OTHER EYE DISEASES

Decide which group your patient belongs to. This will help you to make a definite diagnosis.

2 Taking the visual acuity (Figure 3)

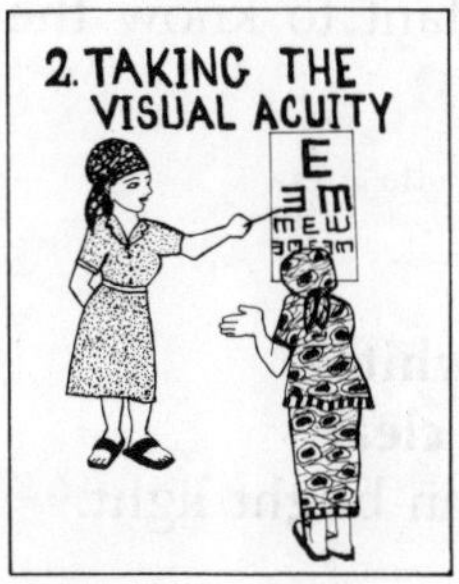

Figure 3
Taking the visual acuity

Having taken the history it is now very important to measure the VISUAL ACUITY in each eye. First the vision in the *right* eye (VR) and then the vision in the *left* eye (VL).

To measure the visual acuity in each eye, follow these steps:
1. The patient should stand or sit 6 metres (6 long steps) from the visual acuity chart.
2. Close the *left* eye with an eye pad or the patient's own hand, so that he can only see with his *right* eye.
3. Now hold the visual acuity or E chart up to the patient at 6 metres and ask him to read, or to point in which direction the 'three legs' go – up, down, right or left. If he can read the 18 line or better at 6 metres he has GOOD VISION in that eye.
4. If he cannot read the 18 line at 6 metres, then try the 60 line, but now at 3 metres from the patient. If he can read the 60 line at 3 metres (but not the 18 line at 6 metres) he has POOR VISION.
5. If he cannot read the 60 line at 3 metres then he is BLIND in that eye.
6. If he is blind then ask him if he is able to see *daylight* or a *bright torch* shone into his eye. If he cannot see light, then he is BLIND TO LIGHT and can probably not be helped.
7. Now repeat this test for the *left* eye, having closed the right eye.
8. Now record the visual acuity in each eye. Here is an example to guide you:
VR = Good vision (6/18 or better)
VL = Blind (less than 3/60, but can see light)

187

There are therefore **four** grades of visual acuity which you should be able to measure:

1	Good vision	Can see the 18 line at 6 metres	= 6/6–6/18
2	Poor vision	Cannot see the 18 line at 6 metres but can see the 60 line at 3 metres	= 6/24–3/60
3	Blind	Cannot see the 60 line at 3 metres, but can see light	= 2/60–PL
4	Blind to light	Cannot see light	= NPL

3 **The normal eye** (Figure 4)

Having taken the HISTORY and measured the VISUAL ACUITY you can now EXAMINE the eyes, but first it is important to know the appearances of the NORMAL EYE.

In the NORMAL EYE:
1 The **eyelids** must **open and close** properly.
2 The **white** of the eye (**conjunctiva**) must be **white**.
3 The **cornea** (the window of the eye) must be **clear**.
4 The **pupil** must be **black,** and become small in bright light.

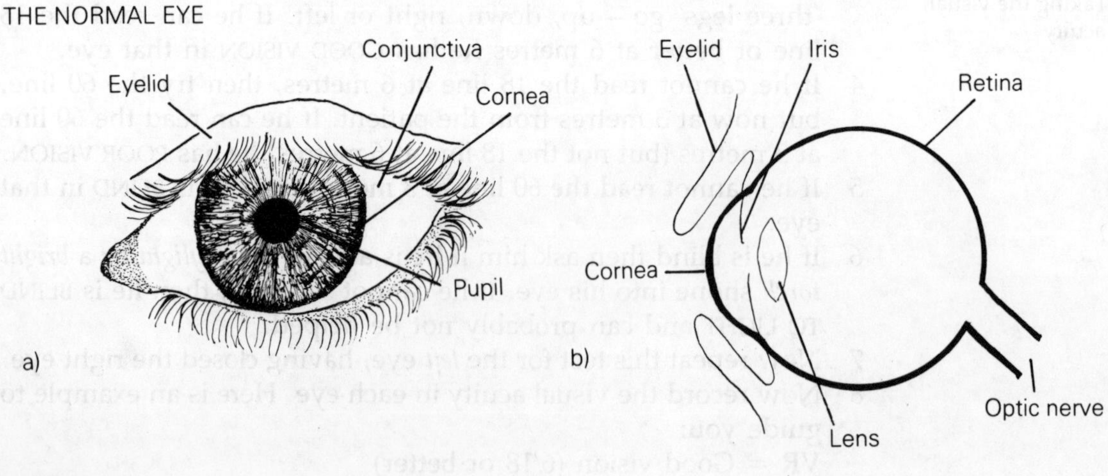

THE NORMAL EYE

Figure 4
The normal eye:
a) front view;
b) side view

188

4 Examination of the eye for abnormalities (Figure 5)

Some of the common abnormalities you should look for in the eyelids, conjunctiva, cornea and pupil are listed below:

4.1 Four abnormalities of the EYELIDS:
1. Cannot close — Lagophthalmos
2. Cannot open — Ptosis
3. Eyelashes turn in — Trichiasis/Entropion
4. Eyelid swelling — Chalazion

4.2 Four abnormalities of the CONJUNCTIVA:
1. It is red — Acute red eye
2. It is growing onto the cornea — Pterygium
3. There is a haemorrhage — Trauma
4. There are white foamy spots (Bitot spots) — Vitamin A deficiency

4.3 Four abnormalities of the CORNEA:
1. There is a white scar — Corneal scar
2. There is a grey spot in a red eye — Corneal ulcer
3. There is a foreign body — Trauma
4. There is a laceration — Trauma

4.4 Four abnormalities of the PUPIL:
1. It is white — Cataract
2. It is irregular in shape — Iritis
3. It is large and does not become small in bright light — Glaucoma
4. There is blood in front of it — Hyphaema/Trauma

Section B deals with the diagnosis and treatment of these abnormalities.

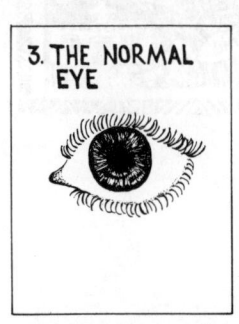

Figure 5 Examining the eye for abnormalites

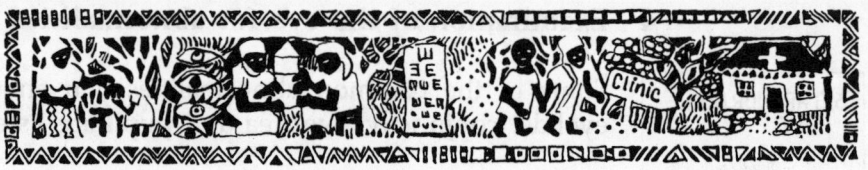

SECTION B:
Making a diagnosis

1 Acute red eye

It is best to think of **four** different groups of patients who may suffer from acute red eye(s):
1 Newborn babies (0–28 days)
2 Children (6 months – 6 years)
3 Patients of any age
4 Following trauma.

1.1 Acute red eyes in newborn babies
Newborn babies may have red, swollen eyes with a pussy discharge which occurs usually a few days after birth. This is called ophthalmia neonatorum (Figure 6). If you see a baby with this problem it is in danger of becoming blind and needs urgent treatment as follows:
1 Clean the pus away from the eyes with a clean cloth and water.
2 Give tetracycline eye ointment every hour into both eyes for four days, then 3 times a day for 10 days more.
3 Give procaine penicillin 60 mgs IM (100,000 IU).

Ophthalmia neonatorum can be easily prevented by cleaning the eyes of all babies as soon as they are born with water and a clean cloth, and then putting tetracycline eye ointment once into both eyes.

1.2 Acute red eyes in young children
Children between the age of six months and six years may become blind from *vitamin A deficiency* (Figure 7) which is sometimes also called xerophthalmia, keratomalacia or blinding malnutrition.

The child is often suffering from general malnutrition and may be very thin or have swollen legs. The child may recently have had measles or severe diarrhoea.

Figure 6
Ophthalmia neonatorum

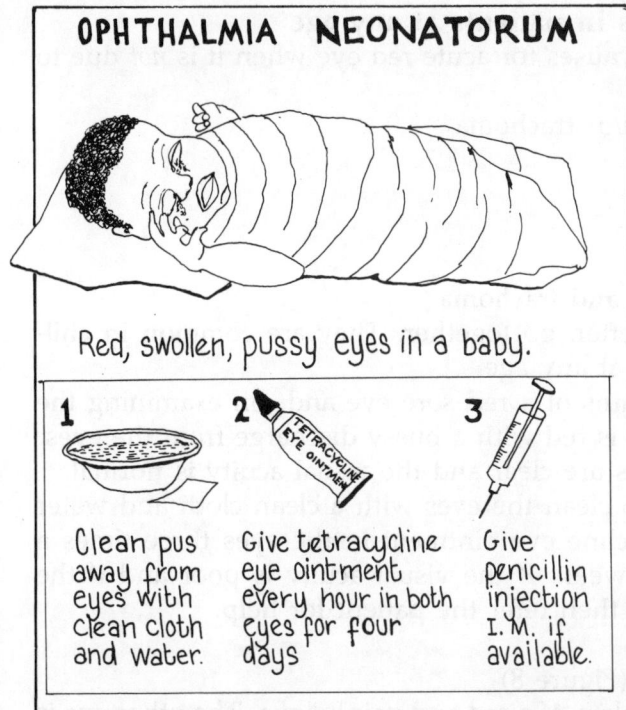

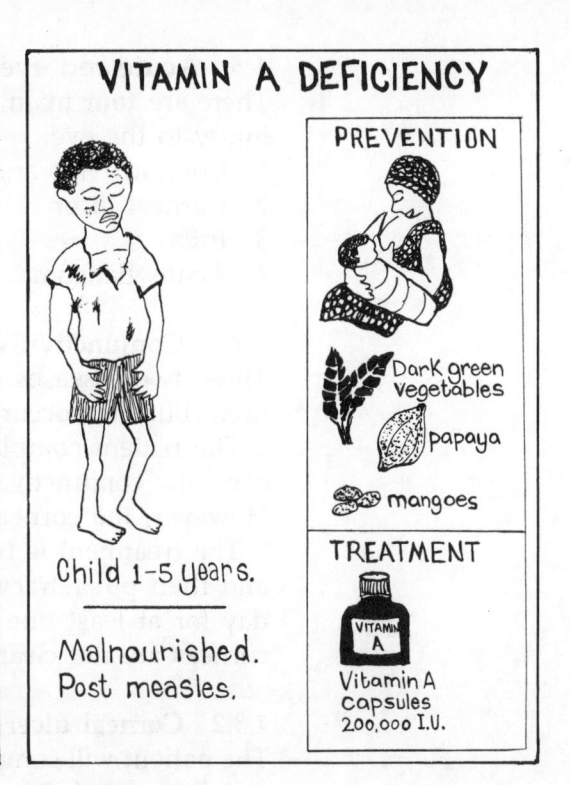

Figure 7
Vitamin A deficiency

When you examine the child it will be difficult to open his eyes, but by gently separating the eyelids you may see *grey spots* on the cornea (corneal ulcer) and sometimes white foamy spots on the lateral conjunctiva (Bitot spots). The treatment is to give Vitamin A 200,000 IU by mouth immediately, and repeat the same the following day and in one week's time.

To prevent blindness from vitamin A deficiency you should encourage mothers to breast feed their children up to 18 months of age, but also to add other foods which have plenty of vitamin A into the child's diet from the age of four months onwards. Such foods are papaya, mangoes and especially dark green leafy vegetables (e.g. spinach).

Children with:
1 Malnutrition
2 Measles
3 Malabsorption (diarrhoea for two weeks or more)
4 Corneal ulcers (grey spots on the cornea),

should all be given one capsule of Vitamin A 200,000 IU by mouth once, in order to prevent vitamin A deficiency, which may lead to blindness and even death of the child. The children with corneal ulcers may also be given another capsule after one day and again after one week. Do not give more than this dosage, as Vitamin A in large doses can harm the child.

1.3 Acute red eyes in patients at any age

There are **four** main causes for acute red eye when it is *not* due to injury to the eye:
1. Conjunctivitis and/or trachoma
2. Corneal ulcer
3. Iritis
4. Acute glaucoma.

1.3.1 Conjunctivitis and trachoma

These two diseases often go together. They are common in children, but may occur at any age.

The patient complains of a red sore eye and, on examining the eyes, the conjunctiva is red with a pussy discharge from the eyes. However, the corneas are clear and the visual acuity is normal.

The treatment is to clean the eyes with a clean cloth and water and then put tetracycline eye ointment in the eyes three times a day for at least one week. If the visual acuity is poor and if the corneas are not clear then refer the patient for help.

1.3.2 Corneal ulcer (Figure 8)

The patient will complain of a red and painful eye. The other eye is usually normal. The visual acuity is poor and the conjunctiva is red. There is a grey spot on the cornea. This is a serious problem and you should give the patient tetracycline eye ointment, an eye pad, and refer the patient for help urgently.

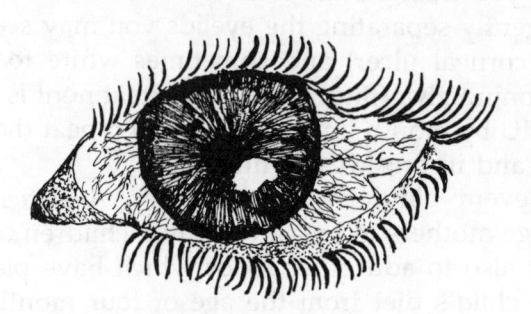

Figure 8
Corneal ulcer

1.3.3 Iritis (Figure 9)

The patient will complain of a red painful eye. There is no discharge but the visual acuity is poor. The conjunctiva is red, but the cornea is clear. However, the pupil is small and may be irregular in shape. This is a serious problem. If you have medicine which makes the pupil large (e.g. atropine), you may apply this and then refer the patient quickly for help.

1.3.4 Acute glaucoma (Figure 10)

In this disease the pressure in the eye goes up very quickly. This causes a red very painful eye, with poor visual acuity (sometimes

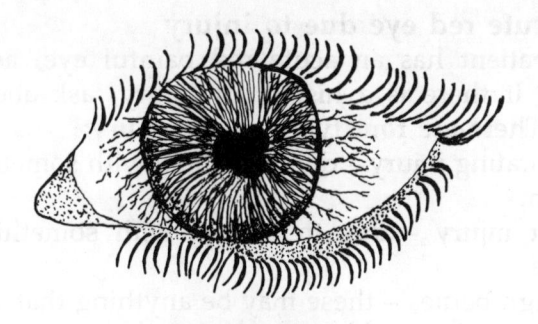

Figure 9
Iritis

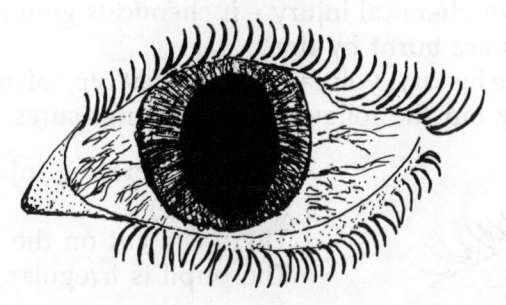

Figure 10
Acute glaucoma

blind). The conjunctiva is red, the cornea is hazy and the pupil is large and does not become small when a bright light is shone into the eye. This is a very serious and painful disease. The patient must be referred for help immediately.

Summary of common causes of acute red eye (no injury)

Disease	Visual acuity	Eye	Cornea	Pupil
Conjunctivitis and trachoma	Good	Both	Clear	Normal
Corneal ulcer	Poor	One	Grey spot	Normal
Iritis	Poor	One	Clear	Small and irregular
Acute glaucoma	Blind	One	Hazy	Large

By carefully taking a history, measuring the visual acuity in each eye and then examining the cornea and pupil you should be able to decide which of the four common causes of acute red eye the patient is suffering from. You will never do any harm by putting simple antibiotic in the eye, e.g. oc tetracycline, but you should **never use any eye medicine containing steroids**. If the problem is in *one eye, with severe pain and loss of vision, you should refer the patient urgently to an eye nurse or doctor.*

1.4 Acute red eye due to injury

If the patient has an acute red painful eye, ask if it has been injured. If there is a history of injury, ask about what type of injury. There are **four** types of eye injury:

1. Perforating injury – due to trauma with something sharp, e.g. a thorn.
2. Blunt injury – due to trauma with something blunt, e.g. a stone.
3. Foreign bodies – these may be anything that goes into the eye.
4. Burns or chemical injury – if chemicals go into the eye or if the eyelids are burnt by fire.

From the history, you can decide what type of injury has occurred. Now carry out the following first aid measures:

1.4.1 Perforating injury
(Figure 11)
There is a cut on the cornea.
The pupil is irregular.

Treatment
– Very gently pad the eye.
– *refer immediately for help.*

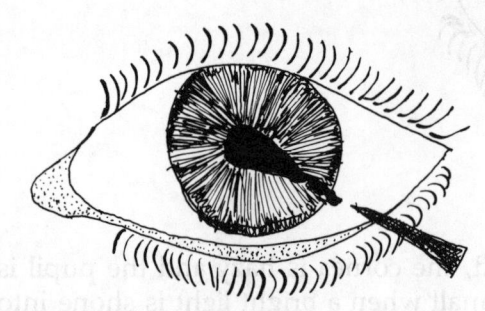

Figure 11 Perforating injury

1.4.2 Blunt injury (Figure 12)
There may be blood behind the cornea – **hyphaema**.

Treatment
– Place an eye pad over the affected eye for two days with complete rest at home.
– If the eye is still very painful or has poor vision after two days then *refer for help.*

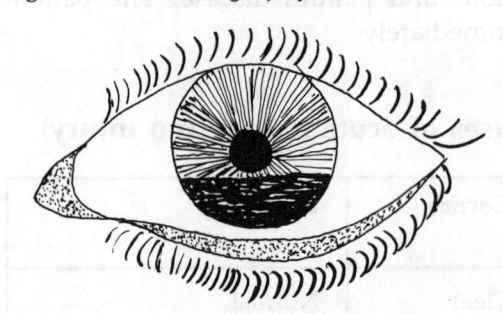

Figure 12 Hyphaema due to blunt injury

1.4.3 Foreign bodies (Figure 13)
Treatment
– If you can see the foreign body on the conjunctiva or under the upper eyelid, then remove it with a piece of cloth or a matchstick, and give tetracycline eye ointment and an eye pad.
– To remove a corneal foreign body remember the **four Ls**:

Lie the patient flat;
Apply Local anaesthetic drops;
Use a good Light;
Lift off with a piece of paper or a matchstick.

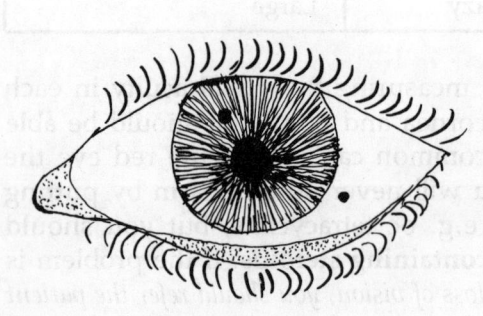

Figure 13 Foreign bodies

1.4.4 Burns or chemical injuries (Figure 14)
Treatment
- If chemicals have gone into the eye, lie the patient flat and pour clean water from a cup gently into the eyes for ten minutes.
- If the eyelids have been burned, give ointment every hour and refer.
- Irrigate chemical injuries with water.
- Lubricate burns to the lids with antibiotic ointment.

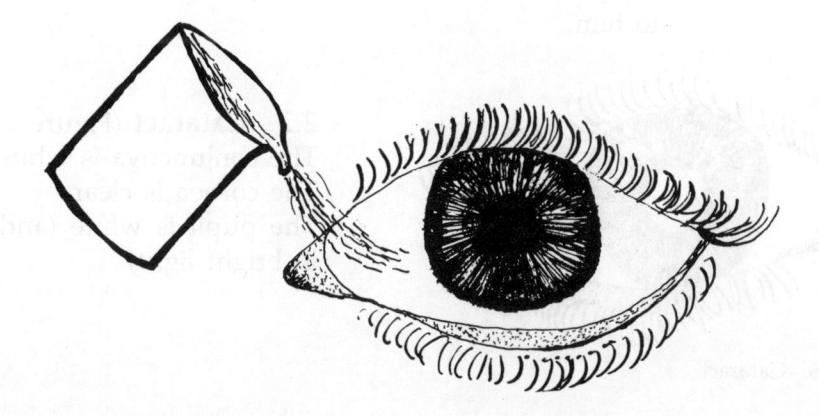

Figure 14
Burns or chemical injuries

2 Blindness

If the patient cannot see the 60 line at 3 metres and he has a white non-painful eye, then he is BLIND in that eye.

From the history and visual acuity find out if he is blind in one or both eyes.

There are **four** common causes of BLIND WHITE EYE(S):
1. Corneal scar – there is a white opacity on the cornea.
2. Cataract – there is an opacity of the lens of the eye.
3. Chronic glaucoma – there is raised pressure in the eye.
4. Other causes – diseases of the retina, optic nerve or need for spectacles.

By carefully examining the cornea and the pupil you can diagnose the common causes of the blindness.

2.1 Corneal scar (Figure 15)
The conjunctiva is white.
The cornea has a white mark on it.
The pupil cannot be seen easily.

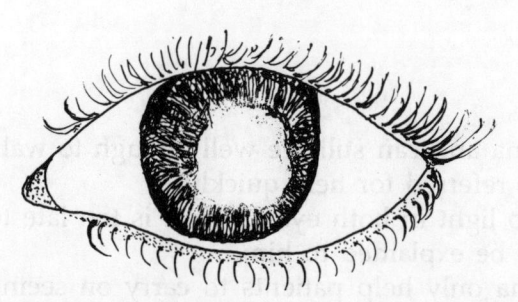

Figure 15 Corneal scar

Management
If the patient has blind vision in both eyes, but can still see light, then he should be referred to a specialist who may be able to help him see again.

If the patient is blind in only one eye but can see with the other, then there is no need to refer him, as he can still see well with one eye.

If he cannot see light at all in both eyes, then there is nothing further that can be done to help him and this should be explained to him.

2.2 Cataract (Figure 16)
The conjunctiva is white.
The cornea is clear.
The pupil is white (and becomes small in bright light).

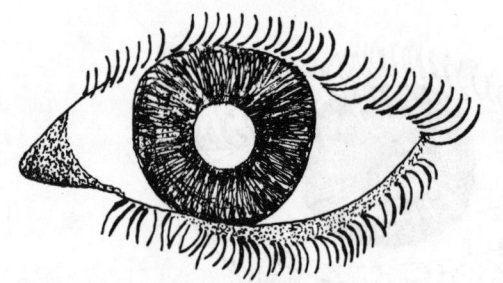

Figure 16 Cataract

Management
If the patient is blind in both eyes, and can still see light, then refer him for an operation which will help him see well again.

If he is blind in one eye only and can see well with the other eye, then he can wait until he is having difficulty seeing with his good eye and then go for help.

2.3 Chronic glaucoma (Figure 17)
The conjunctiva is white.
The cornea is clear.
The pupil is large and does not become small with a bright light.

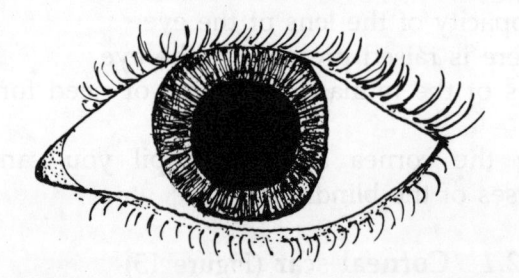

Figure 17 Chronic glaucoma

Management
If the patient has glaucoma and can still see well enough to walk about, then he should be referred for help quickly.

If he is already blind to light in both eyes then it is too late to help him and this should be explained to him.

Operations for glaucoma only help patients to carry on seeing what they can see at present. It does not make them see better.

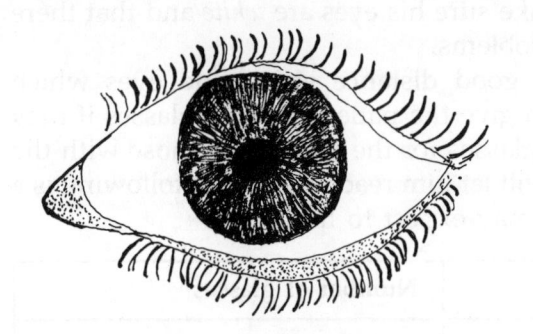

2.4 Other causes (Figure 18)
The conjunctiva is white.
The cornea is clear.
The pupil is normal.

Figure 18 Normal cornea and pupil

Management
If you do not know the cause of blindness, then the patient should be referred for help, especially if the loss of vision is sudden in onset or if the patient is blind in both eyes.

Summary of diagnoses of blindness

Examination of the PUPIL is very useful in deciding on the cause of loss of vision

Pupil	Diagnosis
Pupil not seen	Corneal scar
White pupil	Cataract
Large pupil	Glaucoma
Normal pupil	Other causes

3 Presbyopia – difficulty in reading

Some eye patients will complain that they have difficulty in reading books or in sewing. This occurs as people get older, usually after the age of 40. By carefully examining the patient, you will be able to advise him if he needs READING SPECTACLES or not.

If the patient complains of difficulty in reading there are **four** things you should do:
1. Ask the patient his age. If he is under 40 years of age then he should *not* need reading glasses yet and you can explain this to him.
2. Measure his visual acuity in each eye. You should only continue examining him for reading glasses if he has GOOD VISION in each eye (6/18 or better).

3 Examine his eyes to make sure his eyes are *white* and that there are no other serious problems.
4 If he is over 40, with good distance vision and eyes which appear normal, you can give the patient reading glasses if they are available. The best glasses for the patient are those with the lowest number which will let him read easily. The following is a guideline to what you may expect to find:

Age	Number of glasses
45	plus 1.00
50	plus 1.50
55	plus 2.00
60	plus 2.50
65	plus 3.00

These glasses are *only to be worn for reading* or other close work. They are *not glasses for seeing in the distance. You must explain this carefully to your patient.* If you do not have reading glasses available then you can advise the patient that he/she needs spectacles and, if possible, you can refer him/her to an eye specialist or optician for help.

4 Other eye diseases

If your patient does not have any of the previous eye problems, – i.e. acute red painful eye, blindness, or presbyopia (difficulty in reading) – then we group him in OTHER EYE DISEASES. There are **four** common eye problems of the eyelids and another **four** diseases of the eye itself.

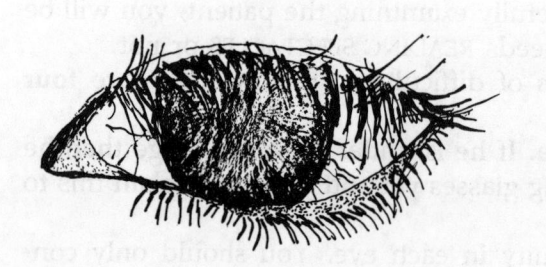

4.1 Four other diseases of the eyelids

4.1.1 Entropion (Trichiasis) (Figure 19)
The eyelashes turn into the eye.
It is caused by trachoma.
It results in corneal scar.

Treatment
– Refer for eyelid surgery *soon*.

Figure 19 Entropion

4.1.2 Lagophthalmos
(Figure 20)
The patient cannot close his eyelids.
It may be due to leprosy.
It can cause a corneal ulcer and scar.

Treatment
- Put tetracycline eye ointment in the eye each night and refer *soon*.

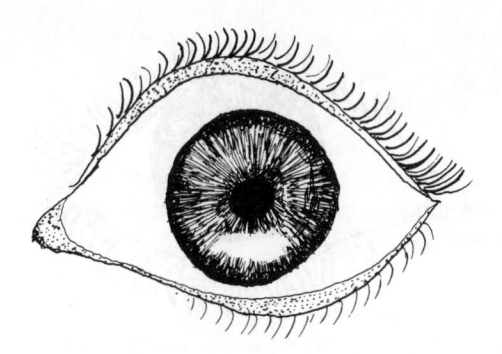

Figure 20 Lagophthalmos

4.1.3 Ptosis (Figure 21)
The patient cannot open his eye.
It may occur in children or adults.

Treatment
- Refer for help *soon*.

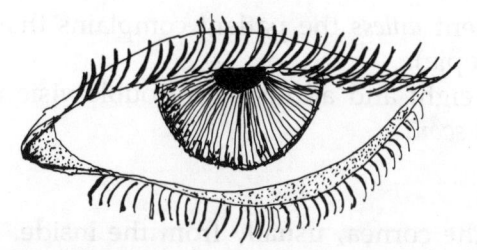

Figure 21 Ptosis

4.1.4 Chalazion (Figure 22)
There is a swelling of the eyelid.
There may be several swellings.

Treatment
- If they are troublesome, refer; *non-urgent*.

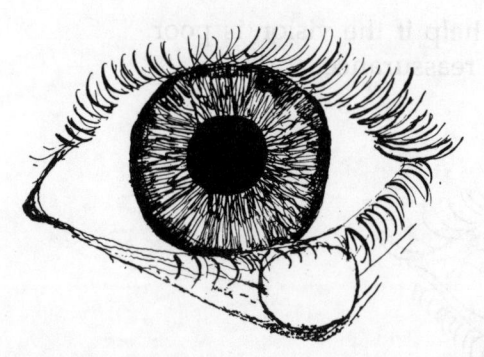

Figure 22 Chalazion

4.2 Four other diseases of the eye itself
4.2.1 Proptosis
The eye is pushed out between the eyelids.
It can occur at any age, and is *always very serious*.
It may cause a corneal ulcer.

Treatment
- Refer *immediately* for help and give tetracycline eye ointment three times a day to the eye, to stop corneal ulceration.

4.2.2 Squint (Figure 23)
The eyes are not straight so that one eye turns *in* or *out*.
It may occur in young children or adults.

199

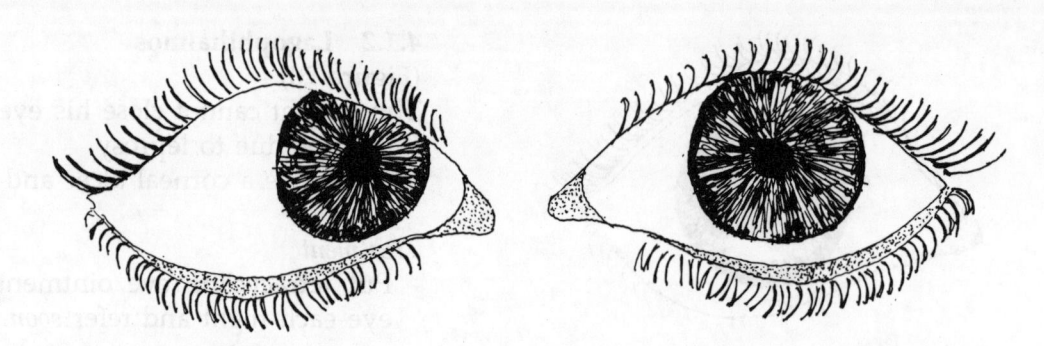

Figure 23 Squint

Treatment
- In adults there is *no* treatment *unless* the patient complains that he sees double vision (diplopia).
- Children under the age of eight and adults with double vision should be referred for help *soon*.

4.2.3 Pterygium (Figure 24)

The conjunctiva grows onto the cornea, usually from the inside. It is common and *not serious*.

Treatment
- Only refer the patient for help if the vision is poor. If the vision is good, give reassurance.

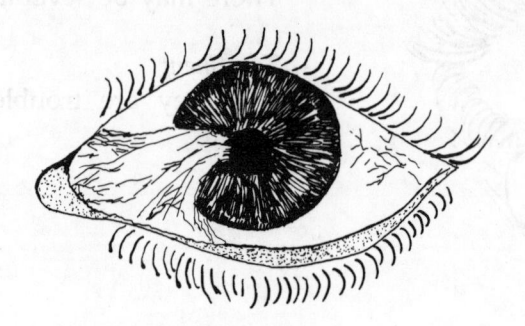

Figure 24 Pterygium

4.2.4 Blind painful eye
Treatment
- If the patient's eye is **blind to light**, and if the eye is **very painful**, then it may be best to remove the eye and stop the pain.
- Refer the patient for help *immediately*.

SECTION C:
How to work in your eye clinic

1 Equipment (Figure 25)

You will need the following equipment to help you examine and treat your eye patients well:
1. Visual acuity charts
2. Torch
3. A room in which to examine patients. Ideally this should be at least six metres long so that you can take visual acuities. It is also good if the room can be darkened, so that it is easier to examine the eyes of your patient with the torch
4. Clean cloth and strapping with which to clean and pad the eye.

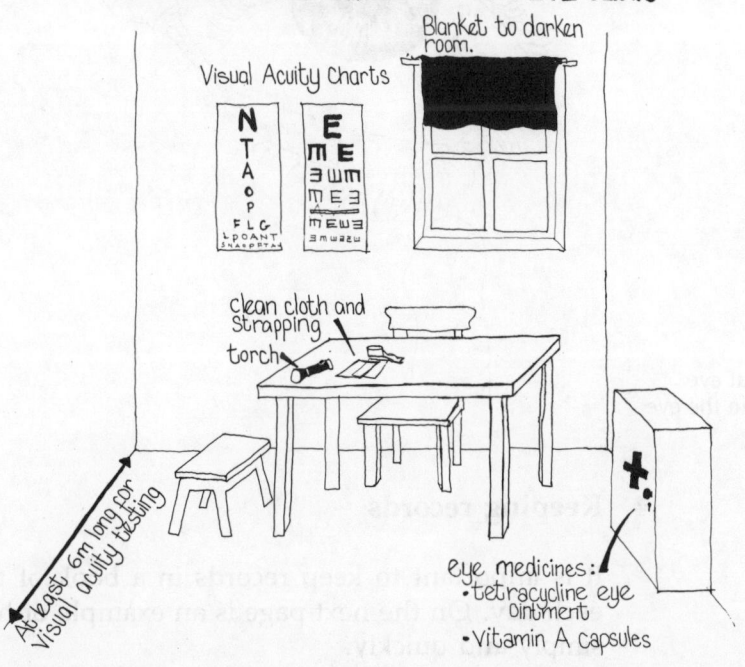

Figure 25
Equipment and drugs for the eye clinic

2 Medicines

There are **two** medicines which are **essential** to your eye work. These are:
1. Tetracycline eye ointment 1%
2. Vitamin A capsules (200,000 I.U.)

There are **two** other eye medicines whch are very useful:
1. Local anaesthetic eye drops
2. Atropine eye ointment

3 How to put eye medicine in the eye (Figure 26)

When putting medicine in the eye, do the following **four** things:
1. Explain to the patient what you will do.
2. Pull the lower lid down so that you can see the conjunctiva.
3. Put a little amount of the medicine at the outer third of the lower conjunctiva, while the patient **looks up**.
4. Close the patient's eye for two minutes to allow the drug to enter the eye well.

It is also very important to learn how to evert (turn outwards) the upper eyelid. This should be learnt practically.

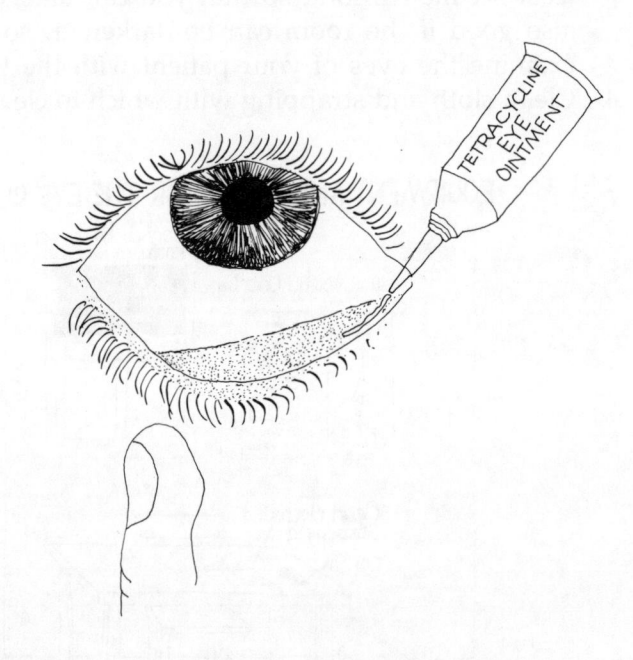

Figure 26
How to put eye medicine in the eye

4 Keeping records

It is important to keep records in a book of the patients you see each day. On the next page is an example of how you may do this simply and quickly.

Record sheet						
Date	Name	Age	Vision VR	VL	Diagnosis	Management
29.3.84	Mathayo	40	g	b	Left cataract	Reassured
29.3.84	Julius	6	g	g	Conjunctivitis	Tetracycline ointment
29.3.84	Rehema	70	b	BL	Cataracts	Refer
30.3.84	John	20	g	g	Normal	Reassured

Key:
g = Good vision
p = Poor vision
b = Blind
BL = Blind to Light

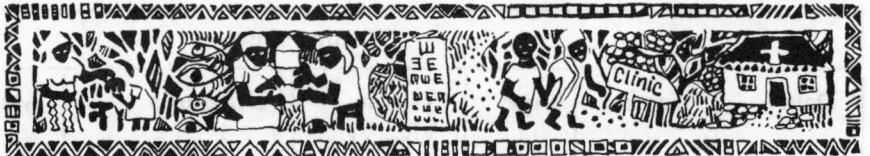

SECTION D:
Health teaching to prevent blindness

There are **four** important facts which you can teach to other people which will help them look after their eyes better, and prevent them from becoming blind (Figure 27).

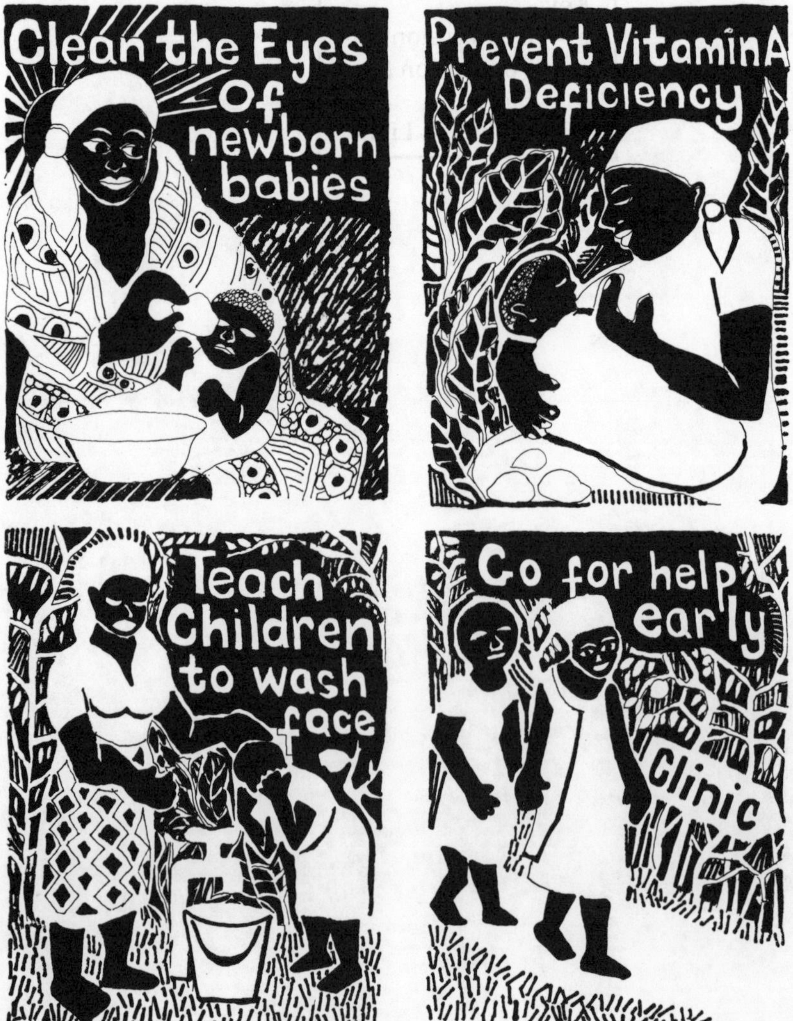

Figure 27
Health teaching to prevent blindness

1. Clean the eyes of all newborn babies as soon as they are born with clean water and a clean cloth. (This prevents ophthalmia neonatorum.) In particular, it should be taught to village midwives (traditional birth attendants).
2. Mothers should make sure their children receive the following foods:

    Age 0-18 months   Breast milk
    Age 4-18 months   Breast milk + papaya/mangoes + dark green leafy vegetables
    Age 18 mths-5 yrs Dark green leafy vegetables + papaya/ mangoes

    Eggs and milk are good for children of all ages. This prevents nutritional blindness from vitamin A deficiency.
3. Washing the face and eyes of all babies, young children and schoolchildren every day should be taught to mothers, teachers and schoolchildren. (This prevents conjunctivitis/trachoma.)
4. When your vision is getting worse, go for help early. When your eyes are red and painful, go for help early. Do not use traditional medicines.

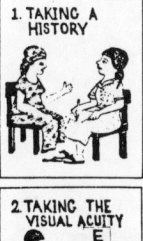

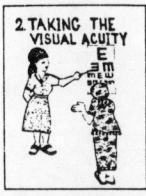

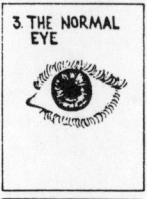

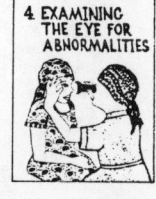

Summary

The eye is red and painful	ACUTE RED EYE
The patient cannot see	BLIND
The patient cannot read clearly	PRESBYOPIA
Any other specific complaint	OTHER EYE DISEASES

Can see 6/18	GOOD VISION
Can see 3/60 but not 6/18	POOR VISION
Cannot see 3/60, can see light	BLIND
Cannot see light	BLIND TO LIGHT

The lids open and close normally
The conjunctiva is white
The cornea is clear
The pupil is black and becomes small in bright light

EYELID	CONJUNCTIVA
Lagophthalmos	Red eye
Ptosis	Pterygium
Entropion	Trauma
Chalazion	Vitamin A deficiency
CORNEA	**PUPIL**
Scar	Cataract
Ulcer	Iritis
Foreign body	Glaucoma
Laceration	Hyphaema

Summary

REMEMBER
1 If both eyes are white,
2 If both eyes have good visual acuity,
3 If he is under 40 (i.e. not presbyopic), and
4 If there is nothing else obviously abnormal

THEN:
Your patient has normal eyes, he does not need treatment, and you should reassure him of this.

PART 3
Lecture notes on common eye diseases for ophthalmic assistants

Contents

Introduction to Part Three	209
Outline	210
SECTION A: *Examination of the eye*	211
Taking a history	211
Taking the visual acuity	211
Basic eye examination	212
Special eye examinations	212
SECTION B: *Basic sciences of the eye*	213
Anatomy	213
Physiology/Optics	216
Pharmacology	220
Pathology	221
SECTION C: *Diagnosis of common eye diseases*	222
Acute red eye	222
Inability to see – blindness	235
Refractive errors	249
Other eye diseases	250
SECTION D: *Management of common eye diseases*	258
Remedy	258
Refer	259
Refract	260
Rehabilitation/Reassurance	261

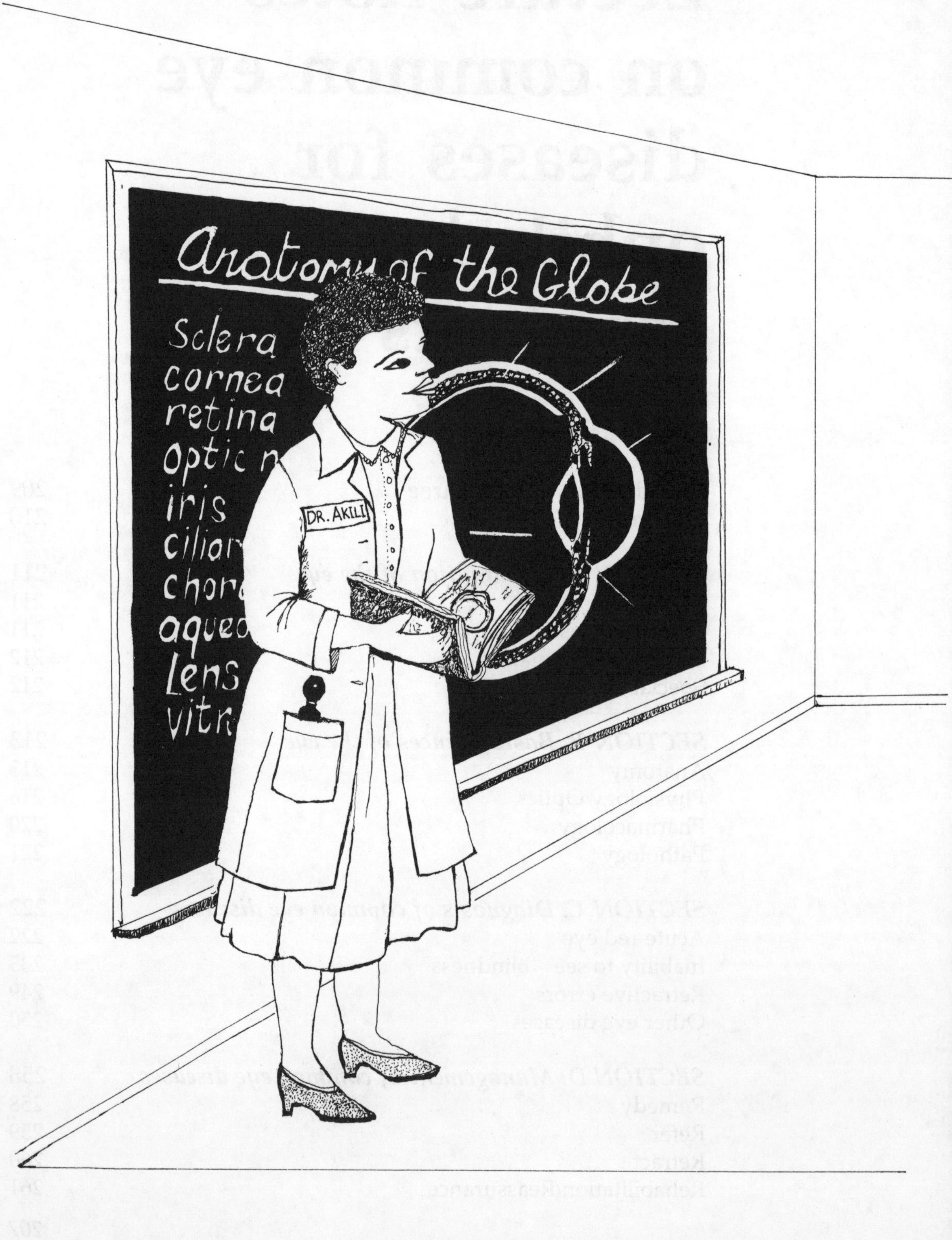
Anatomy of the Globe
Sclera
cornea
retina
iris
Lens
DR. AKILI

Introduction to Part Three

This part of the book is an outline of lecture notes for the thereotical part of teaching ophthalmic assistants and ophthalmic nurses about common eye diseases.

The lecture notes are set out in a problem orientated fashion, based upon common presenting symptoms. For ease of memory the lecture notes use a system of **fours** which is intended to help both the teacher and the student. Needless to say, at times this is rather artificial but, we believe, useful in helping students to examine, diagnose and manage patients in a systematised way.

There are four sections:
A – Examination of the eye
B – Basic sciences of the eye
C – Diagnosis of common eye diseases
D – Management of common eye diseases

In no way are these notes meant to be comprehensive. They are only intended as a teaching aid for use in the classroom. There is no substitute for clinical teaching with patients, which should form the bulk of any course training ophthalmic assistants.

Outline

SECTION A Eye Examination	SECTION B Basic Sciences	SECTION C Diagnosis	SECTION 4 Management
1 HISTORY	ANATOMY	ACUTE RED EYE	REMEDY
Acute red eye Loss of vision Cannot read Other specific symptoms	Globe Orbit	In babies In children At any age Trauma	Use medicines to REMEDY acute red eye(s)
2 VISUAL ACUITY	PHYSIOLOGY	LOSS OF VISION	REFER/ REHABILITATION
Good 6/6-6/18 Poor 6/24-3/60 Blind 2/60-PL Blind to light NPL	Aqueous Vision Tears Optics	Corneal scar Cataract Glaucoma Others	REFER treatable blindness and REHABILITATE non-treatable blindness
3 BASIC EXAMINATION	PHARMACOLOGY	REFRACTIVE ERRORS	REFRACT
Eyelids Conjunctiva Cornea Pupil	Anti-infectives Anti-inflammatory Mydriatics Others	Presbyopia Myopia Hypermetropia Astigmatism	REFRACTIVE ERRORS are treated with spectacles
4 SPECIAL EXAMINATION	PATHOLOGY	OTHER EYE DISEASES	REFER/ REASSURE
Pin hole Tonometry Ophthalmoscopy Slit-lamp etc.	Congenital Inflammations Tumours Degenerations	Orbit Muscles/nerves Eyelids Naso-lacrimal	REFER other serious eye diseases and REASSURE people with normal eyes

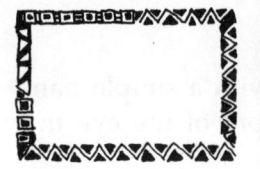

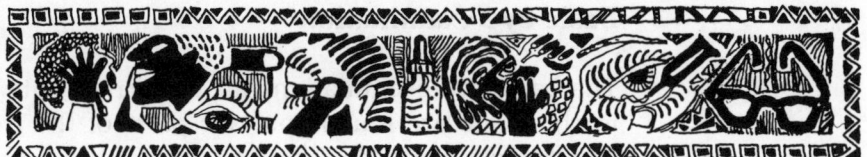

SECTION A:
Examination of the eye

History and examination

The examination of a patient with eye problems can be simply divided into **four** stages:
1 Taking the history.
2 Measurement of visual acuity.
3 Basic examination of the external eye with a torch.
4 Special examinations of the inner parts of the eye.

1 Taking a history

Patients attending an eye clinic can be divided into **four** main groups according to the symptom they complain of.
1.1 Red painful eye(s).
1.2 Cannot see – an inability to see in the distance with one or both eyes.
1.3 Cannot read – an inability to read small print, or see near objects.
1.4 Other specific symptoms – for example diplopia, epiphora, proptosis.

2 Taking the visual acuity

The visual acuity should be assessed in *each* eye of *all* eye patients. The acuity can be measured using the Snellen test chart or the E test type for people who cannot read.
  The visual acuity can be usefully divided into **four** main groups.
2.1 Good vision = 6/6 to 6/18.
2.2 Poor vision = 6/24 to 3/60 (CF3m).
2.3 Blind = 2/60 (CF2m) to PL (perception of light).
2.4 Blind to light = NPL (no perception of light).

3 Basic eye examination

The basic eye examination can be carried out with a simple hand torch. There are **four** important parts of the front of the eye that should be examined:
3.1 The eyelids – do they look and function normally?
3.2 The conjunctiva – is the white of the eye white?
3.3 The cornea – is the cornea clear?
3.4 The pupil – is the pupil black and does it react to light?

4 Special eye examinations

Besides these four basic examinations with a torch there are **four** special examinations which may also be required in examining a patient. The special examinations are:
4.1 Visual acuity with a pin hole (to check for refractive errors).
4.2 Schiotz tonometry (to measure intra-ocular pressure).
4.3 Ophthalmoscopy (preferably after dilation of the pupil).
4.4 Other special examinations – for example slit-lamp microscopy, examination of ocular movements, visual fields. (Any of these special examinations may be required for certain patients.)

Having taken the history, measured the visual acuity and examined the patient one is now in a position to try and make a diagnosis and decide upon the management of the patient.

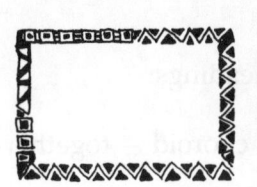

SECTION B:
Basic sciences

In order to better understand how the eye works and how diseases can affect the eye a knowledge of the basic sciences in regard to the eye is required. This is discussed in **four** sections:
1 Anatomy
2 Physiology and optics
3 Pharmacology
4 Pathology.

1 Anatomy

The anatomy of the eye can be considered under two main headings, the anatomy of the globe and the anatomy of the orbit.

ANATOMY OF THE GLOBE

1 Protective coat
Sclera
Cornea

Aqueous
Lens

2 Vascular layer
Iris
Ciliary body
Choroid

3 Visual layer
Retina
Optic nerve

Vitreous

4 Contents
Aqueous
Lens
Vitreous

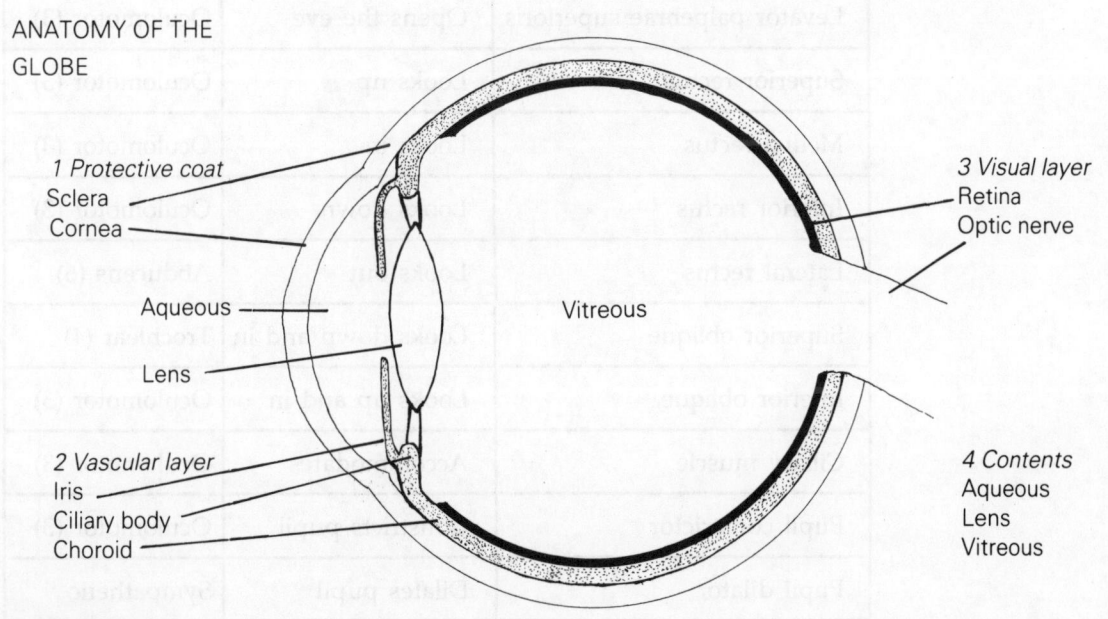

Figure 28
Anatomy of the globe

213

1.1 Anatomy of the globe (Figure 28)

The eye globe can be considered under **four** headings:
- The protective coat – cornea and sclera.
- The vascular layer – iris, ciliary body, and choroid – together called the uvea.
- The visual layer – retina and optic nerve.
- The contents of the eye – aqueous, lens and vitreous.

1.2 Anatomy of the orbit

The structures of the orbit can be considered under **four** headings:

1.2.1 The bones of the orbit
- Roof – frontal bone
- Outside wall – temporal bone
- Floor – maxilla
- Inside wall – ethmoid plate
- Back wall – sphenoid bone

All of these bones (except the temporal) contain an air space known as a SINUS.

1.2.2 The muscles and nerves

Muscles

Muscle	Action	Nerve supply
Orbicularis oculi	Closes the eye	Facial (7)
Levator palpebrae superioris	Opens the eye	Oculomotor (3)
Superior rectus	Looks up	Oculomotor (3)
Medial rectus	Looks in	Oculomotor (3)
Inferior rectus	Looks down	Oculomotor (3)
Lateral rectus	Looks out	Abducens (6)
Superior oblique	Looks down and in	Trochlear (4)
Inferior oblique	Looks up and in	Oculomotor (3)
Ciliary muscle	Accommodates	Oculomotor (3)
Pupil constrictor	Constricts pupil	Oculomotor (3)
Pupil dilator	Dilates pupil	Sympathetic

Nerves

Nerve	Action	Paralysis causes
Optic (2)	Vision	Loss of vision
Oculomotor (3)	Motor to ocular muscles	Ptosis, eye down and out, mydriasis
Trochlear (4)	Superior oblique m.	Diplopia
Trigeminal (5)	Sensation to the eye and face	Corneal anaesthesia
Abducens (6)	Lateral rectus m.	Diplopia with inability to abduct the eye
Facial (7)	Orbicularis oculi m. and facial muscles	Lagophthalmos

1.2.3 The eyelids (Figure 29)

ANATOMY OF THE EYELID

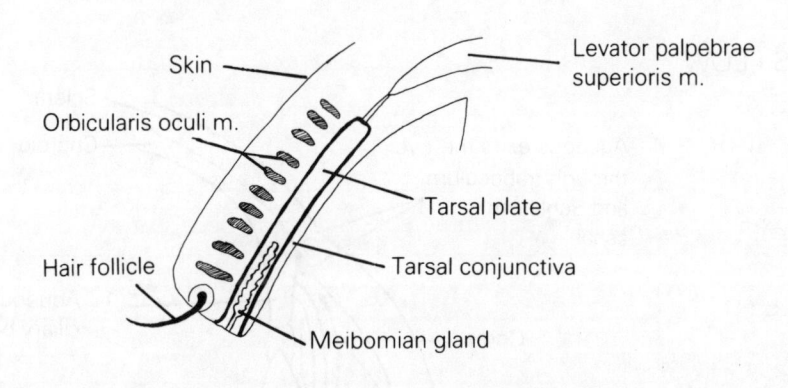

Figure 29
The eyelid

1.2.4 The nasolacrimal apparatus (Figure 30)

ANATOMY OF NASOLACRIMAL APPARATUS

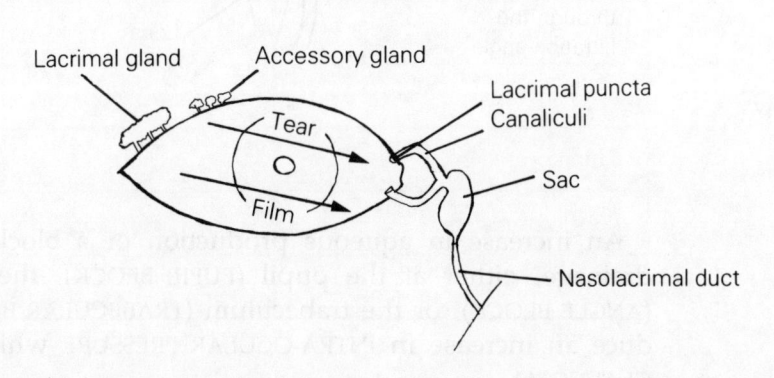

Figure 30
The nasolacrimal apparatus

Diseases of the orbital structures include protrusion of the eye (proptosis), causes of double vision (diplopia), diseases of the eyelids, and causes of a watering eye (epiphora). These diseases are discussed under the section on OTHER DISEASES (page 250).

2 Physiology

There are **four** important parts of eye physiology:
2.1 AQUEOUS production and drainage
2.2 Physiology of VISION
2.3 TEAR production and drainage
2.4 OPTICS of the eye.

2.1 Aqueous (Figure 31)
2.1.1 The aqueous is produced from blood by the ciliary body.
2.1.2 The aqueous flows through the pupil into the anterior chamber.
2.1.3 The aqueous flows from the anterior chamber through the filtration angle of the eye.
2.1.4 The aqueous leaves the eye through the trabeculum to enter the canal of Schlemm and drains to the episcleral veins.

AQUEOUS FLOW

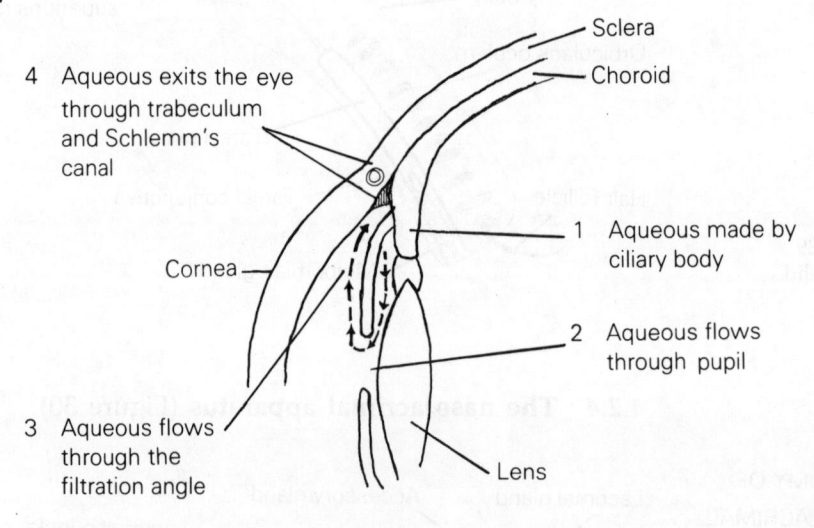

Figure 31
Aqueous flow

An increase in aqueous production or a blockage in aqueous drainage, either at the pupil (PUPIL BLOCK), the filtration angle (ANGLE BLOCK), or the trabeculum (TRABECULAR BLOCK), may produce an increase in INTRA-OCULAR PRESSURE which can result in GLAUCOMA.

2.2 Vision

The eye is the organ of vision and we are able to perceive different forms of vision.

2.2.1 Visual acuity – is the ability to see fine detail. (This is a function of the macula.)

2.2.2 Visual field – is the ability to see to either side in a wide direction. (This is a function of the periphery of the retina.)

2.2.3 Colour vision – is the ability to see different colours. (This again occurs mainly in the macula area.)

2.2.4 Binocular vision – is the ability to see with both eyes at once which gives us a perception of depth.

Each of the different types of vision can be assessed in different ways. However it is the measurement of visual acuity which must always be measured on every patient.

2.3 Tears

2.3.1 Tears are produced by the lacrimal gland (and accessory glands).

2.3.2 Tears flow across the cornea producing the tear film. The tear film is essential for the normal functioning of the cornea.

2.3.3 The tear film consists of a sandwich of three layers. The mucin layer is produced by goblet cells in the conjunctiva, then the aqueous tears and, on the outside, a fatty (lipid) layer produced by the Meibomian glands.

2.3.4 Tears drain from the eye at the lacrimal puncta into the lacrimal sac and on into the nose via the nasolacrimal duct.

2.4 Optics
2.4.1 Refraction in a block of glass and prism

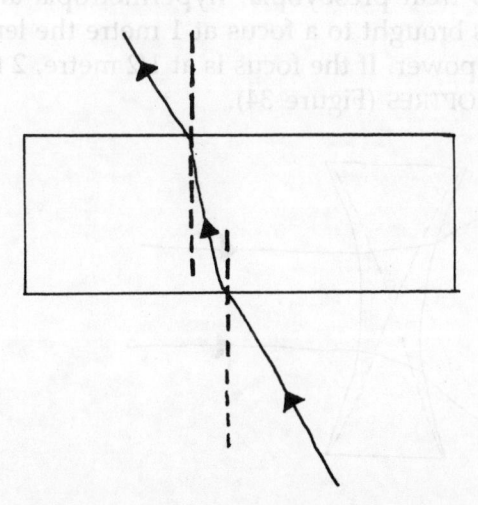

Figure 32
Refraction in a block of glass

As light enters the *glass* from the air, it is displaced towards the vertical. As it leaves the glass it is displaced away from the vertical (Figure 32).

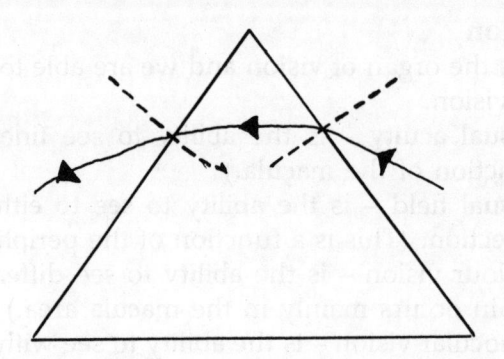

Figure 33
Refraction in a prism

As light passes through a *glass prism* it is displaced towards the base of the prism (Figure 33).

2.4.2 Refraction in convex and concave spheres

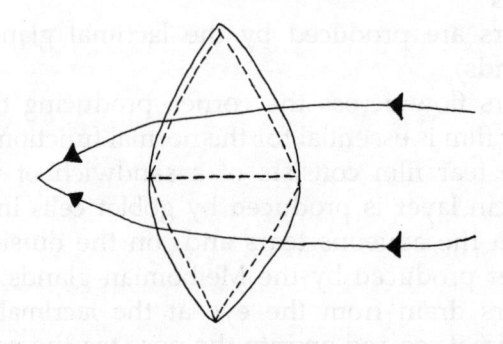

Figure 34
Refraction in a convex lens

A *convex lens* (plus lens) is like two prisms placed base to base. Light passing through a convex lens is converged. Convex lenses are used to treat presbyopia, hypermetropia and aphakia. If parallel light is brought to a focus at 1 metre the lens is said to have 1 DIOPTRE of power. If the focus is at 1/2 metre, 2 DIOPTRES, and a 1/3 metre, 3 DIOPTRES (Figure 34).

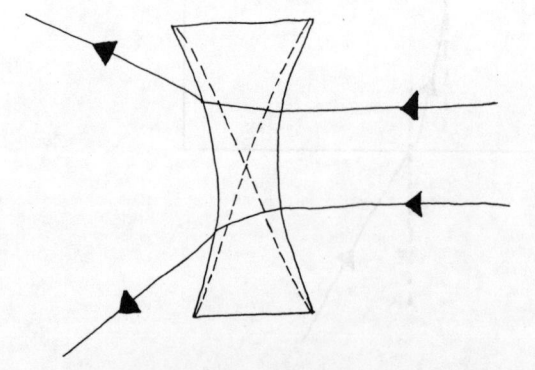

Figure 35
Refraction in a concave lens

A *concave lens* (minus lens) is like two prisms placed apex to apex. Light passing through a concave lens is diverged. Concave lenses are used to treat myopia (Figure 35).

2.4.3 Refraction in cylinders

A cylindrical lens has different powers in the vertical and horizontal axis. Thus, light passing through a cylindrical lens does not focus at one point, but forms two foci, one for the horizontal and the other for the vertical.

Cylindrical lenses may be convex, concave or mixed. They are used to treat astigmatism.

2.4.4 Refraction of the eye

Light entering the eye is converged at the cornea and then the lens acts as a focusing mechanism to converge the light to a point on the retina, so that the object is seen clearly (Figure 36).

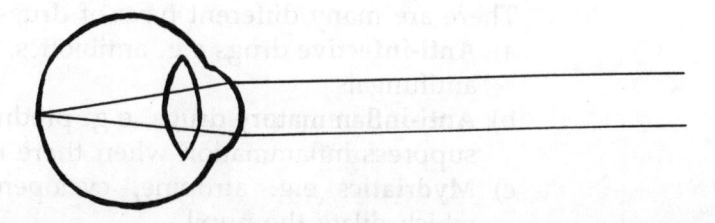

Figure 36
Refraction of the eye

If the object is close to the eye then the lens changes shape so that the light rays can still be focused on the retina. This is called ACCOMMODATION. (The ability to accommodate begins to fail after the age of 40, so that spectacles are needed for close work.) (Figure 37)

Figure 37
Refraction of the eye when the object is close: accommodation

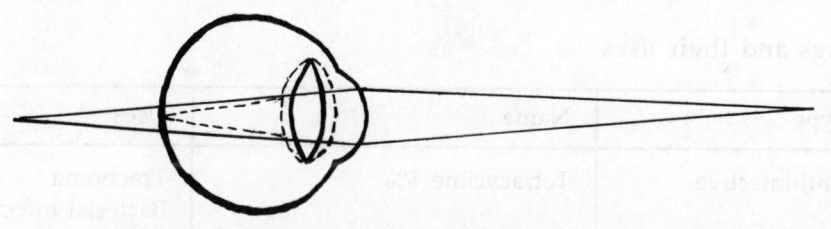

In myopia light rays are focused in front of the retina, so that a *minus* concave lens is needed to diverge the rays (Figure 38). In hypermetropia, it is the opposite, the rays are focused behind the retina so that a *plus* convex lens is needed (Figure 39).

Figure 38
Refraction in the eye: myopia

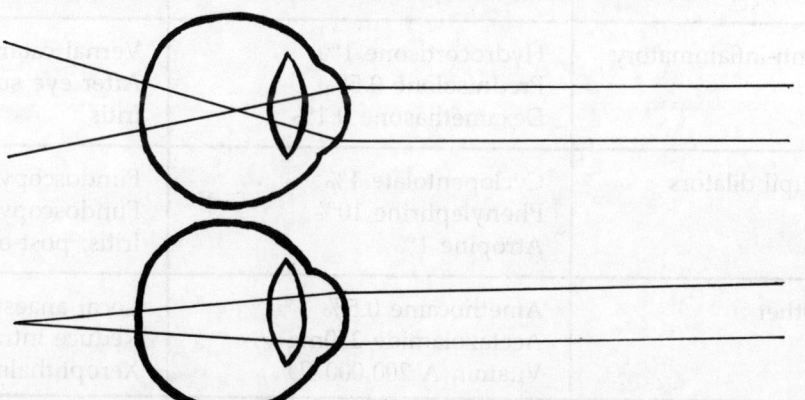

Figure 39
Refraction in the eye: hypermetropia

3 Pharmacology

The common *methods* of applying medications to the eye are as follows:
a) **Drops** – these are particularly useful in in-patients and also may be used to help in the diagnosis of certain diseases.
b) **Ointments** – these tend to be used by patients at home who are being treated as out-patients.
c) **Periocular injections** – these may be subconjunctival or retrobulbar injections around the eye.
d) **Systemic** – sometimes oral therapy, intravenous, or intramuscular injections are required to treat ocular disease.

There are many different *types* of drugs used in eye disease.
a) **Anti-infective** drugs e.g. antibiotics, antivirals, and occasionally antifungals.
b) **Anti-inflammatory** drugs, e.g. prednisolone – these are used to suppress inflammation when there is no infecting organism.
c) **Mydriatics** e.g. atropine, cyclopentolate – these are drugs which dilate the pupil.
d) **Other eye drugs** – this is a miscellaneous group of drugs which includes local anaesthetic drops, drugs which lower the intra-ocular pressure (Diamox), as well as special forms of therapy such as Vitamin A.

Drugs and their uses

Type	Name	Uses
Anti-infective	Tetracycline 1%	Trachoma
		Bacterial infections
	Chloramphenicol 0.5%	Conjunctivitis
		Corneal ulcer
	Gentamicin inj. 20mg.	Bacterial corneal ulcer
	Idoxuridine, Acyclovir	Herpes simplex ulcer
	Econazole 1%, Pimaracin 5%	Fungal ulcer
Anti-inflammatory	Hydrocortisone 1%	Vernal catarrh
	Prednisolone 0.5%	After eye surgery
	Dexamethasone 0.1%	Iritis
Pupil dilators	Cyclopentolate 1%	Fundoscopy, retinoscopy
	Phenylephrine 10%	Fundoscopy
	Atropine 1%	Iritis; post-operative
Other	Amethocaine 0.5%	Local anaesthetic
	Acetazolamide 250mg	Reduce intra-ocular pressure
	Vitamin A 200,000 IU	Xerophthalmia treatment

4 Pathology

Pathology is the study of diseases in man. There are **four** common types of disease processes:

4.1 Congenital abnormalities
These are diseases due to abnormalities in the development of the foetus, which include genetically determined diseases, e.g. congenital cataract or albinism.

4.2 Inflammations
Inflammatory diseases may be due either to infections (bacteria, viruses, fungi, parasites) e.g. trachoma; or inflammation which may be non-infective or may follow injury to the eye, e.g. iritis.

4.3 Tumours
Tumours may be benign (slowly growing and not spreading elsewhere in the body) e.g. lacrimal adenoma; or malignant (usually rapidly growing and tending to spread to other parts of the body), e.g. retinoblastoma.

4.4 Metabolic and degenerative diseases
Many diseases are due to degeneration of the body's tissues with age (and this group includes diseases of blood vessels) e.g. senile macula degeneration and cataract.

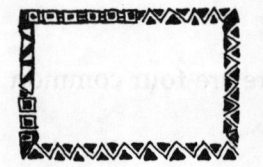

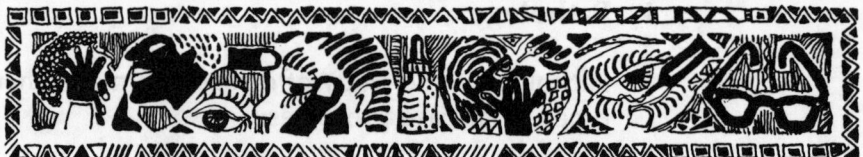

SECTION C:
Diagnosis

The majority of people with eye complaints have common diseases which are usually straightforward to diagnose and treat. In this section notes are given in a systematic form on how to make a diagnosis and treat the common eye conditions, based upon the initial complaint or symptom. The major symptom groups are:
1. Acute red eye
2. Cannot see/loss of vision – for the distance
3. Cannot see near, e.g. reading, sewing
4. Other specific eye symptoms, e.g. diplopia.

1 Acute red eye

Patients presenting with acute red eye may initially be divided into one of **four** groups:
1.1 Acute red eye *in babies* (0-28 days) – ophthalmia neonatorum
1.2 Acute red eye *in children* (6 months-6 years) – this may be due to vitamin A deficiency or measles leading to a corneal ulcer.
1.3 Acute red eye *at any age*:
   1.3.1 Conjunctivitis and trachoma
   1.3.2 Corneal ulcer
   1.3.3 Iritis
   1.3.4 Acute glaucoma.
1.4 Acute red eye due to *injuries*:
   1.4.1 Blunt injuries
   1.4.2 Perforating injuries
   1.4.3 Foreign bodies
   1.4.4 Burns and chemicals.

1.1 Acute red eye in babies – ophthalmia neonatorum
Definition
A sticky eye in any baby during the first twenty eight days of life.

Causes
Neisseria Gonococcus or *Chlamydia Trachomatis*

Diagnosis
a) Eyelids – swollen
b) Conjunctiva – red, swollen and a pussy discharge
c) Cornea – usually clear, but may show a corneal ulcer
d) Pupil – normal

Treatment
a) Clean the eyes with a clean cloth/swab and water.
b) Apply tetracycline eye ointment hourly for four days and then three times a day for ten days.
c) If the ophthalmia neonatorum is very severe, particularly if there is a corneal ulcer, give also antibiotic (e.g. penicillin or chloramphenicol) eye drops every minute for one hour, then every hour for one day then three hourly until there is improvement.
d) Give systemic antibiotics. Example: procaine penicillin 60 mg by IM injection, or other suitable systemic antibiotic.

Prevention
a) Using a clean cloth/swab and water, clean the eyes of each newborn baby immediately at birth even before the baby has opened his eyes.
b) If available, apply tetracycline eye ointment once to a new born baby's eyes (or 1 drop of 1% silver nitrate solution).

1.2 Acute red eye in children – corneal ulcer due to xerophthalmia/measles

As well as the causes of acute red eye which may occur at any age (see page 224), a specific and important cause of red eyes in children is corneal ulcer due to vitamin A deficiency and/or measles.

Definition
Xerophthalmia is dry eyes due to vitamin A deficiency which may lead to corneal ulceration and blindness, particularly during the presence of measles infection.

Causes
Malnutrition – insufficient intake of foods rich in vitamin A
Malabsorption – chronic diarrhoea causing malabsorption of vitamin A
Measles – an increased demand for vitamin A during and after measles infection.

Diagnosis of xerophthalmia
a) Night blindness (XN) – inability to see in dim light e.g. in the evening.

b) Bitot spots (XIB) – white foamy spots on the lateral conjunctiva.
c) Xerosis – dryness of the conjunctiva (XIA) or cornea (X2).
d) Corneal ulcer (keratomalacia) (X3) – ulceration of the cornea.

Treatment of an infant with corneal ulcer
a) Vitamin A 200,000 IU by mouth on the first day, on the second day and after one week.
b) Tetracycline eye ointment three times a day.
c) Atropine eye ointment once a day.
d) An eye pad to stop the child rubbing his eyes and causing perforation.

Prevention of xerophthalmia:
Malnutrition can be prevented by nutrition education. Encourage the use of:
Mother's milk
Mangoes, papaya
More dark green leafy vegetables.
Malabsorption control – oral rehydration solution for diarrhoea.
Measles – immunisation against measles.
Mass Vitamin A supplementation – give Vitamin A capsule (200,000 IU) to children with:
Measles,
Malnutrition,
Malabsorption, or
Any sign of vitamin A deficiency e.g. night blindness or Bitot spots.

1.3 Acute red eye at any age
There are **four** major causes of acute red eye at any age:
1.3.1 Conjunctivitis (this may be acute bacterial infection or chronic chlamydial infection – trachoma)
1.3.2 Corneal ulceration
1.3.3 Iritis
1.3.4 Acute glaucoma.

The differential diagnosis between these common causes of acute red eye can be made by:
a) Assessing the degree of pain and loss of vision
b) Examination of the cornea
c) Examination of the pupil
d) Special diagnostic tests.

1.3.1 Acute conjunctivitis
Definition
Inflammation of the conjunctiva.

Causes
a) Bacterial – *Haemophilus, Streptococcus, Staphylococcus*
b) Viral – *Adenovirus, Herpes simplex, Enterovirus 70*

c) Allergic – Vernal disease
d) Chemical – Cosmetics, smoke, harmful eye practices

Symptoms
a) Little pain
b) Good vision
c) Pus or mucus discharge.

Signs
a) Eyelids – swollen
b) Conjunctiva – redness is maximal in the fornices, often with a discharge
c) Cornea – clear
d) Pupil – normal.

Treatment
a) Bacterial conjunctivitis – tetracycline eye ointment three times a day for one week.
b) Viral conjunctivitis – usually recovers in 7–21 days; tetracycline may be used to stop secondary infection.
c) Severe allergic conjunctivitis (vernal disease) – requires specialist treatment with the minimal and weakest steroid drops needed to relieve symptoms.
d) Chemical conjunctivitis – usually improves once the irritant is removed.

Chronic chlamydial conjunctivitis – Trachoma

Definition
Chronic conjunctivitis due to repeated re-infection with *Chlamydia Trachomatis*.

Causes
There are various environmental factors which favour trachoma and various factors which are important in the repeated transmission of trachoma.
a) **Environment** – features of the environment favouring trachoma:
D̲ry (lack of water)
D̲usty (lack of water)
D̲irty (animal/human faeces)
D̲ischarge (on children's faces).
b) **Transmission** – factors favouring repeated infection with *Chlamydia:*
F̲ingers: eye-finger-eye
F̲lies: eye-fly-eye
F̲omites: eye-cloth/sheet-eye
F̲amily: between mothers, brothers and sisters.

Signs

The signs of trachoma are seen best in the everted upper eyelid and on the cornea. The severity of trachoma depends on the amount of upper eyelid inflammation due to repeated re-infection mainly in childhood.

a) **Active trachoma**
   TF – Trachoma follicles (five or more follicles on the upper tarsal conjunctiva)
   TI – Trachoma intense inflammation (50% or more of the deep tarsal vessels are obscured by papillary hypertrophy)
b) **Inactive**
   TS – Trachoma scars (conjunctival scars)
c) **Trichiasis – entropion**
   TT – Trachoma trichiasis (at least one lash turns in and touches the globe)
d) **Corneal scar**
   CO – Corneal opacity (an opacity which obscures at least part of the pupil margin)

TF and TI is found mainly in pre-school children, the first few years of schooling and in mothers. TS, TT and CO occur more commonly in women than men, starting around the age of 15 and gradually increasing in prevalence.

Treatment

a) Instruct the patient and family in daily face washing.
b) Tetracycline eye ointment two to three times a day for six weeks, for TF and/or TI. Ideally treat the whole family.
c) Systemic treatment with tablets of sulpha or tetracycline for 14 days (this is only required in cases of severe trachoma e.g. severe TI).
d) Epilate for trichiasis, and entropion surgery for entropion.

Prevention

a) Education in the importance of daily face washing, especially for pre-school and school children.
b) Administration of tetracycline eye ointment to any cases of acute red sticky eye, particularly during epidemics of conjunctivitis.

Complications

Severe conjunctivitis from any cause may lead to corneal ulceration, subsequent scarring and blindness.

Inflammation from trachoma leads to conjunctival and tarsal plate scarring which causes the eyelashes to turn in. The lashes rub on the cornea, producing ulceration, scarring and blindness.

1.3.2 Corneal ulceration

Definition

Loss of the corneal epithelium. (Corneal ulceration usually involves the epithelium and stroma of the cornea. Keratitis is an inflammation of the cornea, usually with no loss of corneal epithelium. Corneal abscess is suppuration within the corneal stroma. The term corneal abrasion or corneal erosion is sometimes used for just epithelial loss of the cornea, with or without minor trauma.)

Causes
a) Bacterial – *Staphylococcus, Streptococcus, Gonococcus, Pseudomonas*
b) Viral – *Herpes simplex*, measles
c) Nutritional – Vitamin A deficiency/measles
d) Others – e.g. Harmful eye practices (HEP), trauma

Symptoms
a) Severe pain +++
b) Loss of vision +++

Signs
a) Eyelids – swollen
b) Conjunctiva – redness maximal around the cornea
c) Cornea – there is a grey spot on the cornea
d) Pupil – the pupil is usually normal

Special test
Fluorescein drops or paper applied to the conjunctiva will show green staining of a corneal ulcer when the epithelium is deficient.

Different types of corneal ulceration
a) **Viral** – this is due to *Herpes simplex* virus. The ulcer may be branch-like (DENDRITIC) or may take the appearance of the outline of a country (GEOGRAPHIC, MAP, AMOEBOID) type of ulcer. The treatment of herpetic ulceration is with anti-virals. e.g. idoxuridine ointment × 5/day, trifluorothymidine drops hourly, or acyclovir ointment × 5/day.

b) **Bacterial** – bacterial corneal ulcers may be due to *Staphylococcus, Streptococcus, Pseudomonas,* or *Gonococcus*. They usually present as a stromal ulcer and often produce early **hypopyon** formation. The treatment is with antibiotics. Sub-conjunctival injections of gentamicin 20 mg or chloramphenicol 100 mg are recommended for large corneal ulcers or corneal ulcers with a hypopyon. Combined with this one may give hourly drops of chloramphenicol or tetracycline eye ointment. Smaller ulcers without hypopyon may be treated just with topical antibiotics, example chloramphenicol or gentamicin drops or tetracycline

eye ointment hourly until improvement begins and then slowly reduce the dosage.
c) **Nutritional** – this is due to vitamin A deficiency and is discussed separately (see Section 1.2). The treatment is with Vitamin A.
d) **Fungi** – may also cause a hypopyon ulcer which can be treated with antifungal agents.
e) **Others** – other causes of corneal ulceration include **trauma**, which may cause an abrasion or lead to secondary bacterial infection. The treatment is with antibiotics as for a bacterial ulcer. Another cause of ulceration is the use of **harmful eye practices**, which may cause severe bilateral corneal ulceration with chemical conjunctivitis. The treatment is initially with antibiotics. **Leprosy** may also cause corneal ulceration from exposure of the cornea due to inability to close the eyelids (LAGOPHTHALMOS). This is discussed in the section on leprosy (see Section 2.4.3).

Treatment
The treatment of corneal ulcer is that of the cause – page 227. Atropine ointment 1%, three times/day and an eye pad are usually recommended as well.

Complications
Corneal ulceration may lead to:
a) Diffuse scarring of the cornea
b) Leucoma formation – a dense white scar
c) Perforation of the cornea with adherent iris and possibly staphyloma formation
d) Loss of intra-ocular contents with or without infection (endophthalmitis) leading to phthisis bulbi.

N.B. Staphyloma and endophthalmitis are two of the commonest causes of a blind to light (NPL) painful eye for which the patient may require REMOVAL OF THE EYE. If the patient consents to this procedure, it can be performed in one of two ways:
– **Evisceration** – the cornea and contents of the eye are removed but the scleral shell and optic nerve are left. This is an easy operation and usually produces an acceptable socket which can be fitted with an artificial eye.
– **Enucleation** – the extra-ocular muscles and optic nerve are divided and the whole eye is removed. This is the operation of choice for intra-ocular tumours, e.g. retinoblastoma.

1.3.3 Iritis
Definition
Inflammation of the iris

Causes
a) Trauma/surgery
b) Leprosy
c) Onchocerciasis
d) Others (idiopathic)

Symptoms
a) Pain ++
b) Loss of vision ++
c) Maybe photophobia and lacrimation

Signs
a) Eyelids – normal
b) Conjunctiva – red, with **ciliary injection** around the cornea
c) Cornea – there may be **keratic precipitates** on the inside of the cornea
d) Pupil – the pupil is initially small but on dilation may be irregular due to **posterior synechiae**

Special test
Dilate the pupil in the clinic with cyclopentolate or phenylephrine and look for posterior synechiae which will confirm the diagnosis.

Treatment
a) Dilate the pupil immediately with cyclopentolate and/or phenylephrine.
b) Give atropine ointment three times a day.
c) Give topical steroids as required to reduce the redness and inflammation. (Usually for 1–4 weeks.)
d) Subconjunctival injection of mydriatics or steroids may be required for very severe cases of iritis where drops alone are insufficient to break the posterior synechiae.

Complications
If posterior synechiae develop, the posterior synechiae may cause secondary opacification of the lens leading to **cataract** formation. The posterior synechiae may also occlude the pupil, resulting in a pupil block **glaucoma** with rise in intra-ocular pressure.

1.3.4 Acute glaucoma
Definition
Acute rise in intra-ocular pressure

Causes
a) Primary angle closure
b) Swollen cataract
c) Blunt trauma
d) Iritis

Symptoms
a) Severe pain ++++
b) Vision is markedly reduced ++++
c) Maybe headache and vomiting

Signs
a) Eyelids – often swollen
b) Conjunctiva – red
c) Cornea – hazy due to oedema fluid in the cornea
d) Pupil – the pupil is dilated and does not react to light

Special test
Measurement of intra-ocular pressure with Schiotz tonometer (or digital tonometry)

Treatment
Diamox tablets 500 mg immediately followed by 250 mg four times a day. The patient should be referred for treatment of the cause of the glaucoma, e.g. a swollen cataract will require removal. Primary angle closure can also be treated with pilocarpine drops, but pilocarpine should not be used in acute glaucoma due to swollen cataract, trauma or iritis.

Complications
Persistent elevation in intra-ocular pressure, even for one or two days, will damage the optic nerve causing blindness from optic atrophy.

Summary of acute red eye at any age

	Conjunctivitis	Corneal ulcer	Iritis	Acute glaucoma
Pain and vision loss	+	+++	++	++++
Cornea	Normal	Grey spot	Keratic precipitates	Hazy
Pupil	Normal	Normal	Small and irregular	Dilated and inactive
Special sign	Pus	Fluorescein stain	Irregular pupil after dilation	Raised eye pressure

1.4 Acute red eye due to trauma

There are **four** main types of ocular injury:
1.4.1 Blunt injuries
1.4.2 Perforating injuries
1.4.3 Foreign bodies
1.4.4 Burns or chemicals in the eye.

The type of injury can usually be ascertained from taking the history. The visual acuity in each eye should be measured in all patients with ocular injury.

1.4.1 Blunt injuries to the eye

After taking the history and visual acuity the eye should now be examined.

Examination

a) **Eyelids** – there may be bruising in the eyelids. There is no specific treatment for this and it will gradually resolve over 7–10 days.

There may be a *fracture* of one of the orbital bones. This most commonly affects the medial bone (ethmoid), or the inferior orbital bone (maxilla). The clinical signs of an orbital fracture are:
  i) Bleeding from the nose – epistaxis
  ii) Proptosis of the eye – this may be due to air in the orbit
  iii) Anaesthesia of the lower eyelid – due to damage of the infra-orbital nerve
  iv) Double vision – on looking up due to entrapment of the inferior rectus muscle in an inferior wall fracture; or on looking out – due to entrapment of the medial rectus in a medial wall fracture.

The *management* of a fracture of the orbit depends on the signs. If there is air in the orbit then the patient should be given systemic antibiotics for seven days. If there is double vision, then the patient should be referred to a specialist for possible surgical exploration of the trapped muscle with a view to releasing the muscle from the fracture.

b) **Conjunctiva** – there may be a **sub-conjunctival haemorrhage** due to bleeding under the conjunctiva. There is no specific treatment for this and it will resolve over 7–10 days.

c) **Cornea** – there may be an *abrasion* of the cornea, which will present as an acutely painful eye. This pain will be relieved by local anaesthetic drops and the diagnosis can be confirmed by fluorescein staining of the cornea. The treatment is with antibiotic eye ointment and an eye pad for 24 hours.

d) **Pupil** – the pupil may be *distorted*, or not visible, due to blood in the anterior chamber **(hyphaema).** It is useful to think of hyphaema in two forms. The non-painful variety will usually settle with conservative treatment i.e. bedrest, antibiotic eye ointment and an eye pad for five days. A painful hyphaema may be due to a rise in intra-ocular pressure due to the hyphaema. The eye will be very painful and the pressure will be raised. In this situation, the patient should be given Diamox 250 mg four times a day, and if the hyphaema and glaucoma do not resolve in 48 hours, then surgery may be required to remove the blood from the anterior chamber by paracentesis.

After blunt injury the pupil may be distorted due to *tears in the iris*. This may result in a dilated pupil or an irregular pupil. Occasionally the lens may be damaged by a blunt injury, and there may be **cataract** formation or *dislocation of the lens*. Dislocation of the lens may also cause a rise in intra-ocular pressure, and if this occurs the patient should be referred for possible lens extraction.

The above conditions are the common and more treatable problems arising from blunt injury to the eye. Blunt injury may also damage the posterior segment of the eye and cause vitreous haemorrhage, retinal oedema and haemorrhage, retinal tears and even optic nerve damage. These conditions are less common and usually not easily remediable.

1.4.2 Perforating injury

Having taken a history and visual acuity, which will suggest that the injury is due to a sharp object and may result in perforation of the eye, it is now important to very *gently examine the eye*.

Examination
a) **Eyelids** – there may be lacerations of the eyelids. If these do not involve the lower canaliculus or the lid margin, they can be sutured simply. If the lid margin is involved, then very careful suturing with close apposition of the two edges of the lid margin is required to avoid notching of the margin. If the lower canaliculus has been torn, then the patient will require specialist management to avoid a permanently watering eye from canalicular stenosis.
b) **Conjunctiva** – there may be lacerations of the conjunctiva, but these usually do not require any suturing.
c) **Cornea** – a perforating injury of the eye will usually involve the cornea, and prolapsed uveal tissue will be seen on the surface of the eye.
d) **Pupil** – this will be distorted by the prolapse of iris and the anterior chamber is likely to be shallow. There may also be hyphaema and damage to the lens with cataract formation.

This basic examination of the eye must be undertaken very carefully, making sure that no pressure is placed on the globe as this may result in further prolapse of intra-ocular contents.

Treatment
The first aid management of a perforating injury includes:
a) Administration of tetanus toxoid
b) Antibiotic to the eye (preferably drops)
c) Atropine to the eye (preferably drops)
d) Eye pad.

The patient should then be referred urgently to an eye specialist for admission and treatment. Fresh perforations may be treated surgically by cleaning the wound, excising prolapsed and dead tissue, and resuturing the wound edges with fine sutures followed by reformation of the anterior chamber. With older perforations (after five days) it may be best to treat conservatively with topical antibiotics and atropine.

1.4.3 Foreign bodies
Having taken the history and visual acuity a foreign body may be looked for by performing the following examination.

Examination and treatment
a) **Eyelids** – evert the eyelid and look for a sub-tarsal foreign body on the tarsal conjunctiva. This can be simply removed with cotton wool or a piece of paper.
b) **Conjunctiva** – examine the conjunctiva to see if a foreign body is in the conjunctival sac. This again can simply be removed with cotton wool or a piece of paper.
c) **Cornea** – examine the cornea to see if a foreign body is embedded on the cornea. If the foreign body is superficial, then follow the **four L** practice as follows:
   i) **L**ie the patient flat
   ii) **L**ocal anaesthetic drops are applied
   iii) **L**ight, to give good illumination of the eye
   iv) **L**ift off the foreign body with the corner of a piece of paper, a matchstick or suitable instrument.

The patient should then be given tetracycline eye ointment and an eye pad for 24 hours and seen the next day.

Sometimes the corneal foreign body will be deep, for example a thorn in the cornea. If this is the case it may still be possible to remove the foreign body as above, using a pair of forceps and withdrawing the foreign body in the direction in which it entered the cornea. It is then usually advisable to give a subconjunctival antibiotic injection. If the foreign body is too deeply embedded then it will be necessary to take the patient to the operating theatre and, under full local anaesthesia, perform an operation to remove the foreign body.

d) **Pupil** – occasionally following explosive injuries or an injury where a hammer strikes another piece of metal and a foreign body enters the eye, the foreign body may penetrate the protective layer of the eye and enter right inside. Such an **intra-**

ocular foreign body (IOFB) is of great danger to the eye, but fortunately this is a relatively rare injury. The IOFB may be visible in the anterior chamber; otherwise after dilating the pupil the IOFB may be seen in the lens, vitreous or on the retina. If an intra-ocular foreign body is suspected, the patient should be referred immediately to a specialist after giving topical antibiotics and atropine. If the IOFB can be located it may be possible to remove the IOFB by surgery. However the prognosis for an eye with an intra-ocular foreign body is usually poor.

1.4.4 Burns and chemicals
a) Burns
Burns of the eye may affect the eyelids, conjunctiva or cornea. It is most important to keep the cornea moist and free from exposure. The first aid management is to apply ointment generously all over the conjunctiva, cornea and burned eyelids. An eye pad should *not* be placed over the eye as this may ulcerate the cornea; instead, ointment should be applied every hour to the exposed cornea. The patient should be referred to a specialist who may perform plastic surgery (either a skin graft or tarsorrhaphy) to protect the cornea.

b) Chemicals
The first aid management of chemicals in the eye is immediate and profuse irrigation with water. The patient should lie flat while water is poured into the eye generously for 10–15 minutes. After this time the eye can be examined to see if there is any evidence of corneal ulceration, which can be looked for with fluroescein staining. If there is ulceration, the patient should be given antibiotics, atropine and an eye pad and seen daily.

If concentrated sulphuric acid (car battery acid) or caustic soda (lime) have entered the eye, then this is a much more serious situation. Again the eye should be irrigated profusely for 15 minutes, and then the patient should be immediately referred to hospital for continuous irrigation with a normal saline drip into the eye for 48 hours. Sulphuric acid and lime burns of the eye may lead to severe corneal ulceration, permanent corneal scarring and blindness if they are not vigorously treated.

In summary therefore, **burns** of the eye must be kept *lubricated* and **chemicals** in the eye must be thoroughly *irrigated*.

2 Inability to see – blindness

The symptom of 'cannot see' is a common presenting symptom of eye patients. The causes of loss of vision are many but can, for simplicity, be divided into **four** main groups of diseases.
2.1 Diseases of the cornea – corneal scar.
2.2 Diseases of the lens – cataract.
2.3 Diseases of optic nerve – glaucoma, optic atrophy.
2.4 Other causes of loss of vision:
    2.4.1 Bilateral loss of vision
    2.4.2 Acute unilateral loss of vision
    2.4.3 Leprosy
    2.4.4 Onchocerciasis

The term 'blindness' refers to a loss of vision which results in the patient being unable to continue with a normal lifestyle. Various definitions for blindness are used of which the most common is:
    'Inability to walk by oneself because of loss of vision, usually equivalent to a binocular vision of less than 3/60, less than CF3m.'

The prevalence of blindness varies greatly from country to country and region to region within countries. However, on average it can be said that in industrialised countries 2 people per 1000 are blind compared with 5–20 per 1000 in developing countries. Areas which have blindness from trachoma and onchocerciasis usually have even higher rates of blindness than this, ranging from 10–50 per 1000 total population.

Overall it is estimated that there are as many as 30 million blind people in the world. Nearly half of all the blindness is due to cataract and a quarter of the world's blindness is due to trachoma. Other major causes of blindness are glaucoma, onchocerciasis and xerophthalmia.

The major causes of blindness in both eyes are:
2.1 Corneal scar – trachoma, xerophthalmia, ophthalmia neonatorum, bacterial corneal ulceration, and harmful eye practices
2.2 Cataract
2.3 Optic nerve disease – glaucoma and onchocerciasis
2.4 Other diseases – these include macula degeneration, retinitis pigmentosa, diabetic retinopathy and myopia with its complications.

2.1 Corneal scar
Corneal scarring may account for up to a quarter of all patients with blindness.

The types of scarring can be considered under **four** main groups:
a) Diffuse scar – scar all over the cornea
b) Leucomas – dense white scar in part of the cornea
c) Staphyloma – bulging forward of the cornea
d) Phthisis bulbi – small shrunken eye.

Aetiology
The common causes of *bilateral* corneal scarring are:
a) Ophthalmia neonatorum
b) Vitamin A deficiency
c) Harmful eye practices (HEP)
d) Trachoma.

Common causes of *unilateral* corneal scarring include:
a) Bacterial ulceration
b) Herpetic ulceration
c) Trauma
d) Other rarer causes of corneal ulcer, e.g. fungal infection, leprosy.

Treatment
The management of corneal scar in developing countries is difficult. The majority of patients cannot be helped by medical or surgical treatment. The possibilities for treatment are:
a) **Optical iridectomy** – create an artificial pupil. Optical iridectomy can be performed on *one* eye of a **blind** patient who has a **central leucoma.** It is a relatively simple operation but the visual results are limited.
b) **Corneal grafting** – replaces a corneal scar with a new clear cornea from a donor eye. Corneal grafting can be performed on *one* eye of a **blind** patient with **diffuse scarring** containing only a few or no vessels. It is very difficult to get donor material for corneal grafting and the rejection rate is high, unless there is careful follow-up and the use of long-term topical steroids. For these reasons it is not practical in most situations to undertake corneal grafting in developing countries.
c) **Removal of the eye** – is indicated in patients with a **blind to light painful eye.**
d) The **remainder** of patients with either unilateral corneal scars, phthisis, or scars which do not cause blindness, require no treatment.

Corneal scarring is a major cause of blindness which is difficult to treat. However, the causes of corneal ulcer which lead to scarring are relatively easy to prevent. Corneal scarring accounts on average for 70% of blindness in children in Africa, and 25% of blindness in adults.

2.2 Cataract

Cataract is the single most important cause of blindness in the world. There are an estimated 15 million people blind from cataract in the world of which 3 million live in Africa. On average one in every 200 people is blind from cataract in Africa.

Causes
a) **Congenital** – rubella infection and familial
b) **Traumatic** – perforating and blunt injuries
c) **Secondary** – eye disease (iritis) and systemic diseases (diabetes)
d) **Senile** – no definite cause known

The most common cause of cataract is the senile variety which represents about 85% of all cataracts. There is no proven way of preventing senile cataract, although it is a very treatable disease.

Types of cataract
Cataracts can be classified into different types according to their appearance:
a) **Immature** – this is a partial cataract in which some of the lens has become opaque. It can be further sub-divided into:
 i) Anterior cortical
 ii) Nuclear sclerosis
 iii) Posterior cortical.
b) **Mature** – the total lens has now become opaque.
c) **Intumescent** – all the lens is opaque and the lens is swollen due to absorption of water.
 The intumescent (swollen) cataract may push the iris forward and occlude the angle of the eye causing a **secondary glaucoma.** This will present as an acute red painful eye with a hazy cornea, shallow anterior chamber and fixed dilated white pupil with high intra-ocular pressure.
d) **Hypermature** – the lens is completely opaque but is now small and wrinkled due to loss of water.
 Occasionally the hypermature type of cataract may cause a **secondary iritis** due to leakage of lens protein from the lens into the anterior chamber. This may also lead to a secondary glaucoma due to blockage of the trabecular meshwork with cells and lens protein.

Clinical signs and symptoms
Cataract usually presents as gradual loss of vision in one or both eyes. On examination the visual acuity is reduced, the conjunctiva is white, the cornea is clear, and there is an opacity in the pupil. Immature cataracts cause a grey opacity in the pupil, while mature, intumescent and hypermature cataracts give a white pupil.

Assessment of cataract for surgery

In deciding whether to refer a patient for cataract surgery, the following **four** examinations must be performed:
a) **Visual acuity** – the visual acuity must be accurately measured in each eye.
b) **Pupil reaction** – in cataract there is a normal brisk reaction of the pupil. If the pupil does not react briskly to light, other diseases, for example optic nerve disease, should be suspected as the cause of the loss of vision.
c) **Tonometry** – measurement of the intra-ocular pressure is important to see if the cause of loss of vision may be due to glaucoma.
d) **Ophthalmoscopy** – after dilating the pupil the fundus should be examined with an ophthalmoscope for the red reflex to assess how dense the lens opacity is. This is particularly important in immature cataracts. If it is still easily possible to visualise the optic disc and fundus then the lens opacity is not yet dense enough to warrant cataract extraction.

Treatment of cataract

There are **four** possible treatments:
a) **Cataract extraction** – is indicated in the following circumstances:
  i) To improve the patient's required vision
  ii) To treat a complication of cataract e.g. secondary glaucoma.
b) **Atropine** ointment weekly – this may be indicated in an immature nuclear or posterior cortical cataract which is not yet ready for surgery. The atropine will dilate the pupil and may therefore improve the vision. (There is the possible danger of causing acute glaucoma with atropine, if the anterior chamber is shallow.)
c) **Spectacles** – occasionally the visual loss due to nuclear cataracts is associated with myopia which can be improved by minus (concave) specatacles.
d) **Nil** – in cases of unilateral cataract or bilateral small immature cataracts, no treatment may be indicated at the time but the patient should be reviewed after three to six months.

Management of patients with cataract

Patients presenting with cataract can be considered under **four** groups:
a) **Bilateral cataract** – patients with cataract in both eyes.
b) **Unilateral cataract** – patients with a cataract in one eye and normal lens and vision in the other eye.
c) **Only eye cataract** – patients with a cataract in one eye whose other eye is totally and irremediably blind.
d) **Second eye cataract** – patients who have already had successful cataract surgery in one eye and now have a cataract in the second eye.

Indications for cataract surgery

These correspond to the group the patient is in (opposite). The following are indications for the elderly from rural areas in Africa:

a) **Bilateral cataract** – patients with bilateral cataract should be operated on when the visual acuity is reduced below 6/60 in both eyes i.e. **the vision in both eyes** is **count fingers or less**.

b) **Unilateral cataract** – the indication for surgery in unilateral cataract is to treat, or prevent, possible complications of cataract, as the patient's vision in the other eye is good. The patient's vision will not be improved by operating on a unilateral cataract and prescribing aphakic spectacles. Therefore the indication to operate is **to prevent or treat secondary glaucoma or secondary uveitis.**

c) **Only eye cataract** – surgery should be delayed on patients with only eye cataract until their vision is so poor that they have difficulty in getting about by themselves. This is because of the possible complications that may follow any cataract operation occurring in a patient who is already totally blind in one eye. It is therefore recommended that cataract on an only eye be delayed until the person's vision is severely restricted i.e. **less than count fingers at three metres.**

d) **Second eye cataract** – if the patient is already happy with aphakic spectacles provided after the first cataract operation, then cataract surgery can be considered on the second eye **at any time convenient to the surgeon and patient**. Because the patient can already see with one eye, priority should be given to patients with bilateral cataracts and only-eye cataract, over those requesting surgery on their second eye.

Nursing care of a cataract patient
Pre-operative
a) Explain the operation and ensure patient's consent.
b) Wash the patient's face and cut the eyelashes.
c) Give treatment as ordered:
   i) antibiotics (for 24 hours pre-op)
   ii) dilating drops (1 hour pre-op)
   iii) local anaesthetic drops (1/2 hour pre-op).
d) Label the eye which is to be operated on.
Operative
a) The operation is usually performed under local anaesthetic.
b) A nurse should stay with the patient throughout the operation.
c) The operation is performed under full sterile conditions.
d) An eye pad is placed over the eye at the end of the operation.
Post-operative
a) The patient should remain in bed until next morning when a *first dressing* is performed by the surgeon.
b) After the first dressing, drugs and dressings should be given as ordered by the doctor.

c) The patient is usually discharged between 1 and 10 days after the operation.
d) The patient will require APHAKIC glasses.

Cataract operation
a) The operation is usually performed under local anaesthetic. This consists of giving a facial nerve block to prevent the patient from closing the eye and a retrobulbar nerve block to anaesthetise the eye and also prevent movement of the eye.
b) The cataract can be removed in two ways:
    i) **Intracapsular cataract extraction** in which the whole lens is removed within the capsule of the cataract.
    ii) **Extracapsular cataract extraction** in which the anterior capsule is broken and the nucleus and cortex of the lens removed in pieces leaving the posterior capsule in place.

    Intracapsular cataract extraction is, at present, the preferred method of extraction in developing countries, although extracapsular cataract extraction is safer in younger people, (0–30 years old).

    There are various ways in which the cataract may be removed by intracapsular extraction and these include:
    i) Cryoextraction
    ii) Forceps
    iii) Erisophake
    iv) Expression.
c) After removal of the cataract the corneal section is sutured, usually with nylon or virgin silk sutures. The number of sutures may vary on the size of the incision, but is usually three to seven.

    The patient should rest in bed until the next day when a first dressing is performed.
d) Complications at the time of surgery include:
    i) Accidental rupture of the lens capsule when trying to do an intracapsular extraction resulting in accidental extracapsular extraction.
    ii) Loss of vitreous after removing the cataract.
    iii) Occasionally, bleeding in the eye may be severe and a problem.

Post-operative management
Each day the post-operative cataract patient should be examined and the dressing changed. Early *post-operative complications* include:
a) Infection – **endophthalmitis**. The patient complains of pain in the eye and loss of vision. The eye is red, the cornea hazy and there may be a hypopyon. Treatment is with sub-conjunctival and systemic antibiotics. The prognosis is usually poor.
b) Bleeding – **hyphaema**. There is blood in the anterior chamber. This will usually resolve itself with bed-rest over a few days.

c) Wound leakage – **shallow anterior chamber** and **iris prolapse**. If there is obvious iris prolapse the patient must have another operation, at which the prolapsed iris is excised and the wound resutured. If the anterior chamber is flat, but without iris prolapse, then a firm pad and bandage for 24–48 hours is advised. If this fails and the wound is still leaking aqueous then it will require resuturing.
d) Rise in intra-ocular pressure – **secondary glaucoma**. There are various reasons for the pressure going up after cataract surgery. One of the more common is pupil block with vitreous. The anterior chamber is flat and the pressure high. Full dilation of the pupil will usually break the pupil block glaucoma, and if there is no patent peripheral iridectomy, then it will be necessary to perform this operation as a secondary procedure.
e) Inflammation – **iritis**. Some degree of iritis is common after cataract surgery, which usually resolves itself spontaneously over a few days. The iritis is more severe after extra-capsular cataract surgery or if vitreous has been lost. In these situations it is advisable to give topical steroids for 1–2 weeks after surgery to suppress the iritis.
f) Damage to the corneal endothelium – **striate keratitis**. If the corneal endothelium has been traumatised then there may be visible corneal oedema known as striate keratitis. This does not require treatment and usually settles in 1–5 days.

The post-operative cataract patient should be examined each day with *particular attention* being paid to:
a) **The wound** – to see that it is tight and there is no evidence of iris prolapse.
b) **The cornea** – to see that it is clear.
c) **The anterior chamber** – to examine the depth and also the contents.
d) **The pupil** – to see if it is circular and also whether there is a red reflex.

Cataract patients are usually kept in hospital for 1–10 days and then given a pair of aphakic spectacles (+10). The actual number of glasses required varies from individual to individual, but on average it is around +10.00 for distance and +14.00 for reading. Aphakic spectacles cause some distortions in vision. Objects appear larger and straight edges may appear curved. The field of vision is also limited with aphakic spectacles.

2.3 Glaucoma

There are many causes of optic nerve disease (optic atrophy), but glaucoma is the most important in Africa.

Other causes of optic atrophy include onchocerciasis (see Section 2.4.4), trauma, fevers in childhood, meningitis and occasionally tumours of the orbit or optic chiasma.

Definition
Raised intra-ocular pressure which damages the optic nerve leading to loss of vision. (The pressure may sometimes be recorded as normal.)

Causes
a) Congenital
b) Secondary
c) Primary angle closure
d) Chronic open angle glaucoma

Mechanism
The intra-ocular pressure may rise because of:
a) Increased secretion of aqueous by the ciliary body
b) Decreased drainage of aqueous due to PUPIL BLOCK
c) Decreased drainage of aqueous due to ANGLE BLOCK
d) Decreased drainage of aqueous due to TRABECULAR BLOCK (see Section B 2.1).

Clinical presentation
Glaucoma may present in two clinical forms:
a) **Acute** – an acute rise in intra-ocular pressure leading to a red painful eye with sudden loss of vision, a hazy cornea, shallow anterior chamber, and fixed dilated pupil. This type of glaucoma may be primary or may be secondary to other diseases such as intumescent cataract, trauma, iritis, and other rarer causes.
b) **Chronic** – chronic rise in intra-ocular pressure over a long period of time causes gradual loss of vision in white eyes. This may be due to chronic open angle glaucoma, or secondary to other diseases e.g. blunt injury, or iritis.

The commonest type of glaucoma leading to loss of vision in Africa is chronic glaucoma which is usually open angle. This disease is usually bilateral, but may be asymmetrical. It may occur at any age but is more common after the age of 30. The cause is unknown, but it is believed that the obstruction to drainage is at the level of the trabeculum (trabecular block).

Clinical manifestations
There are **four** important clinical manifestations of chronic glaucoma:
a) **Loss of vision** – this starts as a loss of visual field, followed by a loss of visual acuity, and finally complete loss of light perception.
b) **Abnormal pupil responses** – this begins as a *relative* pupil defect in which one pupil does not react as well as the other to the swinging torch test. Further damage of the optic nerve leads to a *partial* pupil defect in which there is a sluggish response of the pupil, and finally there is a *total* pupil defect in which there is no response at all to light.

c) **Raised intra-ocular pressure** – this can be demonstrated either by digital tonometry which is easy but unreliable, Schiotz tonometry which is relatively easy and fairly reliable, or applanation tonometry, which is more difficult to perform, but which is very accurate. Using a Schiotz tonometer with a 5.5 gm weight, a reading of 2 or less is indicative of high pressure (more than 28 mms Hg), and a reading of 4 or above is indicative of normal pressure (less than 21 mms Hg).

d) **Cupping of the disc** – optic nerve damage can be demonstrated by looking at the optic disc with an ophthalmoscope. In chronic glaucoma the Configuration of the disc is abnormal, with a cup:disc ratio of more than 0.5, the Colour of the disc is pale – not pink, and Comparison of the two eyes of the patient may reveal asymmetry in size and colour between the discs. All these findings suggest glaucoma.

In summary, therefore, chronic glaucoma can be suspected in a patient with loss of vision as demonstrated by the Test Type, an abnormal pupil response demonstrated with a Torch, and raised intra-ocular pressure demonstrated with the Tonometer. Definite cupping of the disc on ophthalmoscopy will confirm the diagnosis and in late cases there may also be a hazy cornea due to corneal oedema.

Management of chronic glaucoma
There are **four** possible managements:
a) **Topical medical therapy** – pilocarpine or timolol. These drugs must be taken regularly for the rest of the patient's life. Their disadvantages are poor patient acceptance and the expense of buying the drugs.
b) **Systemic treatment with Diamox** – this also must be taken four times a day for the rest of the patient's life. It has the disadvantage of causing lethargy and other more serious side effects.
c) **Trabeculectomy** – this relatively simple operation has a reasonable success rate and is the recommended treatment of choice in patients with glaucoma who still have useful vision to save. The operation does not improve the vision but only preserves what remaining vision there is.
d) **Nil** – in patients who are already blind (that is they cannot see to walk by themselves) no therapy will restore the eyesight and no treatment can be recommended.

2.4 Other causes of loss of vision
Discussed under this heading are:
2.4.1 Other causes of *bilateral* visual loss
2.4.2 Causes of *acute* loss of vision in *one* eye
2.4.3 Leprosy
2.4.4 Onchocerciasis.

2.4.1 Other causes of bilateral visual loss
Other causes of loss of vision in both eyes besides corneal scar, cataract and glaucoma include:
a) Refractive errors
b) Uveitis
c) Diseases of the macula of the retina
d) Diseases of the periphery of the retina.

a) **Refractive errors** – can usually be diagnosed from the fact that the visual acuity improves with pin-hole examination. The common refractive errors are:
  i) Myopia
  ii) Hypermetropia
  iii) Astigmatism
  iv) Presbyopia.

These are discussed in more detail later, under 'Refractive errors' (see Section 3, page 249).

b) **Uveitis** – may be unilateral or bilateral and presents as fairly sudden loss of vision over several days in a white eye or, sometimes, a red eye associated with an anterior uveitis. The causes of posterior uveitis are often unknown but may be due to toxoplasmosis or toxocariasis infection. If there is a specific cause, e.g. toxoplasmosis, then treatment with Daraprim and sulphonamides is recommended, otherwise a trial of systemic steroids may be given to see if there is any improvement.

c) **Diseases of the macula** include – senile macular degeneration, chloroquine maculopathy and other less common forms of macular disease. Occasionally infections with toxocara or toxoplasma may affect the macular area.

d) **Diseases of the periphery of the retina** – may cause gradual loss of vision in both eyes. Retinitis pigmentosa is a familial disease which presents as gradual loss of vision in both eyes over several years, often starting in adolescence. The ophthalmoscopic findings are typical, with black pigmentation starting in the periphery and gradually approaching the optic nerve. The pigmentation often follows the distribution of the blood vessels.

In general, diseases of the retina are less common than corneal scar, cataract and chronic glaucoma. Diseases of the retina are usually not treatable.

2.4.2 Acute unilateral loss of vision in a white eye
Occasionally patients may present with sudden loss of vision in one eye. The common causes of this presentation are:
a) Posterior uveitis
b) Retinal detachment
c) Optic neuritis
d) Retinal vessel occlusion.

a) **Posterior uveitis** – this may present as loss of vision over one or two days in a red or a white eye. There may be signs of an anterior uveitis. After dilation of the pupil the vitreous will appear hazy and the view of the fundus is indistinct. Causes of posterior uveitis include toxoplasmosis and toxocariasis. If no specific cause can be identified, a trial of systemic steroids may be used.

b) **Retinal detachment** – the patient may complain of a flash of light, followed by a black floating 'cobweb' in the vision which gradually gives way to a shadow or curtain moving across the vision, eventually causing complete loss of vision in the eye.

After dilation of the pupil, examination with an ophthalmoscope will reveal an abnormal red reflex in one area of the retina, with elevation and abnormal tortuosity of the vessels and retina. Patients diagnosed as having a retinal detachment should be referred urgently to an eye specialist. Retinal detachment is more common in people with high myopia, aphakia or injury to the eye.

c) **Optic neuritis** – this presents as sudden loss of vision in one or both eyes. It sometimes follows the use of drugs or methyl alcohol. Occasionally it occurs without any known cause. Examination reveals severe loss of vision with an absent pupil light reflex. Ophthalmoscopy may show an absolutely normal optic nerve (retrobulbar neuritis) or a swollen optic disc (papillitis). A trial of systemic steroids is justified in severe bilateral cases.

d) **Retinal vessel occlusion** – occlusion of the central retinal artery or central retinal vein may cause sudden loss of vision to the patient. Central retinal artery occlusion reveals a pale oedematous retina on ophthalmoscopy, with a cherry red spot at the macula. Central retinal vein thrombosis on the other hand shows a swollen disc with multiple haemorrhages all over the retina. There is no specific treatment for these conditions, although an underlying cause in the cardiovascular system or blood may be looked for. Central retinal vein thrombosis occasionally causes a secondary glaucoma three months after the thrombosis, which is known as neovascular glaucoma.

2.4.3 Leprosy

Leprosy is a chronic infection of skin and nerves caused by the bacteria *Mycobacterium leprae*.

Leprosy can affect the eyes by damaging the nerves to the eye, or by causing an inflammation in the iris – iritis.

Clinical signs of ocular leprosy

a) **Eyelids** – the most important effect of leprosy on the eyelids is to cause paralysis of the muscle which closes the eye: orbicularis oculi. This muscle is supplied by the facial nerve (seventh cra-

nial nerve) which may be paralysed in leprosy. The inability to close the eye is called **lagophthalmos**. Inability to close the eye leads to exposure of the cornea and resultant corneal ulceration, scarring and blindness.
b) **Conjunctiva** – this is not specifically affected by leprosy.
c) **Cornea** – leprosy may affect the ophthalmic nerve which is a branch of the trigeminal (fifth cranial nerve). This results in **anaesthesia of the cornea**. The patient does not blink as much as usual and may also be unaware of minor trauma to the cornea. This can cause **corneal ulceration**, scarring and blindness. The cornea may also be ulcerated from exposure due to lagophthalmos.
d) **Pupil** – in leprosy there may be acute **iritis** with a red painful eye, and small irregular pupil. This may occur as part of the ENL (Erythema Nodosum Leprosum) reaction when a leprosy patient is treated with anti-leprosy drugs. Leprosy may also cause a chronic silent or quiet iritis in which the pupil is very small and irregular, and will not dilate. The eye is usually white in chronic iritis.

Ocular examination of a leprosy patient
a) Visual acuity – it is always very important to measure the visual acuity in each eye of a leprosy patient.
b) Eyelid closure – ask the patient to gently close his eyes and observe whether there is any lagophthalmos with corneal exposure.
c) Fluorescein staining – using fluorescein, examine the cornea for evidence of exposure keratopathy or corneal ulcer.
d) Dilate the pupil – give short-acting pupil dilators (e.g. cyclopenolate 1%) to examine the pupil for evidence of posterior synechiae due to iritis.

Treatment
a) **Lagophthalmos** – if there is evidence of lagophthalmos it may be necessary to protect the cornea at night when the patient is asleep by applying ointment, and possibly strapping the upper eyelid to the cheek. If the lagophthalmos is severe and permanent, or if there is any evidence of corneal ulceration, then a lateral tarsorrhaphy will be required to protect the cornea. A lateral tarsorrhaphy consists of sewing the upper and lower eyelids together over the lateral third of the eyelid margins.
b) **Corneal anaesthesia** – if there is evidence of corneal anaesthesia without ulceration then the patient should be taught *think-blink*. This requires the patient to consciously think about blinking and so protect the cornea by regularly blinking.
c) **Corneal ulcer** – in the presence of frank corneal ulceration the patient should be treated with topical antibiotics and atropine. If there is lagophthalmos or corneal anaesthesia a lateral tarsorrhaphy should be performed.

d) **Iritis** – in acute iritis the pupil should be dilated immediately and the patient kept on atropine and topical steroids. In chronic iritis it is important to keep the pupil dilated and to maintain the patient on mydriatics for life.

Many leprosy patients become blind from corneal scarring due to exposure of the cornea from lagophthalmos and corneal anaesthesia. This can be prevented by early recognition of the problem, and educating the patient to protect his cornea during the day by blinking, and at night with ointment and strapping of the eyelid to the cheek. If these measures fail to protect the cornea, then a permanent lateral tarsorrhaphy is required. Leprosy patients also become blind because of secondary cataract and secondary glaucoma as a consequence of iritis. If there is any evidence of iritis in a patient with leprosy it is very important to dilate immediately the pupil and keep the patient on atropine for as long as there is any evidence of iritis.

2.4.4 Onchocerciasis

An infection of the skin and eye of man due to *Onchocerca volvulus*.

Natural history (Figure 40)

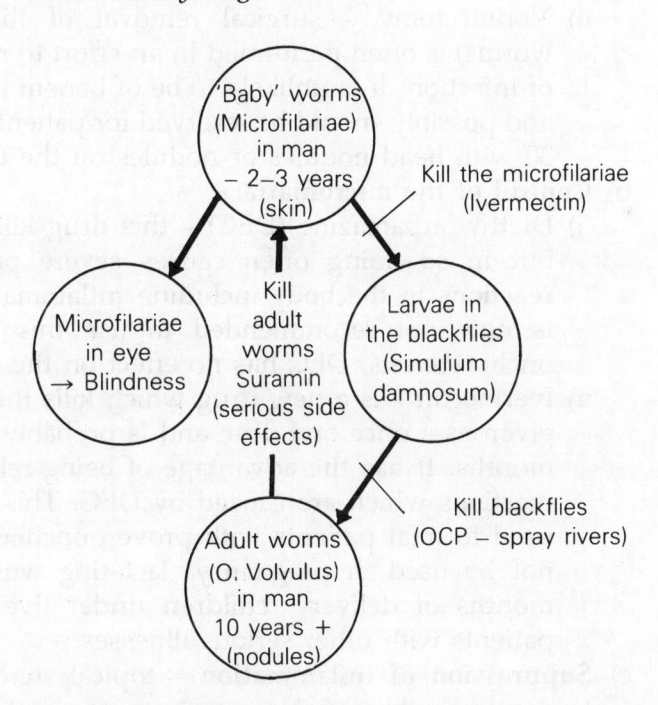

Figure 40
Natural life cycle of onchocerciasis

Skin signs of disease
a) Dermatitis causing roughened skin
b) Dermatitis causing atrophic depigmented skin
c) Dermatitis causing itching
d) Nodules, usually over bony prominences

Eye signs of onchocerciasis
a) Inflammation of the cornea – acute punctate **keratitis**, which may lead on to **sclerosing keratitis** and corneal scar.
b) Inflammation of the iris – **iritis**, which causes posterior synechiae and peripheral anterior synechiae, leading to **secondary glaucoma**.
c) Inflammation of the choroid and retina – **chorioretinitis**, which causes night blindness, with **chorioretinal atrophy** most marked temporal to the macula.
d) Inflammation of the optic nerve – **optic neuritis** leading to secondary **optic atrophy** which is the major cause of visual loss in onchocerciasis.

Control of onchocerciasis infection
There are various forms of possible control of onchocerciasis:
a) **Control of the adult worms:**
   i) Suramin – this drug is given as a weekly intravenous injection over six weeks to kill the adult worms. It is effective but has serious side effects and should only be given to hospitalised patients. It is therefore not a very practical drug for the majority of patients with onchocerciasis.
   ii) Nodulectomy – surgical removal of the nodules (adult worms) is often performed in an effort to reduce the amount of infection. It is unlikely to be of benefit to elderly patients, and possibly should be reserved for patients under the age of 30 with head nodules or nodules on the upper body.
b) **Control of the microfilaria:**
   i) Diethylcarbamazine (DEC) – this drug kills the microfilaria, but in so doing often causes severe pruritus and other reactions in the body including inflammation in the eye. It is now not recommended to use this drug for treating onchocerciasis. DEC has no effect on the adult worm.
   ii) Ivermectin – is a new drug which kills the microfilaria. It is given as a once oral dose and is probably effective for 6–12 months. It has the advantage of being relatively free of the reactions which are caused by DEC. This drug can now be used to treat patients with proven onchocerciasis. It should not be used in pregnancy, lactating women within three months of delivery, children under five years of age, or patients with other serious illnesses.
c) **Suppression of inflammation** – topical steroids may be used to suppress the inflammatory aspects of keratitis and iritis. Systemic steroids are also used in cases of papillitis associated with onchocerciasis.
d) **Vector control** – community programmes for the prevention of blindness from onchocerciasis have mainly focused on reducing the number of Simulium flies by spraying the rivers where the vector breeds. This has been done since 1976 in seven of the

West African countries. This programme, the Onchocerciasis Control Programme, was extended to four other West African countries in 1986.

Management of patients with ocular onchocerciasis
Important aspects in the management of patients with onchocerciasis in order to prevent blindness are:
a) Treatment of patients with Ivermectin 150 ug/kg once/year.
b) Early treatment of iritis and keratitis with topical steroids and atropine.
c) The early diagnosis and management of secondary glaucoma. This may include topical steroids, atropine, Diamox, and possibly trabeculectomy if required.
d) The treatment of active acute papillitis with systemic steroids.

As already mentioned, the value of nodulectomy is questionable, although it is probably reasonable to remove nodules from the head and upper body of younger patients.

3 Refractive errors

Many patients over the age of 40 have difficulty in reading. This condition is called presbyopia. Other refractive errors are more difficult to diagnose and treat. The refractive errors are:
3.1 Myopia
3.2 Hypermetropia
3.3 Astigmatism
3.4 Presbyopia.

3.1 Myopia
The person has difficulty seeing in the distance (reduced visual acuity) but usually no difficulty in seeing near objects. The condition usually starts between ages 5 and 20, and may gradually get worse up to the age of 25. It is corrected by *minus spherical lenses*, which may be different in the two eyes. The spectacles are usually worn for distance and reading. (See Section B 2.4)

3.2 Hypermetropia
This occurs usually in young people who may present in childhood with a **squint**, or in adolescence with headaches and **eyestrain** when reading. The visual acuity is usually normal, although this will begin to fall around the age of 40 if the hypermetropia is not corrected. The treatment is with *plus spherical lenses*, usually worn for distance and reading. (See Section B 2.4)

3.3 Astigmatism
The refractive error of the eye is different in different axis of

direction (e.g. maybe +1.00 vertical and +2.00 horizontal, or −2.50 vertical and +1.00 horizontal). Astigmatism causes a reduction in visual acuity for distance as well as headaches and blurring of vision when doing a lot of close work. It is treated with *cylindrical lenses* of the appropriate power.

3.4 Presbyopia

This is caused by failure of the lens of the eye to change shape (ACCOMMODATION) when focusing from distant objects to near ones. This difficulty usually begins around the age of 40.

Features of Presbyopia
a) The patient complains of difficulty in seeing near objects (e.g. reading, sewing), which is getting worse with increasing age.
b) The patient is usually aged 40 or over.
c) The corrected visual acuity for distance is normal (the patient may or may not have a refractive error for distance – see above).
d) The difficulty in reading is treated by giving *plus spherical lenses* (of equal power to both eyes) usually following these guidelines:
   i) age 45 approximately +1.0
   ii) age 55 approximately +2.0
   iii) age 65 approximately +3.0
   Presbyopic glasses are only worn for close work.

4 Other eye diseases

There are a great many eye diseases which have not been mentioned so far in the text. In this section, a few of the more important eye diseases which affect the ocular adnexae are discussed. Following the system used to describe the anatomy of the orbit, we will discuss these other eye diseases under **four** sections:
4.1 Diseases of the orbital bones and sinuses (Section B 1.2.1).
4.2 Diseases of the muscles and nerves (Section B 1.2.2).
4.3 Diseases of the eyelid (Section B 1.2.3).
4.4 Diseases of the nasolacrimal apparatus (Section B 1.2.4).

4.1 Diseases of the orbital bones and sinuses
4.1.1 Proptosis
Definition
Protrusion of the eye out of the orbit due to a space occupying lesion in the orbit.

Causes:

	Children	Adults
ACUTE (history of less than 3 months)	Retinoblastoma (0–5 yrs) Orbital cellulitis Burkitt's lymphoma (5–15 yrs) Metastases	Orbital cellulitis Pseudotumour Dysthyroid eye disease Lacrimal carcinoma
CHRONIC (history of 3 months or more)	Vascular abnormalities in the orbit Optic glioma	Lacrimal adenoma Frontal mucocoele Meningioma Hydatid cyst

Diagnosis and management

a) **Retinoblastoma** – a malignant tumour of the retina which may be familial and may be bilateral. The first sign can be a squint, followed by a white/yellow reflex in the pupil known as **leucocoria.** Enucleation of the eye or radiotherapy at this stage may save the child's life. If left untreated, the tumour spreads along the optic nerve causing proptosis. The prognosis for life at this stage, even with exenteration of the orbit, is poor.

b) **Orbital cellulitis** – infection may enter the orbit from the sinuses or from trauma. There is a sudden onset of fever with swollen eyelids and proptosis. Treatment is with intensive systemic antibiotics. Orbital cellulitis may lead to cavernous sinus thrombosis with uni- and then bilateral proptosis, venous engorgement and total paralysis of ocular movements. Treatment is with systemic antibiotics.

c) **Burkitt's lymphoma** – this unusual tumour typically occurs between the ages of 5 and 15. The orbit is one of the common sites. There is a rapid onset of usually painless proptosis in which the eye appears relatively normal. Treatment is with cytotoxics, e.g. cyclophosphamide 40 mg/kg IV one dose. This can be repeated after two weeks but only if the blood picture is reasonably normal.

d) **Metastases** – in children the orbit may be the site of secondary deposits from neuroblastoma or acute leukaemia. In adults breast or lung carcinoma may give secondary deposits in the orbit.

e) **Pseudotumour** – this is a condition of unknown cause which typically affects people aged 15–35. Over the course of 1–2 weeks there is uni- or bilateral proptosis with or without paralysis of the extra-ocular muscles. All investigations are normal. The condition responds to high dose systemic steroids which can be tailed off over 4 weeks, although a maintenance dose of prednisolone 5 mg/day may be required for 3–6 months.

f) **Dysthyroid eye disease** – Bilateral or unilateral proptosis may be associated with abnormalities of the thyroid gland. It is more common in middle-aged women. Besides signs of thyroid dysfunction there may be lid retraction and limitation of ocular movements. If the patient is thyrotoxic, this should be treated. If the proptosis threatens vision then systemic steroids may be used and, if this fails, an operation to decompress the orbit can be performed.

g) **Lacrimal carcinoma** – this is a rare malignant tumour of the lacrimal gland usually occuring in elderly people. If diagnosed early surgical removal may be attempted, but the prognosis is poor.

h) **Vascular abnormalities of the orbit** – these may be present at birth, develop during childhood or appear for the first time in adults. They include cavernous and capillary haemangiomas, arterio-venous fistulae and venous varices. Treatment is usually not necessary.

i) **Optic glioma** – this is a slow growing benign tumour of the optic nerve. There is loss of vison with optic atrophy and then unilateral proptosis. Treatment is usually not indicated.

j) **Lacrimal adenoma** – a benign but locally invasive tumour of the lacrimal gland. There is gradual proptosis over months or years with a palpable tumour in the superior-temporal quadrant of the orbit. Treatment is total excision of the tumour with the lacrimal gland.

k) **Frontal mucocoele** – this is a cystic swelling originating from the frontal sinus. There is slowly progressive proptosis with a palpable tumour in the superior-nasal quadrant of the orbit. Treatment is by surgical drainage.

l) **Meningioma** – a benign, slowly growing tumour which may affect the sphenoid bone or the optic nerve. There is gradual proptosis, paralysis of eye movements and loss of vision. There is no satisfactory treatment. Diagnosis can usually be made on the x-ray showing sclerotic appearances.

m) **Hydatid cyst** – in parts of Africa, particularly northern Kenya, hydatid disease is common, and it may cause proptosis. Very careful surgical excision can be performed, but it is important not to rupture the cyst.

In summary, **proptosis** is a fairly uncommon but important and usually serious condition. The age of the patient and rapidity of onset should give an idea as to the diagnosis. Examination of the eye, ocular movements and palpation of the orbital rim for tumours will usually enable a provisional diagnosis to be made. In most situations, further investigations are not possible and the patient should be referred to a specialist if possible, or a trial of therapy may be tried if indicated and if referral is not possible.

4.2 Diseases of the muscles and nerves

Diseases of the muscles and nerves include **four** relatively common conditions:
4.2.1 Strabismus (squint)
4.2.2 Diplopia (double vision)
4.2.3 Ptosis
4.2.4 Lagophthalmos.

4.2.1 Strabismus

Strabismus is when the eyes are not straight. It usually starts in early childhood. The squint may be in-turning (**esotropia**) or out-turning (**exotropia**). If left untreated a squint in childhood can lead to disuse of the eye, with suppression of the visual stimuli leading to loss of vision known as **amblyopia**.

Treatment

It is possible to treat amblyopia and recover vision up to about the age of 8. However, once the child is aged 8 or older the amblyopia will usually remain for life.

If a child is diagnosed as having a squint before the age of 8 he should be referred to a specialist for treatment. Treatment may include:
a) Correction of any refractive error with spectacles.
b) Treatment of any amblyopia with intermittent occlusion of the good eye.
c) Surgery, if required, to straighten the eyes.

If a child, aged 8 or more, or an adult is diagnosed as having a squint and/or amblyopia, then there is no specific treatment. The only reason then for surgery would be to correct the squint to improve the cosmetic appearance.

4.2.2 Diplopia

Diplopia means double vision.

Causes and Treatment

There are many causes, of which some are serious in nature:
a) **A sixth nerve (abducens) palsy** – will cause diplopia with a convergent squint and inability to look out with the affected eye due to paralysis of the lateral rectus muscle. Causes of sixth nerve palsy are hypertension, diabetes mellitus and raised intra-cranial pressure. Treatment is that of the cause.
b) **A third nerve (oculomotor) palsy** – causes ptosis, the eye is displaced down and out and cannot look up or in. The pupil may be dilated. Causes of a third nerve palsy are hypertension, diabetes and brain aneurysms. Treatment is that of the cause.

Patients with definite diplopia should be referred to a specialist quickly.

c) **Myasthenia gravis** – a disease causing weakness of muscles.
d) Any cause of **proptosis**, e.g. thyroid eye disease.

4.2.3 Ptosis
Ptosis is an inability to open the eye normally.

Causes
a) Congenital
b) Traumatic
c) Oculomotor palsy
d) Muscular diseases, e.g. myasthenia gravis

Patients with ptosis should be referred to a specialist to confirm the cause and decide whether ptosis surgery will be of benefit or not.

4.2.4 Lagophthalmos
Lagophthalmos is an inability to close the eye. It is usually due to paralysis of the orbicularis oculi muscle following facial nerve paresis. It is an important sign and complication of leprosy. The management of lagophthalmos is discussed under Section 2.4.3.

4.3 Disease of the eyelids
These are discussed under **four** headings:
4.3.1 Skin tumours
4.3.2 Meibomian cysts/hordeolum
4.3.3 Trichiasis/entropion
4.3.4 Ectropion.

4.3.1 Skin tumours
There are two important skin tumours which can affect the eyelids:

a) The **squamous cell carcinoma** – is a slowly growing malignant tumour which spreads to regional lymph nodes. It is more common in albinos. Squamous cell carcinoma may also arise from the conjunctiva spreading locally to invade the fornices and eyelids.
b) **Basal cell carcinoma** – occurs in elderly people and is more common in light skinned races. It is locally invasive, but rarely metastasises. Treatment is by surgical removal or radiotherapy.

4.3.2 Meibomian cyst and hordeolum
a) Meibomian cyst (**chalazion**) – is a cystic swelling of a Meibomian gland. Multiple cysts often occur and appear as round discrete swellings within the substance of the eyelid. Treatment is required for larger cysts and involves incision and curettage of the cyst from the conjunctival surface under local anaesthetic.
b) **Hordeolum** (stye) – is an infection of a hair follicle on the eyelid. It appears as a tender red swelling on the eyelid margin. Treatment requires removal of the hair follicle and hot bathing

to encourage discharge of the pus. If this fails, antibiotics may be given.

4.3.3 Trichiasis/entropion
Trichiasis is when one or more eyelashes turn in to touch the globe. Entropion is when the eyelid margin turns in so that most or all of the eyelashes turn in on the eye. (The commonest cause in Africa is trachoma.)

Treatment
a) Treatment of **mild trichiasis** is removal of the in-turning eyelashes by epilation. This may have to be repeated every six weeks. Alternatively, the hair follicles may be completely removed by electrolysis.
b) **Entropion** requires corrective lid surgery to return the eyelashes to their normal position. There are many different types of operation including mucous membrane grafting and tarsal plate rotation. Entropion is a major cause of blindness in areas with hyperendemic trachoma. In these situations entropion surgery campaigns are an important way of preventing corneal blindness.

4.3.4 Ectropion
When the eyelid margin is not apposed to the globe the condition is called ectropion. It may follow trauma, burns or deep infections of the eyelids which can also result in scarring and ectropion. In this situation skin grafting after scar excision is required to correct the ectropion.

Ectropion may also be due to lack of tone in the orbicularis oculi muscle and this occurs particularly after facial nerve paresis. If severe, corrective lid surgery can be performed of which the Kuhnt-Zymanowsky operation is the most popular.

4.4 Diseases of the nasolacrimal apparatus
These conditions are discussed under the following **four** headings:
4.4.1 Congenital atresia of the nasolacrimal duct
4.4.2 Dacrocystitis
4.4.3 'The watering eye'
4.4.4 'The dry eye'.

4.4.1 Congenital atresia of the nasolacrimal duct
In some babies, the nasolacrimal duct fails to become patent at birth. Over the first few months the mother notices that the baby's eye waters. A secondary infection may develop with a little discharge of pus at the medial canthus.

In the majority of children, the nasolacrimal duct will open spontaneously by the age of 18 months, so that reassurance and topical antibiotics for any infection is all that is required. If the child still has a watering eye by the age of 2, then probing to open the nasolacrimal duct under general anaesthetic can be performed.

4.4.2 Dacrocystitis

This is inflammation of the lacrimal sac usually due to obstruction of tear drainage through the nasolacrimal duct. It may present as an acute bacterial infection (**acute dacrocystitis**) with a tender red swelling over the lacrimal sac. Treatment is with systemic antibiotics, but if an abscess forms surgical incision and drainage of the abscess will also be necessary.

Chronic dacrocystitis presents as a chronic watering of the eye (**epiphora**). The obstruction is usually in the nasolacrimal duct. Sometimes a lacrimal wash-out can clear a partial obstruction, but if this fails and the patient is greatly troubled by the epiphora, then surgery can be performed. This consists of making an opening between the lacrimal sac and the nose – dacrocystorhinostomy (DCR).

4.4.3 The watering eye

The complaint of watering or tearing is a very common one and, in many cases, there is no serious abnormality. Watering of the eye can be due to:
a) Increased production of tears – lacrimation
b) Obstruction to drainage of tears – epiphora.

a) **Lacrimation** may be due to anything which irritates the eye, so that all the causes of acute red eye also produce lacrimation. These have been discussed in Section 1. Other common causes of lacrimation are pinguecula and pterygium.
   i) **Pinguecula** – a degeneration found in the conjunctiva at either the 3 or 9 o'clock positions. They are slightly raised and often yellow. They may become inflamed. They are of no significance and do not require treatment.
   ii) **Pterygium** – is a wedge of conjunctival tissue usually situated medially which grows onto the cornea. The conjunctiva is raised and may become inflamed causing lacrimation and redness. Most pterygia can be left alone or treated symptomatically with vasoconstrictor drops (e.g. zinc and adrenaline). The only real indication for surgical excison is if the pterygium grows so far across the cornea that it begins to reach the pupil margin and threaten vision. Excision of pterygium can be performed under local anaesthetic, but there is a very high recurrence rate. The simplest operation is to excise the pterygium and to leave an area of bare sclera.
b) **Epiphora** – may be due to any blockage in the lacrimal puncta, canaliculus, sac or nasolacrimal duct. Blockage to the drainage apparatus can usually be confirmed by failure to irrigate saline into the throat of the patient with a lacrimal sac wash-out. If the

epiphora causes a great deal of trouble then surgical bypass of the obstruction may be considered.

4.4.4 The dry eye

There are many conditons which result in a reduction in tears or a poor tear film. Disease of the lacrimal glands may reduce the amount of tears. This occurs more commonly in elderly people and is known as **keratoconjunctivitis sicca**. The patient complains of burning eyes and there is reduced tear production. Treatment is with artificial tears or methylcellulose drops.

Trachomatous conjunctival scarring may also cause lack of tears, and in vitamin A deficiency the goblet cells of the conjunctiva fail to produce mucin resulting in conjunctival and corneal xerosis.

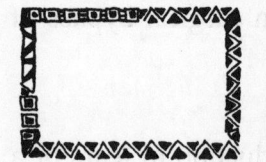

SECTION D:
Management of common eye diseases

The management of common eye diseases has already been covered in Section C. In this section a brief review of the common methods of management available to ophthalmic assistants is made:

1. Diseases causing acute red eye — REMEDY
2. Diseases causing loss of vision — REFER or REHABILITATION
3. Diseases causing difficulty in reading — REFRACT
4. Other eye diseases — REFER or REASSURE

1 Remedy

Medications are particularly used in ophthalmology for treating acute red eyes. They have a small role in the treatment of loss of vision, cannot read or other eye diseases. The medical treatment of glaucoma has very limited value in Africa because of poor patient compliance and the expense of lifelong therapy.

The treatment of conditions causing acute red eye is summarised below. The reader is referred to the text for dosages.

1.1	Acute red eye in babies:	Ophthalmia neonatorum	oc tetracycline 1% penicillin inj. IM
1.2	Acute red eye in children:	Vitamin A deficiency	Vitamin A capsules (200,000 I.U.) oc tetracycline 1%
1.3	Acute red eye at any age:	1.3.1 Conjunctivitis – bacterial – viral – *Chlamydial* (trachoma)	 oc tetracycline 1% oc tetracycline 1% oc tetracycline 1%

		– allergic (mild)	g zinc and adrenaline
		– allergic (vernal)	g prednisolone 0.5%
		– chemical	oc tetracycline 1%
	1.3.2	Corneal ulceration	
		– viral	oc IDU 0.5%
		– bacterial	oc tetracycline 1% g chloramphenicol gentamicin inj. oc atropine 1%
	1.3.3	Iritis	oc atropine 1% g prednisolone 0.5%
	1.3.4	Acute glaucoma	Acetazolamide tabs
1.4 Acute red eye from trauma:	1.4.1	Blunt injuries (with glaucoma)	oc tetracycline 1% ± Acetazolamide tabs
	1.4.2	Perforating injuries	g chloramphenicol g atropine
	1.4.3	Foreign bodies	g amethocaine oc tetracycline 1%
	1.4.4	Burns and chemicals	oc tetracycline 1%

2 Refer

Certain common eye conditions, particularly those which cause **treatable loss of vision**, need to be referred to an eye specialist for intra-ocular surgery.

In addition, some of the **other eye diseases** are not only sight threatening but may also endanger life and should be referred.

Following the order used in Section C, a list of conditions requiring specialist attention is given:

1.3.2 Corneal ulcer – if severe and failing to respond to treatment
1.3.3 Iritis – if severe and failing to respond to treatment
1.3.4 Acute glaucoma
1.4.2 Perforating eye injury
2.1 Corneal scar with bilateral vision less than 3/60
2.2 Cataract 2.2.a) bilateral – with vision less than 6/60
 2.2.b) unilateral – if there is a complication
 2.2.c) only eye – with vision less than 3/60
 2.2.d) second eye – at anytime
2.3 Chronic glaucoma – if travel vision is still present
2.4.1 Sudden bilateral loss of vision – any cause
2.4.2 Sudden unilateral loss of vision due to retinal detachment

4.1.1 Proptosis
4.2.1 Strabismus – age 8 or under
4.2.2 Diplopia
4.2.3 Ptosis
4.3.1 Skin tumours.

The common **surgical procedures** which are performed for eye conditions can be divided into extra-ocular and intra-ocular operations.

Extra-ocular operations
Incision of chalazion
Excision of pterygium
Evisceration
Enucleation
Entropion repair
Ectropion repair
Lateral tarsorrhaphy
Strabismus correction

Intra-ocular operations
Cataract extraction
– intracapsular
– extracapsular
Filtration surgery
– trabeculectomy
– Scheie procedure
Iridectomy
– peripheral, sector, optical
Repair of perforating
injury

Other less common procedures include:
Keratoplasty
Retinal detachment repair/vitrectomy
Oculo-plastic surgery
Orbital exenteration surgery.

Surgical procedures should be learned by watching specialists do the operation, then assisting the surgeon and then being assisted, as one gradually learns the operation technique.

3 Refract

Presbyopia presenting as inability to see close things and other refractive errors causing loss of vision (which can be improved by a pinhole) require spectacles.

Refractive error	Age of presentation	Spectacles
Presbyopia	40 yrs+	plus spheres
Hypermetropia	1–8 yrs or +40 yrs	plus spheres
Myopia	5–20 yrs	minus spheres
Astigmatism	any age	cylinders
Aphakia	post-cataract op	+10 distance

4 Rehabilitation/Reassurance

Patients who are blind in both eyes, for which there is no treatment, should be considered for appropriate education (if children) or rehabilitation (if adults). Children can be taught mobility, basic living skills, agriculture and a handicraft or technical skill. Adults may receive instruction in mobility and basic living skills including cooking for a woman and agriculture for a man.

Untreatable blindness includes:
- Bilateral phthisis
- Bilateral staphyloma
- Bilateral NPL glaucoma
- Blinding onchocerciasis
- Optic atrophy
- Retinitis pigmentosa.

Other patients who, after a careful history and examination, are found not to have a serious eye condition can be **reassured**. If both eyes have good vision, are white, the patient is under 40 and there is no specific symptom then it is likely that there is nothing seriously wrong.

Recommended reading

AHRTAG, *Dialogue on Diarrhoea* (Appropriate Health Resources and Technologies Action Group Ltd, 1 London Bridge Street, London SE9 1SG, England). Newsletter, free to health workers in developing countries.

Bunch, R., *Two Ears of Corn: A guide to people-centred agricultural improvement* (World Neighbours, Oklahoma City, 1985) Obtainable through Hesperian Foundation, Box 1692, Palo Alto, California 94302, USA.

Feuerstein, M.T., *Partners in Evaluation: Evaluating development and community programmes with participants* (Macmillan Publishers, London, 1986) Obtainable through TALC.

Hope, A. and Timmel, S., *Training for Transformation: A handbook for community workers* (book 1–3, Mambo Press, Gweru, Zimbabwe, 1984).

HSDU, *Primary Clinical Care, Book 9: Common eye problems. A manual of important clinical conditions for Primary Health Care Workers in rural and developing areas* (Health Services Development Unit, Department of Community Health, Medical School, University of the Witwatersrand, Johannesburg).

International Centre for Eye Health, *Community Eye Health: An international bulletin to promote eye health worldwide* (International Centre for Eye Health, Institute of Ophthalmology, 27–29 Cayton Street, London EC1V 9EJ) Available free.

Johnston, M.P. and Rifkin, S.B., *Health Care Together: Training exercises for health workers in community based programmes* (Macmillan Publishers, London, 1987) Obtain able through TALC.

Lund, F.J., *The Community-based Approach to Development: A description and analysis of three rural community health projects*. Dissertation 1987, available through Centre for Social Development Studies, University of Natal, Durban, South Africa.

Morley, D., *Paediatric Priorities in the Developing World* (Butterworths, London, 1973) Obtainable through TALC.

Sanders, D. and Carver, R., *The Struggle for Health: Medicine and politics of underdevelopment* (Macmillan, London, 1985) Obtainable through TALC.

Sandford-Smith, J., *Eye Diseases in Hot Climates* (Wright, Bristol, 1986). Obtainable through TALC.

Werner, D. and Bower, B., *Helping Health Workers Learn* (Hesperian Foundation, 1982) Obtainable through TALC.

Wood, C.H., Vaughan, J.P. and de Glanville, H. (Eds), *Community Health* (African Medical Research Foundation, Nairobi, 1981)

World Health Organization and United Nations Children's Fund, *'Alma Ata 1978, Primary Health Care.'* Report of the International Conference on Primary Health Care, Alma Ata, USSR, 6–12 September 1978. (World Health Organization, Geneva, 1978)